WITHDRAWN
University of
Illinois Library
at Urbana-Champaign

Leukocytes and Host Defense

PROGRESS IN LEUKOCYTE BIOLOGY

Series Editor
Sherwood M. Reichard, Medical College of Georgia, Augusta, Georgia

Advisory Board
Hillel S. Koren, Environmental Protection Agency, Chapel Hill, North Carolina
Ronald B. Herberman, National Cancer Institute, Frederick, Maryland
Frank Collins, Trudeau Institute, Saranac Lake, New York
Emil Unanue, Harvard Medical School, Boston, Massachusetts
Philip D. Stahl, Washington University School of Medicine, St. Louis, Missouri
Carleton Stewart, Los Alamos National Laboratory, Los Alamos, New Mexico
Emil Skamene, Montreal General Hospital, Montreal, Quebec, Canada
Dolph O. Adams, Duke University Medical Center, Durham, North Carolina
Joost J. Oppenheim, National Cancer Institute, Frederick, Maryland
Siamon Gordon, Oxford University, Oxford, England
Ralph van Furth, University Hospital, Leiden, The Netherlands
Klaus Resch, Hannover Medical School, Hannover, FRG
Michael Feldman, Weizmann Institute of Science, Rehovot, Israel
David S. Nelson, Royal North Shore Hospital, Sydney, Australia

TITLES IN THE SERIES

Volume 1
Viral Mechanisms of Immunosuppression
Norbert Gilmore and Mark A. Wainberg, *Editors*

Volume 2
The Physiologic, Metabolic, and Immunologic Actions of Interleukin-1
Matthew J. Kluger, Joost J. Oppenheim, and
Michael C. Powanda, *Editors*

Volume 3
Genetic Control of Host Resistance to Infection and Malignancy
Emil Skamene, *Editor*

Volume 4
Macrophage Biology
Sherwood Reichard and Mizu Kojima, *Editors*

Volume 5
Leukocytes and Host Defense
Joost J. Oppenheim and Diane M. Jacobs, *Editors*

Leukocytes and Host Defense

Proceedings of the 17th Meeting of the International Leukocyte
Culture Conference, held jointly with the 22nd National Meeting
of the Reticuloendothelial Society, Ithaca, New York, August 3–8, 1985

Editors

Joost J. Oppenheim
Laboratory of Molecular Immunoregulation
National Cancer Institute
Frederick, Maryland

Diane M. Jacobs
Department of Microbiology
State University of New York
Buffalo, New York

Alan R. Liss, Inc., New York

Address all Inquiries to the Publisher
Alan R. Liss, Inc., 41 East 11th Street, New York, NY 10003

Copyright © 1986 Alan R. Liss, Inc.

Printed in the United States of America

Under the conditions stated below the owner of copyright for this book hereby grants permission to users to make photocopy reproductions of any part or all of its contents for personal or internal organizational use, or for personal or internal use of specific clients. This consent is given on the condition that the copier pay the stated per-copy fee through the Copyright Clearance Center, Incorporated, 27 Congress Street, Salem, MA 01970, as listed in the most current issue of "Permissions to Photocopy" (Publisher's Fee List, distributed by CCC, Inc.), for copying beyond that permitted by sections 107 or 108 of the US Copyright Law. This consent does not extend to other kinds of copying, such as copying for general distribution, for advertising or promotional purposes, for creating new collective works, or for resale.

Library of Congress Cataloging-in-Publication Data

International Leucocyte Culture Conference (17 :
   1985 : Cornell University)
   Leucocytes and host defense.

   (Progress in leukocyte biology ; v. 5)
   Includes bibliographies and index.
   1. Leucocytes—Congresses. 2. Lymphocytes—Congresses. 3. Immunity—Congresses. I. Oppenheim, Joost J., 1934–   . II. Jacobs, Diane M.,
III. Reticuloendothelial Society. National Meeting (22nd : 1985 : Cornell University) IV. Titl.
V. Series.
QR185.8.L48I67   1985   612'.112   85-23770
ISBN 0-8451-4104-X

Contents

Contributors xiii

Preface
Joost J. Oppenheim and Diane M. Jacobs xxiii

Acknowledgments xxv

Section I. Development and Differentiation of T Lymphocytes

Mature and Immature Thymocytes: Surface Phenotype, Immune Function and Intrathymic Location
Ken Shortman, Roland Scollay, Anne Wilson, Paul Andrews, Richard Boyd, Eugene Butcher, and Irving Weissman 3

Studies of Adoptive Transfer of Thymic Rudiments
David A. Crouse and Reg K. Jordan 11

New Approaches to the Assessment of the Role of Thymic Stromal Cells in Development of T Cell Restriction Specificities
Ada M. Kruisbeek 21

Development of T Cell Receptor Expression in Fetal Thymus Organ Cultures
Willi Born, Neal Roehm, Janice White, Ella Kushnir, Edward Palmer, John Kappler, and Philippa Marrack 29

The Components of the Murine T Cell Antigen Receptor Complex
Lawrence E. Samelson, Joe B. Harford, and Richard D. Klausner 37

T Cell Markers and Subsets Involved in T Cell Differentiation
Bonnie J. Mathieson and Charles A. Janeway, Jr. 47

Section II. Effect of Interleukins on T and B Lymphocytes

Regulation of Human Interleukin 2 Gene Expression
Raymond Kaempfer and Shimon Efrat 57

IL 2 and Autoimmunity. Hyperproduction of IL 2 in Obese Strain Chickens With Spontaneous Autoimmune Thyroiditis Is Due to a Defect in Non-Specific Suppressor Mechanisms
Konrad Schauenstein, Guido Krömer, and Georg Wick 69

Biochemical Mechanism(s) of Interleukin 2 Regulation of
Lymphocyte Growth
*William L. Farrar, Stuart W. Evans, Francis W. Ruscetti, Ezio Bonvini,
Howard A. Young, and Maria C. Birchenall-Sparks* 75

Regulation of C-*myc* Expression and T Lymphocyte Proliferation
by Interleukin 2 and Inhibitors
*John C. Reed, Michael B. Prystowsky, Brian V. Jegasothy,
Richard G. Hoover, and Peter C. Nowell* 83

Patterns of Protein Synthesis Following IL 2 Stimulation of
Cloned T Helper Lymphocytes
Daniel E. Sabath and Michael B. Prystowsky 89

Identification and Characterization of a Released Form of the
Interleukin 2 Receptor
*Laurence A. Rubin, Carole C. Kurman, M. Elizabeth Fritz,
Robert Yarchoan, and David L. Nelson* 95

Evidence of Interleukin 2-Independent Proliferation of Non-
Transformed T Cells
Jay P. Siegel, D. Bruce Burlington, and Theresa L. Gerrard 103

Interleukin 2 Is a Growth Factor for B Lymphocytes
*John W. Lowenthal, Rudolf H. Zubler, Noboru Hashimoto,
Markus Nabholz, and H. Robson MacDonald* 109

Interleukin 1 (IL 1) as a Possible Autocrine Signal: Existence of
Specific IL 1 Receptors on Human Epstein Barr Virus
Transformed B Lymphocytes
Kouji Matsushima 115

Section III. Growth Regulation in Normal and Abnormal Leukocytes

Sodium Ion Influx: An Essential Early Signal in Lymphocyte
Proliferation
A. Severini, K.V.S. Prasad, W.L. Greer, and J.G. Kaplan 123

Calcium Mobilization by Specific Recombinant Ligands in IL 2
and IL 3 Dependent Cell Lines
Jeffrey L. Rossio, William L. Farrar, and Frank W. Ruscetti 131

Requirements for the Initial Activation and Cell Cycle
Progression of Naive T Cells
Laurie Davis and Peter E. Lipsky 137

Structure and Some Functional Aspects of hnRNP Complexes in
Lectin-Stimulated Lymphocytes
Birgit Henrich, Helmut Werr, Hans-Erich Wilk, and Klaus P. Schäfer . . *143*

Chromosome and Genetic Changes in Leukemia
Peter C. Nowell, Beverly S. Emanuel, and Carlo M. Croce *153*

Biochemical Changes Leading to Oncogenesis
Herbert L. Cooper and Robert H. Bassin *167*

Modulation of Immune Response in the Acquired Immuno-
deficiency Disease Syndrome
*Susanna Cunningham-Rundles, Bijan Safai, Craig E. Metroka, and
Michael Lange* *175*

Section IV. Neuroendocrine-Immune Interactions

Immunotransmitters: A New Class of Neuroactive Peptides
Produced by the Lymphoid System That Modulate Both Immune
and Neuroendocrine Circuits
*Nicholas R. Hall, Bryan L. Spangelo, John M. Farah, Jr.,
Thomas L. O'Donohue, and Allan L. Goldstein* *187*

Integration of Activated Immune Cell Products in Immune-
Endocrine Feed-Back Circuits
Hugo O. Besedovsky, A. del Rey, and E. Sorkin *197*

Some Immunological Effects of Methionin-Enkephalin in Man:
Potential Therapeutical Use
Joseph Wybran and Liliane Schandene *205*

Inhibition of Macrophage In Vivo Activiation by Pharmacologic
Blockade of Prolactin Release
*Edward Bernton, Dan Hartmann, Micheal Gilbreath, John Holaday, and
Monte S. Meltzer* *213*

Immunoregulatory Molecules Modulate Glial Cell Growth
Etty N. Benveniste, Sally Kutsunai, and Jean E. Merrill *221*

The Association of Nerves and Plasma Cells in a Tear Gland
Benjamin Walcott, Kent T. Keyser, and Patrick A. Sibony *227*

Section V. Development and Differentiation of Macrophages

Regulation of the Production, Cloning of the Complementary
(cDNA), and Functions of Human Macrophage Growth
Factor, CSF-1
Peter Ralph *235*

Biochemical Mechanism of Signal Transmittance by Fc Receptors for IgG2a at the Surface of a Murine Macrophage-Like Cell Line, P388D1: Activation of Adenylate Cyclase by IgG2a-Binding Proteins
Tsuneo Suzuki and Rafael Fernandez-Botran 243

Molecular Bases for Activation of Cytotoxic Macrophages
Luigi Varesio, Michael A. Clayton, Elisabetta Blasi, Ezio Bonvini, and Danuta Radzioch 253

Activated Macrophage Mediated Iron Removal From Enzymes With Iron-Sulfur Clusters in Tumor Target Cells: A Possible Mechanism for Selective Inhibition of Metabolic Pathways
John B. Hibbs, Jr., and Jean-Claude Drapier 261

Aconitase, a Krebs Cycle Enzyme With an Iron-Sulfur Center, Is Inhibited in Tumor Target Cells After Cocultivation With Cytotoxic Activated Macrophages
Jean-Claude Drapier and John B. Hibbs, Jr. 269

Establishment of Macrophage Cell Lines by In Vitro Infection of Mouse Bone Marrow (BM) Cells With a Retrovirus Containing v-*raf* Plus v-*myc* Oncogenes
Elisabetta Blasi, Ulf Rapp, and Luigi Varesio 275

Differences in Functional, Phenotypical and Physical Properties of Human Peripheral Blood Monocytes (Mo) Reflect Their Various Maturation Stages
Carl G. Figdor, Anje A. te Velde, Jack Leemans, and Willy S. Bont 283

Monoclonal Antibodies Reactive With Different Stages in Murine Macrophage Differentiation
P.J.M. Leenen, U. Willmer, F.W. Falkenberg, A.M.A.C. Jansen, and W. van Ewijk 289

Surface Antigen Analysis of Human Macrophage Maturation and Heterogeneity
Reinhard Andreesen, Klaus J. Bross, and Frank Emmrich 295

Antibodies to LFA-1 and Related Molecules Inhibit Conjugate Formation Between Human Peripheral Blood Monocytes and Melanoma Cells
Anje A. te Velde, Gerrit D. Keizer, Jan E. de Vries, and Carl G. Figdor . 301

The Cytokinetic Behavior of Resident Pulmonary Alveolar Macrophage in Splenectomized-Strontium 89 Monocytopenic Mice
Richard T. Sawyer 307

Section VI. Microbial-Host Interactions

Macrophages and Host Defense: Induction of Antimicrobial
Effector Reactions of Activated Macrophages
*Carol A. Nacy, Monte S. Meltzer, Anne H. Fortier, Micheal G. Gilbreath,
and David L. Hoover* 315

Biological Functions In Vitro and In Vivo of Cloned Autoreactive
T Cells From *Mycobacterium bovis* BCG-Infected Mice
I. Müller, A. Rolink, N. Freudenberg, and S.H.E. Kaufmann 325

Protection Against *Listeria monocytogenes* With a Clonotypic
Antiserum
*Stefan H.E. Kaufmann, Klaus Eichmann, Ingrid Müller, and
Laura J. Wrazel* 331

The Synthetic Analoga of Bacterial Lipoprotein Are Potent
Immunoadjuvants in Combination With or Covalently Linked to
Antigen
*W.G. Bessler, A. Lex, B. Suhr, A. Ortmann, S. Schlecht, H. Bühring,
C. Muller, J. Metzger, K.H. Wiesmüller, and G. Jung* 337

Section VII. Role of Leukocytes in Host Defense

Mast Cells in Host Defense
John Bienenstock and Dean Befus 347

The Role of the Eosinophil in Host Defense
D.G. Colley, S.J. Stewart, E.K. Duncan, and W.E. Secor 357

Platelet-Neutrophil Interactions in the Eicosanoid Pathway
*Aaron J. Marcus, Lenore B. Safier, Harris L. Ullman,
M. Johan Broekman, Naziba Islam, Thomas D. Oglesby,
Robert R. Gorman, and Clemens von Schacky* 365

Role of GTP-Binding Proteins in the Regulation of the Human
Neutrophil
*Pramod M. Lad, Charles V. Olson, Iqbal S. Grewal, Marianne Frolich,
Paula A. Smiley, and Stephen J. Scott* 373

Chemotactic Properties of Synthetic Collagen-Like Peptides
Debra L. Laskin and Richard A. Berg 379

Concomitant Expression of Chemiluminescence and Bacterial
Killing by Bovine Neutrophils
Charles J. Czuprynski and Holly L. Hamilton 385

Section VIII. Regulation and Functions of Cells With Natural Killer Activity

Stimulation of Natural Killer and Activated Killer Cell Cytotoxicity by Interferons and Interleukins
J.R. Ortaldo, A. Mason, J. Langer, and R. Overton 393

Regulation of Viral Infections by Large Granular Lymphocytes
Raymond M. Welsh, Christine A. Biron, Jack F. Bukowski, Kim W. McIntyre, Robert J. Natuk, and Hyekyung Yang 403

NK Susceptibility of Human Cells May Be Regulated by Genes in the HLA Region of Chromosome 6
Annick Harel-Bellan, Anne Quillet, Carmen Marchiol, Robert De Mars, and Didier Fradelizi 411

Activation of Alveolar Macrophage Intracellular Microbicidal Activity by a Preformed LGL Cytokine
Arnold H. Greenberg, Jose Gomez, Bill Pohajdak, Shane O'Neill, and John Wilkins 417

Role of Laminin and Laminin Receptors in Natural Killer Cell Recognition of Tumor Metastases
John C. Hiserodt, Dan M. Hyder, Katherine A. Laybourn, and James Varani 423

Section IX. Tumor-Host Interactions

Tumorigenesis and Immune Surveillance
Zvi Grossman 433

Cytostatic Factors Produced by Lymphocytes in Response to Tumor Cells
T.J. Sayers, J.H. Ransom, A.C. Denn III, H.M. Shepard, R.B. Herberman, and J.R. Ortaldo 441

The Role of Cytotoxins in Monocyte/Macrophage Tumor Cytotoxicity In Vitro
Jim Klostergaard 447

Chemoimmunotherapy of Advanced Murine Renal Carcinoma
R.R. Salup and R.H. Wiltrout 457

Tumor-Induced Suppression of Cell-Mediated Immunity: Selective Effects on Lymphokine Production and Lymphocyte Transformation and Independence of Cyclophosphamide-Sensitive Suppressor Cells
Lesley C. McIntosh, Lora M. Morrice, Yasuhiro Udagawa, and Angus W. Thomson 465

Section X. Thymocyte Development

Phenotypic Properties and In Vitro Growth of Immature
Lyt-2$^-$/L3T4$^-$ Thymocytes
Rh. Ceredig and H.R. MacDonald *473*

Index *479*

Contributors

Reinhard Andreesen, Medizinische Klinik I, D-7800 Freiburg, West Germany [295]

Paul Andrews, Lymphocyte Differentiation Unit, The Walter and Eliza Hall Institute of Medical Research, Melbourne 3050, Australia [3]

Robert H. Bassin, Laboratory of Tumor Immunology and Biology, National Cancer Institute, Bethesda, MD 20205 [167]

Dean Befus, Department of Microbiology and Immunology, University of Alberta, Calgary, Alberta, Canada [347]

Etty N. Benveniste, Department of Neurology, University of California, Los Angeles, CA 90024 [221]

Richard A. Berg, Department of Biochemistry, Rutgers Medical School, Piscataway, NJ 08854 [379]

Edward Bernton, Walter Reed Army Institute of Research, Washington, DC 20307 [213]

Hugo O. Besedovsky, Schweiz. Forschungsinstitut, Medizinische Abteilung, CH-7270 Davos, Switzerland [197]

W.G. Bessler, Arbeitsbereich Mikrobiologie und Immunologie, Institut für Organische Chemie, and Medizinische Klinik der Universität, Tübingen, and Max-Planck-Institut für Immunbiologie, Freiburg, West Germany [337]

John Bienenstock, Department of Pathology, McMaster University, Hamilton, Ontario, Canada [347]

Maria C. Birchenall-Sparks, Laboratory of Molecular Immunoregulation, BRMP, DCT, National Cancer Institute, NIH, Frederick Cancer Research Facility, Frederick, MD 21701 [75]

Christine A. Biron, Department of Pathology, University of Massachusetts Medical School, Worcester, MA 01605 [403]

Elisabetta Blasi, Laboratory of Molecular Immunoregulation, BRMP, DCT, NCI-FCRF, Frederick, MD 21701 [253,275]

Willy S. Bont, Division of Immunology, The Netherlands Cancer Institute, Plesmanlaan 121, 1066 CX Amsterdam, The Netherlands [283]

Ezio Bonvini, Bureau of Biologics, National Institutes of Health, Bethesda, MD 20892 [75,253]

Willi Born, Department of Medicine, National Jewish Center, University of Colorado Health Sciences Center, Denver, CO 80206 [29]

Richard Boyd, Department of Pathology and Immunology, Monash University Medical School, Melbourne 3168, Australia [3]

The number in brackets is the opening page number of the contributor's article.

M. Johan Broekman, Department of Medicine, Division of Hematology-Oncology, New York Veterans Administration Medical Center, New York, NY 10010 [365]

Klaus J. Bross, Medizinische Klinik I, D-7800 Freiburg, West Germany [295]

H. Bühring, Arbeitsbereich Mikrobiologie und Immunologie, Institut für Organische Chemie, and Medizinische Klinik der Universität, Tübingen, and Max-Planck-Institut für Immunbiologie, Freiburg, West Germany [337]

Jack F. Bukowski, Department of Pathology, University of Massachusetts Medical School, Worcester, MA 01605 [403]

D. Bruce Burlington, Division of Virology, Office of Biologics Research and Review, Center for Drugs and Biologics, Food and Drug Administration, Bethesda, MD 20205 [103]

Eugene Butcher, Department of Pathology, Stanford University School of Medicine, Stanford, CA 94305 [3]

Rh. Ceredig, John Curtin School of Medical Research, Canberra, Australia [473]

Michael A. Clayton, Laboratory of Molecular Immunoregulation, BRMP, DCT, NCI-FCRF, Frederick, MD 21701 [253]

D.G. Colley, VA Medical Center, Vanderbilt University School of Medicine, Nashville, TN 37203 [357]

Herbert L. Cooper, Laboratory of Tumor Immunology and Biology, National Cancer Institute, Bethesda, MD 20205 [167]

Carlo M. Croce, Wistar Institute of Anatomy and Biology, Philadelphia, PA 19104 [153]

David A. Crouse, Department of Anatomy, University of Nebraska Medical Center, Omaha, NE 68105 [11]

Susanna Cunningham-Rundles, Department of Immunohematology, Memorial Sloan-Kettering Cancer Center, New York, NY 10021 [175]

Charles J. Czuprynski, Department of Pathobiological Sciences, University of Wisconsin School of Veterinary Medicine, Madison, WI 53706 [385]

Laurie Davis, The Harold C. Simmons Arthritis Research Center, and the Department of Internal Medicine, University of Texas Health Science Center at Dallas, Dallas, TX 75235 [137]

A. del Rey, Schweiz. Forschungsinstitut, Medizinische Abteilung, CH-7270 Davos, Switzerland [197]

Robert De Mars, Genetic Building, University of Wisconsin, Madison, WI 53706 [411]

A.C. Denn III, Biological Therapeutics Branch, BRMP, DCT, National Cancer Institute, Frederick, MD 21701 [441]

Jan E. de Vries, Division of Immunology, The Netherlands Cancer Institute, Plesmanlaan 121, 1066 CX Amsterdam, The Netherlands [301]

Jean-Claude Drapier, VA Medical Center and Department of Medicine, Division of Infectious Diseases, University of Utah School of Medicine, Salt Lake City, UT 84148 [261,269]

E.K. Duncan, Department of Microbiology, Vanderbilt University School of Medicine, Nashville, TN 37203 **[357]**

Shimon Efrat, Department of Medical Virology, The Hebrew University-Hadassah Medical School, 91010 Jerusalem, Israel **[57]**

Klaus Eichmann, Max-Planck-Institut für Immunbiologie, 7800 Freiburg, West Germany **[331]**

Beverly S. Emanuel, Department of Pediatrics, Children's Hospital of Philadelphia, Philadelphia, PA 19104 **[153]**

Frank Emmrich, Max-Planck-Institut für Immunbiologie, D-7800 Freiburg, West Germany **[295]**

Stuart W. Evans, Laboratory of Molecular Immunoregulation, BRMP, DCT, National Cancer Institute, NIH, Frederick Cancer Research Facility, Frederick, MD 21701 **[75]**

F.W. Falkenberg, Department of Medical Microbiology and Immunology, 4630 Bochum 1, West Germany **[289]**

John M. Farah, Jr., Experimental Therapeutics Branch, NINCDS, Bethesda, MD 20205 **[187]**

William L. Farrar, Laboratory of Molecular Immunoregulation, BRMP, DCT, National Cancer Institute, NIH, Frederick Cancer Research Facility, Frederick, MD 21701 **[75,131]**

Rafael Fernandez-Botran, Department of Microbiology, University of Kansas Medical Center, Kansas City, KS 66103 **[243]**

Carl G. Figdor, Division of Immunology, The Netherlands Cancer Institute, Plesmanlaan 121, 1066 CX Amsterdam, The Netherlands **[283,301]**

Anne H. Fortier, Department of Immunology, Walter Reed Army Institute of Research, Washington, DC 20307 **[315]**

Didier Fradelizi, Laboratoire d'Immunologie, Institut Gustave Roussy, 94805 Villejuif, France **[411]**

N. Freudenberg, Institut für Pathologie, Universität Freiburg, Freiburg, West Germany **[325]**

M. Elizabeth Fritz, Immunophysiology Section, Metabolism Branch, National Cancer Institute, National Institutes of Health, Bethesda, MD 20205 **[95]**

Marianne Frolich, Kaiser Regional Research Laboratory, Los Angeles, CA 90027 **[373]**

Theresa L. Gerrard, Division of Virology, Office of Biologics Research and Review, Center for Drugs and Biologics, Food and Drug Administration, Bethesda, MD 20205 **[103]**

Micheal Gilbreath, Walter Reed Army Institute of Research, Washington, DC 20307 **[213,315]**

Allan L. Goldstein, Department of Biochemistry, The George Washington University School of Medicine, Washington, DC 20037 **[187]**

Jose Gomez, Department of Medicine, University of Manitoba, Winnipeg, Canada R3E OV9 **[417]**

Robert R. Gorman, Department of Medicine, Division of Hematology-Oncology, New York Veterans Administration Medical Center, New York, NY 10010 **[365]**

Arnold H. Greenberg, Department of Pediatrics, University of Manitoba, Winnipeg, Canada R3E OV9 **[417]**

W.L. Greer, Department of Biochemistry, University of Alberta, Edmonton T6G 2H7, Canada **[123]**

Iqbal S. Grewal, Kaiser Regional Research Laboratory, Los Angeles, CA 90027 **[373]**

Zvi Grossman, School of Mathematical Sciences, Tel Aviv University, Tel Aviv, Israel, and National Cancer Institute, Frederick Cancer Research Facility, Frederick, MD 21701 **[433]**

Nicholas R. Hall, Department of Biochemistry, The George Washington University School of Medicine, Washington, DC 20037 **[187]**

Holly L. Hamilton, Department of Pathobiological Sciences, University of Wisconsin School of Veterinary Medicine, Madison, WI 53706 **[385]**

Annick Harel-Bellan, Laboratoire d'Immunologie, Institut Gustave Roussy, 94805 Villejuif, France **[411]**

Joe B. Harford, Cell Biology and Metabolism Branch, National Institute of Child Health and Human Development, National Institutes of Health, Bethesda, MD 20892 **[37]**

Dan Hartmann, Department of Pathology, Georgetown University School of Medicine, Washington, DC 20007 **[213]**

Noboru Hashimoto, Swiss Institute for Experimental Cancer Research, 1066 Epalinges, Switzerland **[109]**

Birgit Henrich, Ruhr-Universität Bochum, Lehrstuhl für Biochemie, D-4630 Bochum 1, West Germany **[143]**

R.B. Herberman, Biological Therapeutics Branch, BRMP, DCT, National Cancer Institute, Frederick, MD 21701 **[441]**

John B. Hibbs, Jr., VA Medical Center and Department of Medicine, Division of Infectious Diseases, University of Utah School of Medicine, Salt Lake City, UT 84148 **[261,269]**

John C. Hiserodt, Department of Pathology, University of Michigan, Ann Arbor, MI 48109 **[423]**

John Holaday, Walter Reed Army Institute of Research, Washington, DC 20307 **[213]**

David L. Hoover, Department of Immunology, Walter Reed Army Institute of Research, Washington, DC 20307 **[315]**

Richard G. Hoover, Department of Pathology, University of Pennsylvania, Philadelphia, PA 19104 **[83]**

Dan M. Hyder, Department of Pathology, University of Michigan, Ann Arbor, MI 48109 **[423]**

Naziba Islam, Department of Medicine, Division of Hematology-Oncology, New York Veterans Administration Medicine Center, New York, NY 10010 **[365]**

Charles A. Janeway, Jr., Department of Pathology, Yale University School of Medicine, New Haven, CT 06510 **[47]**

A.M.A.C. Jansen, Department of Cell Biology and Genetics, Erasmus University, 3000 DR Rotterdam, The Netherlands **[289]**

Brian V. Jegasothy, Department of Dermatology, University of Pennsylvania, Philadelphia, PA 19104 **[83]**

Contributors xvii

Reg K. Jordan, Department of Anatomy, University of Newcastle-upon-Tyne, Newcastle NE2 4HH, England **[11]**

G. Jung, Arbeitsbereich Mikrobiologie und Immunologie, Institut für Organische Chemie, and Medizinische Klinik der Universität, Tübingen, and Max-Planck-Institut für Immunbiologie, Freiburg, West Germany **[337]**

Raymond Kaempfer, Department of Molecular Virology, The Hebrew University-Hadassah Medical School, 91010 Jerusalem, Israel **[57]**

J.G. Kaplan, Department of Biochemistry, University of Alberta, Edmonton T6G 2H7, Canada **[123]**

John Kappler, Department of Medicine, National Jewish Center, University of Colorado Health Sciences Center, Denver, CO 80206 **[29]**

S.H.E. Kaufmann, Max-Planck-Institut für Immunbiologie, Freiburg, West Germany **[325,331]**

Gerrit D. Keizer, Division of Immunology, The Netherlands Cancer Institute, Plesmanlaan 121, 1066 CX Amsterdam, The Netherlands **[301]**

Kent T. Keyser, Department of Psychiatry, School of Medicine, State University of New York, Stony Brook, NY 11794 **[227]**

Richard D. Klausner, Cell Biology and Metabolism Branch, National Institute of Child Health and Human Development, National Institutes of Health, Bethesda, MD 20892 **[37]**

Jim Klostergaard, Department of Tumor Biology, University of Texas, M.D. Anderson Hospital and Tumor Institute, Houston, TX 77030 **[447]**

Guido Krömer, Institute of General and Experimental Pathology, University of Innsbruck, School of Medicine, A-6020 Innsbruck, Austria **[69]**

Ada M. Kruisbeek, Medicine Branch, National Institutes of Health, Bethesda, MD 20205 **[21]**

Carole C. Kurman, Immunophysiology Section, Metabolism Branch, National Cancer Institute, National Institutes of Health, Bethesda, MD 20205 **[95]**

Ella Kushnir, Department of Medicine, National Jewish Center, University of Colorado Health Sciences Center, Denver, CO 80206 **[29]**

Sally Kutsunai, Department of Neurology, University of California, Los Angeles, CA 90024 **[221]**

Pramod M. Lad, Kaiser Regional Research Laboratory, Los Angeles, CA 90027 **[373]**

Michael Lange, Department of Infectious Diseases, St. Luke's Roosevelt Hospital Center, New York, NY 10025 **[175]**

J. Langer, Roche Institute of Molecular Biology, Nutley, NJ **[393]**

Debra L. Laskin, Department of Pharmacology and Toxicology, Rutgers Medical School, Piscataway, NJ 08854 **[379]**

Katherine A. Laybourn, Department of Pathology, University of Michigan, Ann Arbor, MI 48109 **[423]**

Jack Leemans, Division of Immunology, The Netherlands Cancer Institute, Plesmanlaan 121, 1066 CX Amsterdam, The Netherlands **[283]**

P.J.M. Leenen, Department of Cell Biology and Genetics, Erasmus University, 3000 DR Rotterdam, The Netherlands [289]

A. Lex, Arbeitsbereich Mikrobiologie und Immunologie, Institut für Organische Chemie, and Medizinische Klinik der Universität, Tübingen, and Max-Planck-Institut für Immunbiologie, Freiburg, West Germany [337]

Peter E. Lipsky, The Harold C. Simmons Arthritis Research Center, and The Department of Internal Medicine, University of Texas Health Science Center at Dallas, Dallas, TX 75235 [137]

John W. Lowenthal, Ludwig Institute for Cancer Research, Lausanne Branch, 1066 Epalinges, Switzerland [109]

H. Robson MacDonald, Ludwig Institute for Cancer Research, Lausanne Branch, 1066 Epalinges, Switzerland [109,473]

Carmen Marchiol, Laboratoire d'Immunologie, Institut Gustave Roussy, 94805 Villejuif, France [411]

Aaron J. Marcus, Department of Medicine, Division of Hematology-Oncology, New York Veterans Administration Medical Center, New York, NY 10010 [365]

Philippa Marrack, Department of Medicine, National Jewish Center, University of Colorado Health Sciences Center, Denver, CO 80206 [29]

A. Mason, Biological Therapeutics Branch, BRMP, DCT, National Cancer Institute, Frederick, MD 21701 [393]

Bonnie J. Mathieson, Monoclonal Antibody/Hybridoma Section, Biological Therapeutics Branch, BRMP, DCT, NCI, Frederick Cancer Research Facility, Frederick, MD 21701 [47]

Kouji Matsushima, Laboratory of Molecular Immunoregulation, Biological Response Modifiers Program, DCT, NCI, Frederick, MD 21701 [115]

Lesley C. McIntosh, Department of Pathology, University of Aberdeen, Aberdeen Royal Infirmary, Foresterhill, Aberdeen AB9 2ZD, Scotland [465]

Kim W. McIntyre, Department of Pathology, University of Massachusetts Medical School, Worcester, MA 01605 [403]

Monte S. Meltzer, Walter Reed Army Institute of Research, Washington, DC 20307 [213,315]

Jean E. Merrill, Department of Neurology, University of California, Los Angeles, CA 90024 [221]

Craig E. Metroka, Department of Immunohematology, Memorial Sloan-Kettering Cancer Center, New York, NY 10021 [175]

J. Metzger, Arbeitsbereich Mikrobiologie und Immunologie, Institut für Organische Chemie, and Medizinische Klinik der Universität, Tübingen, and Max-Planck-Institut für Immunbiologie, Freiburg, West Germany [337]

Lora M. Morrice, Department of Pathology, University of Aberdeen, Aberdeen Royal Infirmary, Foresterhill, Aberdeen AB9 2ZD, Scotland [465]

C. Muller, Arbeitsbereich Mikrobiologie und Immunologie, Institut für Organische Chemie, and Medizinische Klinik der Universität, Tübingen, and Max-Planck-Institut für Immunbiologie, Freiburg, West Germany **[337]**

I. Müller, Max-Planck-Institut für Immunbiologie, Freiburg, West Germany **[325,331]**

Markus Nabholz, Swiss Institute for Experimental Cancer Research, 1066 Epalinges, Switzerland **[109]**

Carol A. Nacy, Department of Immunology, Walter Reed Army Institute of Research, Washington, DC 20307 **[315]**

Robert J. Natuk, Department of Pathology, University of Massachusetts Medical School, Worcester, MA 01605 **[403]**

David L. Nelson, Immunophysiology Section, Metabolism Branch, National Cancer Institute, National Institutes of Health, Bethesda, MD 20205 **[95]**

Peter C. Nowell, Department of Pathology and Laboratory Medicine, University of Pennsylvania, Philadelphia, PA 19104 **[83,153]**

Thomas L. O'Donohue, Experimental Therapeutics Branch, NINCDS, Bethesda, MD 20205 **[187]**

Thomas D. Oglesby, Department of Medicine, Division of Hematology-Oncology, New York Veterans Administration Medical Center, New York, NY 10010 **[365]**

Charles V. Olson, Kaiser Regional Research Laboratory, Los Angeles, CA 90027 **[373]**

Shane O'Neill, Department of Medicine, University of Manitoba, Winnipeg, Canada R3E OV9 **[417]**

J.R. Ortaldo, Biological Therapeutics Branch, BRMP, DCT, National Cancer Institute, Frederick, MD 21701 **[393,441]**

A. Ortmann, Arbeitsbereich Mikrobiologie und Immunologie, Institut für Organische Chemie, and Medizinische Klinik der Universität, Tübingen, and Max-Planck-Institut für Immunbiologie, Freiburg, West Germany **[337]**

R. Overton, Program Resources, Inc., NCI-FCRF, Frederick, MD 21701 **[393]**

Edward Palmer, Department of Medicine, National Jewish Center, University of Colorado Health Sciences Center, Denver, CO 80206 **[29]**

Bill Pohajdak, Department of Pediatrics, University of Manitoba, Winnipeg, Canada R3E OV9 **[417]**

K.V.S. Prasad, Department of Biochemistry, University of Alberta, Edmonton T6G 2H7, Canada **[123]**

Michael B. Prystowsky, Department of Pathology, University of Pennsylvania, Philadelphia, PA 19104 **[83,89]**

Anne Quillet, Laboratoire d'Immunologie, Institut Gustave Roussy, 94805 Villejuif, France **[411]**

Danuta Radzioch, Laboratory of Molecular Immunoregulation, BRMP, DCT, NCI-FCRF, Frederick, MD 21701 **[253]**

Peter Ralph, Department of Cell Biology, Cetus Corporation, Emeryville, CA 94608 **[235]**

J.H. Ransom, Litton Bionetics, Inc., Rockville, MD 20850 [441]

Ulf Rapp, Laboratory of Viral Carcinogenesis, NCI-FCRF, Frederick, MD 21701 [275]

John C. Reed, Department of Pathology, University of Pennsylvania, Philadelphia, PA 19104 [83]

Neal Roehm, Department of Medicine, National Jewish Center, University of Colorado Health Sciences Center, Denver, CO 80206 [29]

A. Rolink, Basel Institute for Immunology, Basel, Switzerland [325]

Jeffrey L. Rossio, Program Resources, Inc., NCI-Frederick Cancer Research Facility, Frederick, MD 21701 [131]

Laurence A. Rubin, Immunophysiology Section, Metabolism Branch, National Cancer Institute, National Institutes of Health, Bethesda, MD 20205 [95]

Francis W. Ruscetti, Laboratory of Molecular Immunoregulation, BRMP, DCT, National Cancer Institute, NIH, Frederick Cancer Research Facility, Frederick, MD 21701 [75,131]

Daniel E. Sabath, Department of Pathology and Laboratory Medicine, University of Pennsylvania, Philadelphia, PA 19104 [89]

Bijan Safai, Dermatology Service, Department of Medicine, Memorial Sloan-Kettering Cancer Center, New York, NY 10021 [175]

Lenore B. Safier, Department of Medicine, Division of Hematology-Oncology, New York Veterans Administration Medical Center, New York, NY 10010 [365]

R.R. Salup, Program Resources, Inc., Frederick Cancer Research Facility, Frederick, MD 21701 [457]

Lawrence E. Samelson, Cell Biology and Metabolism Branch, National Institute of Child Health and Human Development, National Institutes of Health, Bethesda, MD 20892 [37]

Richard T. Sawyer, Division of Basic Medical Science, Mercer University School of Medicine, Macon, GA 31207 [307]

T.J. Sayers, Biological Therapeutics Branch, BRMP, DCT, National Cancer Institute, Frederick, MD 21701 [441]

Klaus P. Schäfer, Ruhr-Universität Bochum, Lehrstuhl für Biochemie, D-4630 Bochum 1, West Germany [143]

Liliane Schandene, Department of Immunology, Hematology and Transfusion, Erasme Hospital, Université Libre de Bruxelles, 1070 Brussels, Belgium [205]

Konrad Schauenstein, Institute of General and Experimental Pathology, University of Innsbruck, School of Medicine, A-6020 Innsbruck, Austria [69]

S. Schlecht, Arbeitsbereich Mikrobiologie und Immunologie, Institut für Organische Chemie, and Medizinische Klinik der Universität, Tübingen, and Max-Planck-Institut für Immunbiologie, Freiburg, West Germany [337]

Roland Scollay, Lymphocyte Differentiation Unit, The Walter and Eliza Hall Institute of Medical Research, Melbourne 3050, Australia [3]

Stephen J. Scott, Kaiser Regional Research Laboratory, Los Angeles, CA 90027 **[373]**

W.E. Secor, Department of Microbiology, Vanderbilt University School of Medicine, Nashville, TN 37203 **[357]**

A. Severini, Department of Biochemistry, University of Alberta, Edmonton T6G 2H7, Canada **[123]**

H.M. Shepard, Genentech, Inc., San Francisco, CA 94080 **[441]**

Ken Shortman, Lymphocyte Differentiation Unit, The Walter and Eliza Hall Institute of Medical Research, Melbourne 3050, Australia **[3]**

Patrick A. Sibony, Department of Ophthalmology and Neurology, School of Medicine, State University of New York, Stony Brook, NY 11794 **[227]**

Jay P. Siegel, Division of Virology, Office of Biologics Research and Review, Center for Drugs and Biologics, Food and Drug Administration, Bethesda, MD 20205 **[103]**

Paula A. Smiley, Kaiser Regional Research Laboratory, Los Angeles, CA 90027 **[373]**

E. Sorkin, Schweiz. Forschungsinstitut, Medizinische Abteilung, CH-7270 Davos, Switzerland **[197]**

Bryan L. Spangelo, Department of Biochemistry, The George Washington University School of Medicine, Washington, DC 20037 **[187]**

S.J. Stewart, VA Medical Center, Vanderbilt University School of Medicine, Nashville, TN 37203 **[357]**

B. Suhr, Arbeitsbereich Mikrobiologie und Immunologie, Institut für Organische Chemie, and Medizinische Klinik der Universität, Tübingen, and Max-Planck-Institut für Immunbiologie, Freiburg, West Germany **[337]**

Tsuneo Suzuki, Department of Microbiology, University of Kansas Medical Center, Kansas City, KS 66103 **[243]**

Anje A. te Velde, Division of Immunology, The Netherlands Cancer Institute, Plesmanlaan 121, 1066 CX Amsterdam, The Netherlands **[283,301]**

Angus W. Thomson, Department of Pathology, University of Aberdeen, Aberdeen Royal Infirmary, Foresterhill, Aberdeen AB9 2ZD, Scotland **[465]**

Yasuhiro Udagawa, Department of Pathology, University of Aberdeen, Aberdeen Royal Infirmary, Foresterhill, Aberdeen AB9 2ZD, Scotland **[465]**

Harris L. Ullman, Department of Medicine, Division of Hematology-Oncology, New York Veterans Administration Medical Center, New York, NY 10010 **[365]**

W. van Ewijk, Department of Cell Biology and Genetics, Erasmus University, 3000 DR Rotterdam, The Netherlands **[289]**

James Varani, Department of Pathology, University of Michigan, Ann Arbor, MI 48109 **[423]**

Luigi Varesio, Laboratory of Molecular Immunoregulation, BRMP, DCT, NCI-FCRF, Frederick, MD 21701 **[253,275]**

Clemens von Schacky, Department of Medicine, Division of Hematology-Oncology, New York Veterans Administration Medical Center, New York, NY 10010 [365]

Benjamin Walcott, Department of Anatomical Sciences, School of Medicine, State University of New York, Stony Brook NY 11794 [227]

Irving Weissman, Department of Pathology, Stanford University School of Medicine, Stanford, CA 94305 [3]

Raymond M. Welsh, Department of Pathology, University of Massachusetts Medical School, Worcester, MA 01605 [403]

Helmut Werr, Ruhr-Universität Bochum, Lehrstuhl für Biochemie, D-4630 Bochum 1, West Germany [143]

Janice White, Department of Medicine, National Jewish Center, University of Colorado Health Sciences Center, Denver, CO 80206 [29]

Georg Wick, Institute of General and Experimental Pathology, University of Innsbruck, School of Medicine, A-6020 Innsbruck, Austria [69]

K.H. Wiesmüller, Arbeitsbereich Mikrobiologie und Immunologie, Institut für Organische Chemie, and Medizinische Klink der Universität, Tübingen, and Max-Planck-Institut für Immunbiologie, Freiburg, West Germany [337]

Hans-Erich Wilk, Ruhr-Universität Bochum, Lehrstuhl für Biochemie, D-4630 Bochum 1, West Germany [143]

John Wilkins, Department of Medicine, University of Manitoba, Winnipeg, Canada R3E OV9 [417]

U. Willmer, Department of Medical Microbiology and Immunology, 4630 Bochum 1, West Germany [289]

Anne Wilson, Lymphocyte Differentiation Unit, The Walter and Eliza Hall Institute of Medical Research, Melbourne 3050, Australia [3]

R.H. Wiltrout, Biological Therapeutics Branch, Biological Response Modifiers Program, DCT, NCI, Frederick, MD 21701 [457]

Laura J. Wrazel, Max-Planck-Institut für Immunbiologie, 7800 Freiburg, West Germany [331]

Joseph Wybran, Department of Immunology, Hematology and Transfusion, Erasme Hospital, Université Libre de Bruxelles, 1070 Brussels, Belgium [205]

Hyekyung Yang, Department of Pathology, University of Massachusetts Medical School, Worcester, MA 01605 [403]

Robert Yarchoan, Clinical Oncology Program, National Cancer Institute, National Institutes of Health, Bethesda, MD 20205 [95]

Howard A. Young, Laboratory of Molecular Immunoregulation, BRMP, DCT, National Cancer Institute, NIH, Frederick Cancer Research Facility, Frederick, MD 20892 [75]

Rudolf H. Zubler, Swiss Institute for Experimental Cancer Research, 1066 Epalinges, Switzerland [109]

Preface

Over the past 20 years interested scientists have met informally to exchange the latest research findings obtained in in vitro studies of leukocytes at a series of Leukocyte Culture Conferences (LCC). The 17th meeting of the International LCC met at the Ithaca, New York campus of Cornell University from August 3 until August 8, 1985. Because of shared scientific interests, this conference was held jointly with the 22nd National Meeting of the Reticuloendothelial Society (RES).

The first LCC was held in 1965 to discuss and resolve problems of in vitro leukocyte culture and lymphocyte transformation. Early conferences were primarily small, technically oriented workshops. As techniques developed and became more widely used in addressing particular scientific problems, the meetings have evolved into multidisciplinary conferences which focus on lymphocyte biology and include participants whose interests range from immunology, biochemistry, cell biology, molecular biology, hematology, physiology, oncology, pathology to pharmacology. These conferences have been sustained by a group of scientists who value their continuation by continued participation of the international scientific community. A loosely organized Steering Committee provides continuity and guidance and meets during each conference to select the organizer and location for future meetings. Meetings have been held almost annually (17 meetings in 20 years) and the site alternates between North America and Europe (including Israel).

The RES Society was founded in 1954 and incorporated in 1965. The current focus of the society is on two basic elements: monocyte and macrophage function and cellular cooperation in host defences, and to advance the exchange of information on the inflammatory process and its control, including cell production and distribution, chemotaxis, mediators, and pharmacological modulation. In pursuit of these goals, the RES has held annual national meetings since the first in 1964. In addition, the RES publishes the Journal of Leukocyte Biology (formerly the Journal of the Reticuloendothelial Society).

The objectives of this meeting were to provide a forum for discussion of current research on the cells involved in host defense systems and their modulation in normal and neoplastic states. The timeliness and usefulness of this meeting was based on its appreciation of the variety of leukocytes responsible for host defense and their modulation in pathological states and by pharmacologically active factors. By focusing on host defense systems, a number of related topics could be considered and permitted the development of a biological perspective.

Over 500 scientists engaged in scientific interchanges over a five-day period at symposia, poster sessions, and workshop discussions. The meeting attracted investigators concerned with the basic mechanisms and clinical problems of host defense from such diverse disciplines as immunology, pathology, pharmacology, cell biology, oncology, infectious diseases, and neuroendocrinology. The format of the meeting included symposia on major themes presented by invited speakers. The role of lymphocytes, macrophages, NK cells, granulocytes and platelets and the mechanism of their activation were presented. The development and differentiation of lymphocytes and macrophages were also discussed by symposia speakers. The symposia were supplemented by poster sessions followed by discussions on related topics to permit participants to discuss their recent research findings in small groups. Parallel workshops considered the effects of lymphokines, bacterial products, and biological response modifiers. The role of effector leukocytes in host defense and their modulation by lymphokines, neuroendocrine, microbial, and tumor cell-derived signals were emphasized. The meeting promoted increased understanding of the role of inflammation and the immune response in infectious diseases and malignancy, and the control of the host defenses by the neuroendocrine system.

It is the intent of this book to communicate the highlights of the proceedings to the scientific community. Selected symposium speakers and two to three of the most appropriate presentations from each of the 16 workshops were chosen by the session chairpersons to contribute concise articles to this volume. These articles have been organized into ten themes which reflect the major topics considered at the meeting. Consequently this volume contains a selection of research papers and reviews largely dealing with in vitro evaluation of the many vital roles of leukocytes in host defense.

Joost J. Oppenheim
Diane M. Jacobs

Acknowledgments

Obviously a meeting of this scope and size requires a group effort. Many devoted individuals contributed to the success of the conference and the resultant creation of this book.

We have ambivalent feelings towards the LCC steering committee for nominating us to organize this meeting. In retrospect it has been a worthwhile and productive experience, albeit marked by periods of considerable anxiety concerning the ways and means of managing such a large unfunded undertaking.

Our special thanks go to Dr. Ronald B. Herberman whose support fostered this joint meeting of the RES Society with the LCC. We are particularly grateful for the managerial skills and budgetary acumen of Dr. Sherwood Reichard and his staff who were responsible for the successful organization and support of the meeting. In addition, we are very grateful for the secretarial support of Ms. Bobbie Unger and Louise Shaw who dealt with the voluminous correspondence generated in organizing the meeting.

The local host committee led by Dr. Virginia Utermohlen was responsible for the special ambience of the meeting. She together with Dr. S. Gordon Campbell, who headed the workshop committee, with the assistance of Drs. Robin G. Bell, Douglas Antczak, Barbara A. Baird, Richard H. Jacobson, and Donald L. Wasson and a number of devoted Cornell undergraduate and graduate students organized the scientific sessions, provided succor and assistance to participants, arranged for transportation, good weather, entertainment, paraphernalia and all the necessary logistical support that led to an efficient and pleasant conference.

All of the participants also enjoyed the banquet presentation by Dr. James Larrick of Cetus Immune Laboratories on "The Waorani Indians of the Ecuadorian Amazon Rain Forest."

We are grateful to those scientists who advised us concerning the choice of symposia speakers, namely: Drs. Herbert L. Cooper, William Farrar, Ronald B. Herberman, Bonnie J. Mathieson, Francis Ruscetti, Carleton C. Stewart, Luigi Varesio, Robert H. Wiltrout, and Dorothea Zucker-Franklin.

Acknowledgments

In addition, we were aided by the heroic assistance of Drs. Peter Ralph, Thomas S. Edgington, and Priscilla A. Campbell who read, rated, and organized over 350 submitted abstracts into 16 coherent poster sessions followed by workshops. The workshop discussions were organized by selected chairpersons who also chose the workshop contributors to this volume as follows: Drs. Priscilla A. Campbell, Stanley Cohen, Philip Davies, Thomas S. Edgington, Bonnie J. Mathieson, Herman Friedman, Ronald H. Goldfarb, Warner C. Greene, Zvi Grossman, Stephen Haskill, Stephen M. Hedrick, Christopher S. Henney, Diane M. Jacobs, Charles A. Janeway, Jr., J. Gordin Kaplan, David A. Lawrence, Robert I. Lehrer, Peter Lipsky, Walter Pierpaoli, Richard J. Robb, Ross E. Rocklin, Frank Fitch, Stephen W. Russell, Kathy Kelly, Shagra Segal, Ethan M. Shevach, Novera H. Spector, Carleton C. Stewart, Osias Stutman, J. Brice Weinberg, Robert H. Wiltrout, and David D. Wood.

Finally, we are grateful to the following government and non-profit organizations and pharmaceutical firms for the financial support that made this meeting possible:

> Abbott Laboratories
> Ayerst Laboratories Research Inc.
> Boehringer Ingelheim Pharmaceuticals Inc.
> Bristol-Myers Company
> Cetus Corporation
> CIBA-GEIGY Corporation
> Cutter Laboratories
> E.I. Du Pont de Nemours & Company
> Eli Lilly and Company
> Genentech, Inc.
> Hoffman-La Roche, Inc.
> Monsanto Company
> National Institutes of Health
> The Noble Foundation
> Pfizer Central Research
> Sandoz, Inc.
> Schering Corporation
> Serono Laboratories, Inc.
> Smith Kline French Laboratories
> E.R. Squibb & Sons, Inc.
> Upjohn Company

The Reticuloendothelial Society also acknowledges the continuing financial support provided by our Corporate Members for 1985:

> AB Astra
> A.H. Robbins Company
> Abbott Laboratories
> Accurate Chemical & Scientific Corporation
> American Cyanamid
> Amgen
> Bristol-Myers
> Burroughs Wellcome
> E.I. De Pont de Nemours & Company
> Eli Lilly and Company
> Hoffman-La Roche, Inc.
> ICI, PLC
> Pfizer, Inc.
> Norwich Eaton Pharmaceuticals
> Schering Corporation
> Smith Kline French Laboratories
> Syntex
> Upjohn Company
> Wyeth Laboratories

Support for the Symposia and Awards was provided in part by the Office of Naval Research.

Support for Symposium II was provided in part by Serono Symposia, USA.

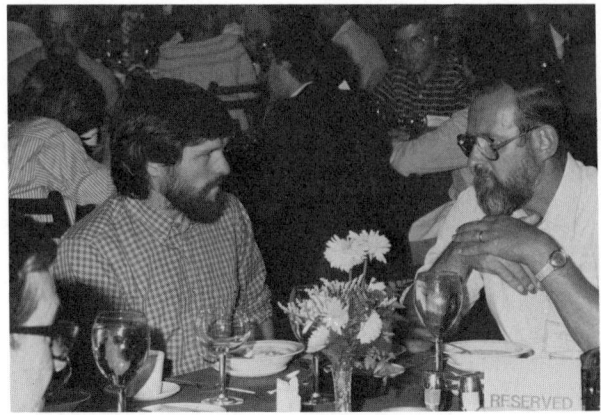

Dr. James W. Larrick (left) discussing his keynote address on the Waorani Indians of the Amazon with Dr. Joost J. Oppenheim.

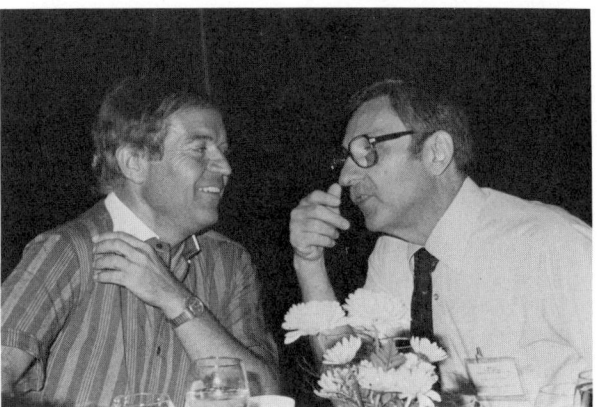

J.C. Mani (l.) from Montpellier, France, organizer of the 18th Leukocyte Culture Conference, to be held in La Grande Motte, June 1987, getting inside information from Dr. S. Reichard, Program Coordinator for the Reticuloendothelial Society.

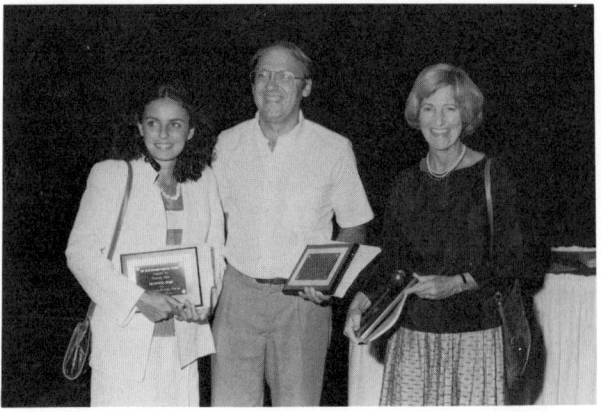

Winners of the Reticuloendothelial Society awards (l. to r.) Elisabetta Blasi (Presidential Award) and Craig W. Reynolds (Young Investigator Award) with RES president Dr. Dorothea Zucker-Franklin.

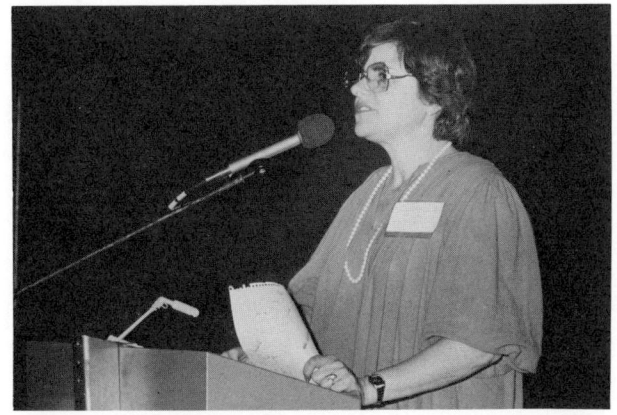
Dr. Diane Jacobs delivering her welcome speech at the Awards Banquet.

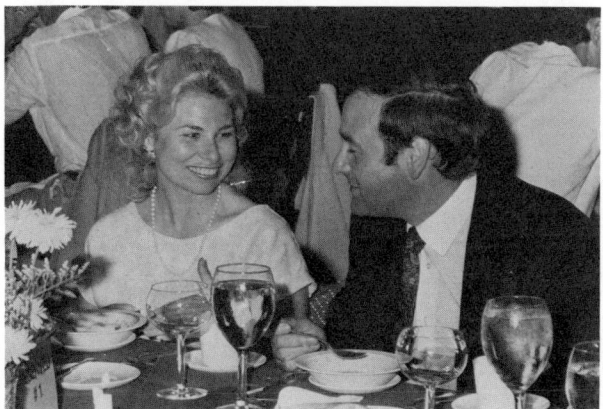
Marie T. Bonazinga, in whose honor the Marie T. Bonazinga Annual Research Award is named, in conversation with Dr. Phillip Davies.

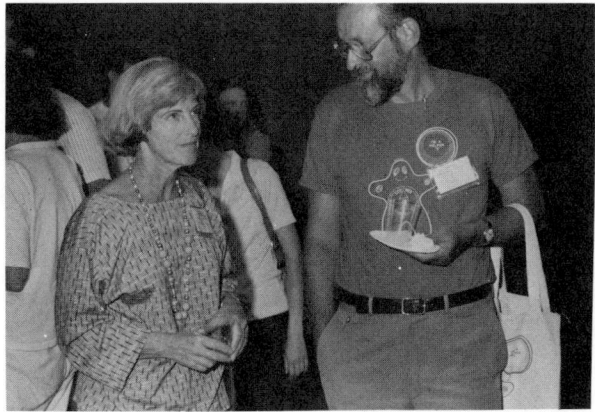
Dr. Zucker-Franklin contemplating a question posed by Dr. Oppenheim, who is sporting the LCC/RES T-shirt and bag.

Section I. Development and Differentiation of T Lymphocytes

MATURE AND IMMATURE THYMOCYTES : SURFACE PHENOTYPE, IMMUNE FUNCTION AND INTRATHYMIC LOCATION

Ken Shortman, Roland Scollay, Anne Wilson, Paul Andrews, Richard Boyd*, Eugene Butcher** and Irving Weissman**
The Walter and Eliza Hall Institute of Medical Research, Melbourne, Australia 3050; *Department of Pathology and Immunology, Monash University Medical School, Melbourne, Australia 3168; **Department of Pathology, Stanford University School of Medicine, Stanford, California 94305, U.S.A.

The search for stages of T-cell development within the thymus usually involves, as a first step, the sorting out of those thymocytes considered to be "mature" [meaning already immunologically functional and like peripheral T cells in surface characteristics] and those considered to be "immature" [meaning non-functional and different from peripheral T cells in surface characteristics]. The use of different criteria for making this primary division has led to many different views on what constitutes the immediate pool of "late" thymocytes for export to the periphery, and on what constitutes the generative pool of "early" thymocytes that serve as the ultimate source of peripheral T cells. This article summarises our experience with murine thymocytes using different approaches to this problem.

The traditional classification of thymocytes is into two populations, those of "cortical" phenotype and those of "medullary" phenotype, using markers such as peanut agglutinin [PNA] binding, Thy 1 level or H-2K level. This is best done by multiparameter flow cytometric analysis [Scollay and Shortman, 1983]. The major population, located in the cortex, is PNA^+ high Thy 1 and low H-2 and is thus different from peripheral T cells. Limit-dilution precursor-frequency analysis [Ceredig et al., 1982; Chen et al., 1982; Kisielow et al., 1982] has confirmed the earlier findings that these cells are not immunocompetent [Table 1]. On the basis of such evidence these cortical cells have been termed "immature thymocytes". This term carries the built-in assumption that these cells will later mature and give rise to medullary thymocytes and then to peripheral T cells.

TABLE 1. The Level of Immunocompetent Precursor T Cells Within the Conventional Cortical [PNA$^+$] and Medullary [PNA$^-$] Thymus Subpopulations

	Precursor frequency per Thy 1^+ cell	
	PTL-p	CTL-p
Spleen	.98 ± .15	.29 ± .02
Thymus	.080 ± .004	.034 ± .002
PNA$^-$ thymus	.46 ± .03	.117 ± .003
PNA$^+$ thymus	.0023 ± .0002	.0008 ± .0001

However, kinetic studies show the majority of cortical thymocytes are not the immediate precursors of medullary cells [Shortman and Jackson, 1974; Fathman et al., 1975] and it now seems clear that the majority of cortical thymocytes die in the thymus [McPhee et al., 1979; Scollay et al., 1980] as Metcalf [1966] originally suggested. Are any of the cells of this "immature" phenotype capable of developing into functional mature T cells? We have cultured PNA$^+$ thymocytes in the presence of high levels of T-cell produced lymphokines or purified IL-2 [Chen et al., 1983], or in the presence of a series of thymus hormone preparations, or in the presence of potent stimulators such as phorbol ester [Andrews et al., 1985]. In no case did any of the small cortical thymocytes, or any of the cortical blasts, produce any detectable increase in functional precursors. We consider it unlikely that any of these typical cortical thymocytes are on direct pathway leading to mature peripheral T cells. They represent what appears to be a "dead-end" pathway, and their significance is still obscure.

Does the minor population of low PNA binding "mature" or "medullary" phenotype cells correspond precisely to the thymocytes located within the medulla, and are these the immediate source of peripheral T cells? Most cells within the thymic medulla are of mature surface phenotype by most criteria. The issue is whether there also exists within the cortex a small subset of cells of "mature" or "medullary" phenotype which are the real source of thymus migrants. An argument for this is the existence within the cortex of a small subset of cells bearing high levels of the lymphocyte homing-receptor, detected by the monoclonal antibody MEL-14 [Reichert et al., 1984]; normally only mature peripheral T cells bear such high levels of the MEL-14 antigen. In addition, it is clear that the CBA mouse thymus contains more PNA⁻ thymocytes [14.5% average] than there are thymocytes actually located within the medulla [11.5% average] [Shortman et al., 1985]. However, a complicating factor is that many of the early blast cells in the cortex [discussed later] are also PNA⁻ and MEL-14⁺, and these blast cells are clearly immature. In an attempt to detect true mature phenotype cells in the cortex, we first selectively labeled outer-cortical thymocytes by dipping the intact thymus in fluorescent dyes, and then used either functional assays or multiparameter flow-cytometry to analyse these trans-capsular labeled cells in subsequent thymus cell suspensions. We were unable to detect any significant level of functionally mature cells, or of cells of full mature phenotype, in the outer cortex [Shortman et al., 1985]. However, this still leaves the possibility that such a population of mature cells exists within the inner cortex.

Are all the PNA⁻ "medullary" phenotype cells functionally mature? Our earlier studies [Chen et al., 1983] showed that, although all immunocompetent precursors are concentrated within the PNA⁻ thymocyte fraction, these cells still lack the almost 100% cloning efficiency of splenic T cells. Table 1 gives an example, where proliferative T-lymphocyte precursors [PTL-p] represent all cells able to form a clone measured by ^{3}H-TdR uptake in response to concanavalin A as stimulus, and cytotoxic T-lymphocyte precursors [CTL-p] represent all cells able to form a clone lysing P815 tumor target cells in the presence of phytohemagglutinin. We estimate that, allowing for losses on labeling and sorting, only about 70% of "medullary" phenotype cells are immunocompetent, and this implies that about 30% must be incompetent or "immature". We have recently confirmed this conclusion by directly separating functional from non-functional PNA⁻ thymocytes, based on their expression of the lymphocyte homing receptor. These results are summarised in Figure 1. About 70% of PNA⁻ thymocytes are MEL-14 antigen positive, although their level of expression is less than that of peripheral T cells. About 30% are MEL-14 negative. When PNA⁻ thymocytes were sorted into various fractions based on MEL-14 level, then assayed for all CTL-p, activity was

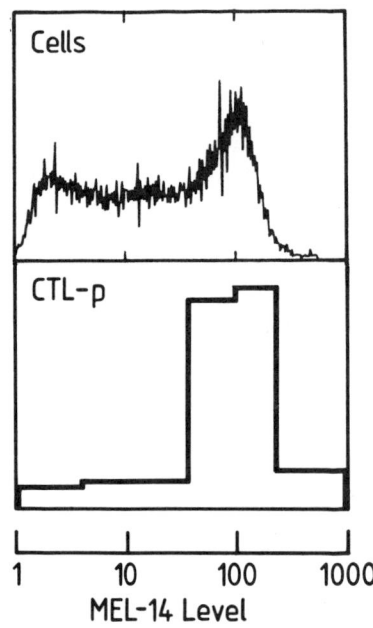

Figure 1. A comparison of the distribution of MEL-14 antigen on all cells and on all cytotoxic precursor cells in the PNA⁻ thymocyte fraction.

associated with the MEL-14$^+$ but not with the MEL-14$^-$ cells. We now require the results of a comparable PTL-p assay, and a knowledge of the distribution of Ly 2$^+$ and L3T4$^+$ cells, to fully interpret these findings. However it is clear that what was originally classed as one "mature" subpopulation can be divided, on the basis of function and MEL-14 expression, into "mature" and "immature" subsets.

A quite different way of distinguishing putative "mature" and "immature" thymocytes is based on their expression of the lineage-specific and function-associated surface antigens Ly 2 and L3T4. This type of separation was first carried out for human thymocytes using the T8 and T4 markers [Reinherz et al., 1980]. Murine thymocytes give comparable results [Ceredig et al., 1982; Scollay et al., 1984]. The majority of thymocytes differ from mature T cells in simultaneously expressing both Ly 2 and L3T4; these are the small cortical thymocytes and the more typical cortical blasts. Whether this double-expression represents an "immature" state, or merely the matured end-state of a dead-end pathway, is subject to the same arguments as those above for these same cells defined as PNA$^+$ and high Thy 1.

These $Ly\ 2^+\ L3T4^+$ cells are not immunocompetent. However the thymus does contain lineage-committed cells expressing only one or the other marker in the manner of mature T cells. These $Ly\ 2^+\ L3T4^-$ and $Ly\ 2^-\ L3T4^+$ cells are functional, and are found primarily in the medulla. Thus they can be classed as "mature", and we believe these markers provide a less ambiguous definition than PNA binding or Thy 1 level. However, we have not as yet attempted to subdivide these two "mature" subsets by MEL-14 antigen level.

This analysis also reveals a fourth $Ly\ 2^-\ L3T4^-$ subpopulation, representing about 4% of adult murine thymocytes. These are large blast cells located in the cortex, especially in the outer cortex [Scollay et al., 1984]. We believe these $Ly\ 2^-\ L3T4^-$ blasts, rather than the $Ly\ 2^+\ L3T4^+$ cortical cells, do have the necessary credentials for classification as "immature", or "early" thymocytes; in particular they include the intrathymic precursor cells able to reconstitute an irradiated thymus [Fowlkes et al., 1984]. They are discussed in more detail by Ceredig elsewhere in this volume. The aspect we wish to emphasise here is that the 4% $Ly\ 2^-\ L3T4^-$ cells are far from representing a single subpopulation. We have found they can be subdivided on the basis of B2A2, Thy 1 and Ly 1 expression, of PNA binding and more recently of MEL-14 antigen expression [Scollay et al., 1984; Scollay and Shortman, 1985]. Such a degree of complexity might be expected if key developmental decisions are being made within this group of putative early precursor cells. We can expect a continuing debate concerning degrees of maturity or immaturity as we attempt to align these subsets into a developmental sequence.

Our final approach to thymocyte classification is based, not just on location in the cortex or medulla, but on an intimate association with thymic epithelial cells. Wekerle and Ketelsen [1980] first observed, in enzymic digests of the thymus, large complexes consisting of epithelial cells enclosing many thymocytes, and called these "nurse cells". They appear to reflect pre-existent and closed microenvironments in the outer cortex [Kyewski and Kaplan, 1982; Andrews and Boyd, 1985], and include only about 1% of all thymocytes. As the imaginative name implies, "nurse cells" could be a site where immature thymocytes are nurtured to maturity, and the nature of the thymocytes within them is therefore of interest.

The intra-nurse cell thymocytes have been reported to be like other cortical cells in surface phenotype. However, several reports suggested they had both helper [Vakharia and Mitchison, 1984] and cytotoxic precursor [Fink et al., 1984] function. The picture was thus of an intermediate form of cortical cell, in the process of maturing to immunocompetence. We have recently tested intra-nurse-cell thymocytes for their level of functional precursors, in a way that should allow a total balance sheet of functional and non-functional cells [Andrews et al., 1985]. In this study we micromanipulated individual nurse-cells from enriched preparations, and so were able to ensure, by microscopic inspection, the complete absence of any contaminating exogenous cells. The individual nurse cells were incubated in micro-culture to release their contents, the freed lymphoid cells counted and then assayed in limit dilution culture at the level of one cell per culture. The results are summarised in Table 2.

The majority of intra-nurse cell thymocytes did not form clones in response to concanavalin A in our cultures, although side-by-side assays on other mature cell sources gave high cloning efficiencies. However about one intra-nurse-cell thymocyte in 30, or 2-6 thymocytes per nurse cell, did form a clone. This frequency was around 10-fold higher than that of PNA^+ cortical cells in general. However not one of these clones, out of hundreds tested, was cytolytic. We are currently assessing if the PTL-p were mature cells of the helper lineage, or if they represented early cycling blast cells that merely continued to proliferate in our cultures. The overall conclusion is that most intra-nurse-cell thymocytes are non-functional or "immature" like most other cortical cells, but the nurse-cell might contain some functional or "mature" cells of the helper, $L3T4^+$, lineage.

TABLE 2. The Limited Immunocompetence of Nurse Cell Lymphocytes

	Precursor frequency	
	PTL-p	CTL-p
Cortisone-resistant (medullary) thymocytes	0.88 ± 0.04	0.13 ± 0.03
PNA^+ (cortical) thymocytes	0.003 ± 0.001	0.0008 ± 0.0002
Nurse cell lymphocytes	0.030 ± 0.008	0.0000 ± 0.0000

REFERENCES

Andrews P, Boyd R (1985). The murine thymic nurse cell: An isolated thymic microenvironment. Eur J Immunol 15:36-42.

Andrews P, Boyd R, Shortman K (1985). The limited immunocompetence of thymocytes within murine thymic nurse cells. Eur J Immunol (in press).

Andrews P, Shortman K, Scollay R, Potworowski EF, Kruisbeek AM, Goldstein G, Trainin N, Bach J-F (1985). Thymic hormones do not induce proliferative ability or cytolytic function in PNA$^+$ cortical thymocytes. Cell Immunol 91:455-466.

Ceredig R, Glasebrook AL, MacDonald HR (1982). Phenotypic and functional properties of murine thymocytes. I. Precursors of cytolytic T lymphocytes and interleukin-2 producing cells are contained within a subpopulation of "mature" thymocytes as analysed by monoclonal antibodies and flow microfluorometry. J Exp Med 155:358-379.

Ceredig R, Dialynas DP, Fitch FW, MacDonald HR (1983). Precursors of T-cell growth factor producing cells in the thymus: Ontogeny, frequency and quantitative recovery in a subpopulation of phenotypically mature thymocytes defined by monoclonal antibody GK-1.5. J Exp Med 158:1654-1671.

Chen W-F, Scollay R, Shortman K (1982). The functional capacity of thymus subpopulations: Limit-dilution analysis of all precursors of cytotoxic lymphocytes and of all T cells capable of proliferation in subpopulations separated by the use of peanut agglutinin. J Immunol 129:18-24.

Chen W-F, Scollay R, Clark-Lewis I, Shortman K (1983). The size of functional T-lymphocyte pools within thymic medullary and cortical cell subsets. Thymus 5:179-195.

Fathman CG, Small M, Herzenberg LA, Weissman IL (1975). Thymus cell maturation. II. Differentiation of three "mature" subclasses in vivo. Cell Immunol 15:109-128.

Fink PJ, Weissman IL, Kaplan HS, Kyewski BA (1984). The immunocompetence of murine stromal cell-associated thymocytes. J Immunol 132:2266-2272.

Fowlkes B-J, Edison L, Mathieson B, Chused TM (1984). In Sercarz E, Cantor H, Chess L (eds): "Regulation of the Immune System; UCLA Symposium on Molecular and Cellular Biology, New Series," New York: Alan R. Liss, pp 285-293.

Kisielow P, von Boehmer H, Haas W (1982). Functional and phenotypic properties of subpopulations of murine thymocytes. I. The bulk of peanut agglutinin-positive Lyt-1, 2, 3 thymocytes lacks precursors of cytotoxic T lymphocytes responsive to interleukin-2 (T cell growth factor). Eur J Immunol 12:463-467.

Kyewski RA, Kaplan HS (1982). Lymphoepithelial interactions in the mouse thymus: Phenotypic and kinetic studies on thymic nurse cells. J Immunol 128:2287-2294.

McPhee D, Pye J, Shortman K (1979). The differentiation of T lymphocytes: Evidence for intrathymic death of most thymocytes. Thymus 1:151.

Metcalf D (1966). The nature and regulation of lymphopoiesis in normal and neoplastic thymus. In Wolstenholme GWE, Porter R (eds): "The Thymus: Experimental and Clinical Studies," CIBA Foundation Symposium, London:Churchill, p 242.

Reichert RA, Gallatin WM, Butcher EC, Weissman IL (1984). A homing receptor-bearing cortical thymocyte subset: Implications for thymus cell migration and the nature of cortisone-resistant thymocytes. Cell 38:89-99.

Reinherz EL, Kung PC, Goldstein G, Levey RH, Schlossman SF (1980). Discrete stages of human intrathymic differentiation. Analysis of normal thymocytes and leukemic lymphoblasts of T cell lineage. Proc Natl Acad Sci USA 77:1588-1592.

Scollay R, Butcher E, Weissman I (1980). Thymus migration: Quantitative studies on the rate of migration of cells from the thymus to the periphery in mice. Eur J Immunol 10:210-218.

Scollay R, Bartlett P, Shortman K (1984). T cell development in the adult murine thymus: Changes in the expression of the surface antigens Ly 2, L3T4 and B2A2 during development from early precursor cells to emigrants. Immunol Rev 82:79.

Scollay R, Shortman K (1983). Thymocyte subpopulations: An experimental review, including flow cytometric cross-correlations between the major murine thymocyte markers. Thymus 5:245-295.

Scollay R, Shortman K (1985). Identification of early stages of T lymphocyte development in the thymus cortex and medulla. J Immunol (in press).

Shortman K, Jackson H (1974). The differentiation of T-lymphocytes. I. Proliferation kinetics and inter-relationships of subpopulations of mouse thymus cells. Cell Immunol 12:230-246.

Shortman K, Mandel T, Andrews P, Scollay R (1985). Are any functionally mature cells of medullary phenotype located in the thymus cortex? Cell Immunol 93: (in press).

Vakharia DD, Mitchison NA (1984). Helper T cell activity demonstrated by thymic nurse cell T cells (TNC-T). Immunol 51:269-273.

Wekerle H, Ketelsen UP (1980). Thymic nurse cells - Ia bearing epithelium involved in T-lymphocyte differentiation. Nature 283:402-404.

STUDIES OF ADOPTIVE TRANSFER OF THYMIC RUDIMENTS

David A. Crouse and Reg K. Jordan

Departments of Anatomy, University of Nebraska Medical Center, Omaha, Nebraska 68105 (D.A.C.), and University of Newcastle-upon-Tyne, Newcastle, England NE2 4HH (R.K.J.)

INTRODUCTION

Since the observation that thymectomy of newborn mice causes a severe impairment in cell mediated function (Miller, 1962) there has been little doubt that the thymus plays a pivotal role in the development of a competent T-lymphocyte system. Events such as the rearrangement of T-lymphocyte receptor genes (Born et al., 1985), the expression of antigen specific receptors (Snodgrass et al., 1985), as well as the emergence of heterogeneity and functional specialization within the thymocyte and peripheral T-lymphocyte populations (Fowlkes and Mathieson, 1985; Scollay et al., 1984) are all accepted as features of the ontogeny of the immune system. Many of these characteristics are described in detail elsewhere in the proceedings of this symposium.

The broad objective of the studies reported here was to investigate the nature and consequences of cell interactions within the thymic microenvironment which lead to T-lymphocyte differentiation. In our working hypothesis, we have envisaged the thymus as providing the primary site for the amplification of T-cell clones physiologically capable of functioning with the host self-environment. Such a view presupposes a series of interactions between the thymic epithelial matrix and the colonizing lymphohematopoietic cells which ultimately supply, at a minimum, T-progenitors, macrophages and dendritic cells. The rationale employed in the design of the experiments is based upon the _in vitro_ isolation of the thymic epithelial matrix and its subsequent controlled recombination with other elements of the thymic microenvironment in both in vivo and in vitro models. In earlier studies (Jordan et al., 1979) we used monolayer cultures of thymic "epithelial" cells and have described their limitations. More recently, two different treatment protocols which employ the organ culture of 14 d fetal thymus have provided suitable preparations of thymic epithelial matrix free of lymphoid cells or their precursors. In this report we summarize a comparison of these two methods and the capacity of the epithelial preparations to provide functional reconstitution in two different immunodeficient mouse models.

METHODS

Epithelium from 14 d gestational age fetal mouse thymus was purified by two methods. Firstly, we used low temperature organ culture (LTOC) treatment (7 d at 24°C then 7 d at 37°C) as previously described (Jordan et al., 1985a) and modeled after the pancreas islet allograft studies of Lacy et al., (1979). Secondly, we used 1.35 mM deoxyguanosine (DGUO) treatment in 37°C organ cultures of similar embryonic materials as described by Jenkinson et al., (1982).

We also employed two immunodeficient mouse models to evaluate the morphological, marker and functional reconstitution elicited by grafting of the purified epithelial matrix. For our first model, we prepared adult thymectomized (8 wk old), lethally irradiated (8.5 Gy, Co^{60} γ) and fetal liver (2×10^7 16 day fetal liver cells i.v., 24 hr post-exposure) reconstituted mice as immunodeficient (ATxFL) radiation chimeras. As a second model, we used the nude (nu/nu) mouse which has a congenital thymic dysplasia resulting in a profound T-cell immunodeficiency. For each set of experiments, groups of ATxFL or nu/nu mice were grafted (Jordan et al., 1985a) with two lobes of thymic epithelium depleted of lymphoid cells and their precursors as described above. Other age matched groups of the same mice were grafted with fresh 16 d fetal thymic lobes or left ungrafted as positive and negative controls respectively. In the studies with ATxFL hosts, all grafting was conducted one week post-hemopoietic reconstitution. Although mice were sampled over a wide range of time points, the data presented here represent results from studies at 30-60 days post-grafting. At the time of sacrifice, some grafts along with the lymphocyte depleted materials sampled at the time of grafting, were prepared and evaluated histologically using routine light and electron microscopic methods. The grafted mice, as well as positive and negative controls were evaluated for reconstitution by enumeration of the frequency of T-cell surface marker positive populations in the graft and spleen and by various routine *in vivo* or *in vitro* immunological functional assays (mitogens, MLR, CTL, DTH and antibody production) using methods previously described (Jordan et al., 1985a & 1985b; Crouse et al., 1984b).

RESULTS AND DISCUSSION

Both LTOC and DGUO Treatment Provide Morphologically Equivalent Lymphocyte Depleted Thymic Epithelium

In agreement with previous studies in our laboratory and elsewhere, using morphological or marker analysis, no lymphoid cells could be detected in any of the lymphocyte depleted thymic preparations (i.e. LTOC or DGUO) even after being returned to normal culture conditions (Crouse et al., 1984a; Jordan et al., 1985a; Jenkinson et al., 1982). In our hands, both the LTOC and DGUO derived thymic epithelial lobes were morphologically quite similar. Each was composed of a compact epithelial matrix with abundant tonofilaments and desmosomes. Interspersed in the epithelial mass were cystic areas typically lined by a more darkly staining epithelial cell population with stubby microvilli and occasional cytoplasmic vesicles compatible with a secretory function.

Characterization of Repopulating Lymphohematopoietic Cells

Upon grafting of ATxFL or nu/nu immunodeficient hosts (ATxFL or nu/nu) with LTOC prepared thymic epithelium, we have previously shown that the repopulating lymphoid and Ia+ adherent cells were of host origin (Crouse et al., 1984a; Jordan et al., 1985b;) and demonstrated a surface marker phenotype (TL, Thy 1, Ly 1, Lyt 2) characteristic of a normal young adult thymocyte population. Although no two color studies were performed, the presence of high percentages (>90%) of cells with each marker would be in keeping with a typical double positive cortical population dominating the heterogeneous thymocyte population (Scollay et al., 1984; Fowlkes and Mathieson, 1985). Unfortunately, in the absence of two color fluorescence techniques, relative frequency of double negative cells could not be accurately determined. In addition to surface marker phenotype, the intragraft population displayed a mitogen response to Con A and a mixed lymphocyte response against allogeneic cells which was in keeping with their thymocyte nature. The low but reproducible levels of these responses in normal thymus have been attributed to the small "mature" T-cell population associated with the medulla. The similarities of the intragraft and control thymic cells, with respect to surface marker defined populations and functional capacities, is compatible with the classification of the intragraft cells as thymocytes.

Splenic Reconstitution in LTOC Thymic Grafted ATxFL Mice

The apparently normal repopulation of the LTOC thymic epithelial graft would, of course, be expected to precede the peripheralization of surface marker identifiable and immunologically functional T-cells. Surprisingly, this was not the case. Over the course of greater than 100 days post-grafting, we were unable to demonstrate peripheral reconstitution in the ATxFL mouse grafted with LTOC thymus. These data are partially summarized in Table 1. The ATxFL radiation chimeras grafted with fresh 16 d fetal thymus, though not restored to full function, show a significant return toward the normal range of markers and response and the ATxFL ungrafted negative controls show very little return of the splenic T-cell populations and remain profoundly immunodeficient. We have speculated that the lack of peripheral reconstitution may be related to the altered frequency of ectodermally versus endodermally derived thymic epithelium as a potential consequence of the LTOC treatment

TABLE 1. Summary of reconstitution of T-cell markers and functions in spleens of ATxFL mice with or without thymic grafts

Group	% Thy 1+	Lyt2	L3T4	PHA	LPS	anti-SRBC
Normal Control	100[a]	100	100	100	100	100
ATxFL	16	26	27	13	117	25
ATxFL + 16 d FT[b]	51	60	49	125	93	–
AtxFL + LTOC	24	39	–	15	121	15

a. All values are normalized to the control which is expressed as 100%.
b. Fresh thymus from 16 d gestational age fetal mice.

(Crouse et al., 1984). We must also, however, consider the well documented long term immunological deficiencies frequently observed in radiation chimeras bearing an intact thymus (Gratama et al., 1984; Ueda et al., 1984) and the additional limitations placed on the model by orthotopically grafting a culture manipulated fetal thymus. Although the fetal liver used to reconstitute the irradiated host will provide adequate hemopoietic progenitor populations, it has been shown that the very early embryonic thymic anlagen is populated by successive waves of progenitors (LeDourain et al., 1984) and that both intra- and extra-embryonic sources contribute to the early thymic migratory populations (Kau and Turpen, 1983) It is conceivable that the use of later embryonic materials along with a fully depleted epithelial matrix does not provide the complement of thymic migrants which will allow full and/or efficient repopulation of the peripheral T-cell compartments.

Splenic Reconstitution in nu/nu Mice Grafted with LTOC or DGUO Thymus

In a series of discussions at the Kyoto International Congress of Immunology we learned that at least two groups of researchers were able to reconstitute the peripheral T-cell compartments of nu/nu hosts following grafting with thymic materials depleted by LTOC or similar <u>in vitro</u> manipulations (Cohen, 1983). In the past 18 months, we also have been able to demonstrate significant immunological reconstitution of nu/nu hosts grafted with either LTOC or DGUO prepared thymic epithelium. These results are summarized in Table 2 below.

TABLE 2. Summary of reconstitution of T-cell markers and functions in spleens of nu/nu mice with or without thymic grafts

Group	% Thy 1^+	ConA	CTL	DTH	anti-OVA
Normal Control	100^a	100	100	100	100
nu/nu	2	<5	<5	<5	<5
nu/nu + 16 d FT^b	62	37	178	61	–
nu/nu + LTOC	56	34	97	52	56
nu/nu +DGUO	69	–	88	54	–

a. Normalized to the control which is expressed as 100%.
b. Fresh thymus from 16 d gestational age fetal mice.

Both T-cell marker frequencies and a battery of functional assessments supported a return of splenic T-lymphocyte populations to levels which were comparable to that attained following fresh thymus grafting. Other laboratories have also reported on the reconstitution of the T-lymphocyte pool in similar nu/nu models (Ready et al., 1984; VonBoehmer and Shubiger, 1984).

These results left us with the need to explain the paradoxical findings of our own reconstitution studies using thymic epithelial grafts in ATxFL hosts versus nu/nu mice. In the former, we were unable to demonstrate significant promotion of peripheral T-cell function beyond that emerging in the absence of thymic influence, while in the latter, reconstitution of a wide range of peripheral T-cell functions was easily obtained. We previously suggested a possible explanation based on a deficient microenvironmental component of the low temperature treated fetal thymus (Crouse et al., 1984a) compensated for by the nude recipient's own dysplastic primarily endodermal thymic rudiment (an hypothesis we do not as yet exclude). As previously stated, an alternative explanation may be related to the hemopoietic perturbations imposed in the ATxFL system versus the "intact" hemopoietic system of the nu/nu host. Just over five years ago, most investigators would have adhered to the view that on the pathway from hemopoietic stem cell to mature T-lymphocyte, traffic of T-progenitors through the thymic microenvironment was an obligatory step (Stutman, 1978). With the demonstration that in the absence of normal thymic influence, some function can be induced by appropriate exogenous stimulation (Gillis et al., 1979; Hunig, 1983) and that alternative extrathymic pathways of precursor differentiation may exist, the predominant view became one in which the thymus was simply the preferred site for T-cell differentiation and expansion. This view however relegates the extrathymic pathway to a minor role in the normal intact animal, being demonstrable only in mutant and experimentally manipulated models. While not entirely discarding this view, we now believe that an alternative conceptual framework, such as the one proposed by Dosch et al. (1985), where an extrathymic T-precursor pool matures under the influence of thymic emigrants or their products, is worth more consideration. The contribution of such an extrathymic T-cell precursor population to the mature peripheral T-cell pool may have been underestimated and should be examined in other model systems.

It has been shown that thymectomized, bone marrow reconstituted radiation chimeras (ATxBM) develop CTLp that can respond to antigen only if ConA supernatant is added to the culture, indicating that a T-helper cell deficit may be a major cause of non-responsiveness in these chimeras (Duprez et al., 1984). Thus, following thymectomy, irradiation and hemopoietic reconstitution in our ATxFL model, putative extrathymic precursor pools may be perturbed, contributing to their failure to reconstitute even though low temperature organ culture thymic grafts show intragraft "thymocytes" regenerate. This would not be an attendant problem in the nude mouse which would have both precursor pools intact and lack only the thymic microenvironment necessary for the maturation of regulatory thymic emigrants. In this context it is interesting to speculate that an analogous situation may exist following irradiation and autologous reconstitution of bone marrow transplant patients who often fail to show full recovery of immune function (Gratama et al., 1984; Ueda et al., 1984). Furthermore, other long standing paradoxes should be reappraised from this view of dual pathways of T-dependent differentiation. Significant among these is the role of the thymus in dictating the MHC restriction specificity of the T-cell repertoire. Initially, some experiments employing radiation chimeras coupled with thymic transplantation suggested that commitment of T-lymphocytes to MHC components is determined during an intrathymic stage of differentiation (Bevan and Fink, 1978; Zinkernagel, 1980). Other experiments, however, indicated that MHC restriction could be imposed as a consequence of immunization, occurring at the level of antigen presentation (Miller, 1980). In the former once again there was attendant hemopoietic perturbation and the requirement for differentiation of the test responder population from precursors, while in the latter mature peripheral T-cells from unmanipulated donors were assayed, albeit after negative depletion of alloreactivity. More recently in studies using either nu/nu recipients (Kast et al., 1984) or radiation chimeras (Kruisbeek et al., 1983) , thymus appears to exert a major influence on T-cells restricted to Class II molecules, whereas its role with respect to Class I restricted T cells is limited. These observations can be interpreted as strengthening the argument that extrathymic precursor maturation may play a significant part in the generation of the T-cell repertoire.

REFERENCES

Bevan MJ, Fink PJ (1978). Influence of thymus H-2 antigens on the specificity of maturing killer and helper cells. Immunol Rev 42:3-19.

Born W, Yague J, Palmer E, Kappler J, Marrak P (1985). Rearrangement of T-cell receptor B-chain genes during T-cell development. Proc Natl Acad Sci USA 82:2925-2929.

Cohen J (1983). Differentiation and development of T-cells. Questions of intrathymic ancestry. Immunology Today 4:302-303.

Crouse DA, Perry GA, Jordan RK (1984a). Transplantation of lymphoid free thymic epithelium in syngeneic and allogeneic immunodeficient mice. In Cantor H, Chess L, Sercarz E (eds): "Regulation of the Immune System," New York: Alan R. Liss, pp 231-242.

Crouse DA, Jordan RK, Sharp JG (1984b). Thymic microenvironment. Biblthca Haemat 48:293-320.

Dosch H-M, White D, Grant C (1985). Reconstitution of nude mouse T cell function *in vivo*: IL2-independent effect of human T cells. J Immunol 134:336-342.

Duprez V, Maziarz R, Weinberger O, Burakoff SJ (1984). Thymectomized irradiated, and bone marrow-reconstituted chimeras have normal cytolytic T-lymphocyte precursors but a defect in lymphokine production. J Immunol 132:2185-2189.

Fowlkes BJ, Mathieson BJ (1985). Intrathymic differentiation: Thymocyte heterogeneity and the characterization of early T-cell precursors. Surv Immunologic Res 4:96-109.

Gillis SH, Union NA, Baker PE, Smith KA (1979). The *in vitro* generation and sustained culture of nude mouse cytolytic T-lymphocytes. J Exp Med 149:1460-1476.

Gratama JW, Naipal A, Oljans P, Zwaan FE, Verdonck LF, deWitte T, Vossen JMJJ, Bolhuis RLH, deGast GC, Jansen J (1984). T lymphocyte repopulation and differentiation after bone marrow transplantation. Early shifts in the ratio between T4+ and T8+ T lymphocytes correlate with the occurrence of acute graft-versus-host disease. Blood 63:1416-1423.

Hunig T (1983). T-cell function and specificity in athymic mice. Immunol Today 4:84-87.

Jenkinson EJ, Franchi LL, Kingston R, Owen JJT (1982). Effect of deoxyguanosine treatment on lymphopoiesis in the developing thymus *in vitro*: Application in the production of chimeric thymic rudiments. Eur J Immunol 12:583-587.

Jordan RK, Crouse DA, Owen JJT (1979). Studies on the thymic microenvironment: Nonlymphoid cells responsible for transferring the microenvironment. J Reticuloendothel Soc 26:373-383.

Jordan RK, Bentley AL, Perry GA, Crouse DA (1985a). Thymic epithelium I. Lymphoid-free organ cultures grafted in syngeneic intact mice. J Immunol 134:2155-2160.

Jordan RK, Robinson JH, Hopkinson NA, House KC, Bentley AL (1985b). Thymic epithelium and induction of transplantation tolerance in nude mice. Nature 314:454-456.

Kast WM, deWaal LP, Melief CJM (1984). Thymus dictates major histocompatibility complex (MHC) specificity and immune response gene phenotype of class II MHC-restricted T cells but not of class I MHC-restricted T cells. J Exp Med 160:1752-1766.

Kau C-L, Turpen JB (1983). Dual contribution of embryonic ventral blood island and dorsal lateral plate mesoderm during ontogeny of hemopoietic cells in Xenopus Laevis. J Immunol 131:2262-2266.

Kruisbeek AM, Sharrow SO, Singer A (1983). Difference in the MHC-restricted self-recognition repertoire of intra-thymic and extra-thymic cytotoxic T lymphocyte precursors. J Immunol 130:1027-1032.

Lacy PE, Davie JM, Finke EH (1979). Prolongation of islet allograft survival following in vitro culture (24°C) and a single injection of ALS. Science 204:312-313.

LeDouarin NM, Dieterlen-Lievre F, Oliver PD (1984). Ontogeny of primary lymphoid organs and lymphoid stem cells. Am J Anat 170:261-299.

Miller JFAP (1962). Effect of neonatal thymectomy on the immunological responsiveness of the mouse. Proc Roy Soc B 156:415-428.

Miller JFAP (1980). MHC restrictions in cell cooperation. In Fougereau M, Dausset J (eds): "Immunology 80: Progress in Immunology IV," London: Academic Press, pp 359-374.

Ready AR, Jenkinson EJ, Kingston R, Owen JJT (1984). Successful transplantation across major histocompatibility barrier of deoxyguanosine-treated embryonic thymus expressing class II antigens. Nature 310:231-233.

Scollay R, Bartlett P, Shortman K (1984). T-cell development in the adult murine thymus: Changes in the expression of the surface antigens Ly2, L3T4 and B2A2 during development from early precursor cells to emigrants. Immunol Rev 82:79-103.

Snodgrass HR, Dembic Z, Steinmetz M, VonBoehmer H (1985). Expression of T-cell antigen receptor genes during fetal development in the thymus. Nature 315:232-233.

Stutman O (1978). Intrathymic and extrathymic T-cell maturation. Immunol Rev 42:138-174.

Ueda M, Harada M, Shiobara S, Nakao S, Kondo K, Odaka K, Matsue K, Mori T, Hattori K-I (1984). T-lymphocyte reconstitution in long-term survivors after allogeneic and autologous marrow transplantation. Transplantation 37:552-556.

VonBoehmer H, Schubiger K (1984). Thymocytes appear to ignore class I major histocompatibility complex antigens expressed on thymic epithelial cells. Eur J Immunol 14:1048-1052.

Zinkernagel RM (1980). T cell differentiation and restriction. In Fougereau M, Dausset J (eds): "Immunology 80: Progress in Immunology IV," London: Academic Press, pp 338-350.

ACKNOWLEDGEMENTS

We wish to thank Drs. JG Sharp, JB Turpen, JH Robinson, GA Perry and AL Bentley for their discussions and involvement in the studies reported here. Supported by NIH-AI15819.

NEW APPROACHES TO THE ASSESSMENT OF THE ROLE OF THYMIC STROMAL CELLS IN DEVELOPMENT OF T CELL RESTRICTION SPECIFICITIES

Ada M. Kruisbeek

Medicine Branch, National Institutes of Health, Building 10, Room 12N226, Bethesda, MD 20205

INTRODUCTION

Major histocompatibility complex (MHC) - restricted recognition is not an inherent property of T cells, but is a learned event which is dictated by the MHC-determinants expressed by the non-lymphoid elements in the thymus (1,2). Thus, the receptor specificities which T cells express when they have become functionally competent are determined by the MHC phenotype of the thymus in which they differentiate, rather than by the MHC phenotype of the T cells themselves. Although the intrathymic events that establish MHC-restriction specificities are largely unknown, it is now appreciated that class I-MHC- and class II-MHC-specific T cells may undergo different differentiation pathways. The self-MHC specificity and immune response (Ir)-gene phenotype of class II-specific T cells is determined strictly intrathymically, i.e., class II-specific T cells can only self-recognize class II-molecules expressed on nonlymphoid thymic elements (3-6). Class I-specific T cells, on the other hand, appear to be capable of recognizing class I-molecules expressed both in the thymic and in the extrathymic environment (1,2,5,6). Much attention has been focussed on the exact nature of the nonlymphoid thymic stromal elements involved in development of MHC restriction specificities. What follows is a review of studies which explore the relationship between thymic stromal cells and development of T cell restriction specificities.

IDENTIFICATION OF DISTINCT MHC-ANTIGEN BEARING THYMIC STROMAL CELLS

Indirect evidence from studies in chimeras and thymus-grafted nude mice show that selection of T cell specificities is greatly influenced by MHC-antigens expressed by (radioresistant) thymic stromal cells (e.g., 1-6). These findings led to the yet unproven hypothesis that interactions between the T cell receptor on thymocytes and MHC-antigens on stromal cells constitute the primary signals responsible for receptor diversification and imposition of MHC-restriction specificities. The isolation of various types of lympho-stromal complexes, thought to represent the specific in vivo association of thymocytes with certain stromal cells, has lent further credence to this view (7,8).

The characterization of thymic stromal cells with respect to their intrathymic localization, MHC-antigen expression and lympho-stromal interaction should provide us with tools for further assessment of the role of the individual cell types in regulation of T cell differentiation. The major stromal component of the thymus is epithelial in nature. It is now generally accepted that the epithelium is composed of two epithelia of different embryological origins: ectodermally and endodermally derived epithelium (9). Absence of the ectodermal component (as observed in nude mice (10) and in chickens in which the cephalic neural crest population is ablated (11)) leads to incomplete thymus development. More importantly for this discussion, epithelial cells and other stromal cells express high levels of class I and class II antigens.

CLASS II-BEARING EPITHELIAL CELLS

Both cortical and medullary epithelial cells are stained with reagents specific for class II-antigens in the mouse and the human thymus (12-14). Several studies suggest a function for the class II-molecules on epithelial cells in T cell development. First, the embryonic nude mouse thymic rudiment lacks class II-antigen bearing stromal cells (15, 16) whereas expression of class I-antigens is normal (15). While many reports document the presence of class I-specific T cells in nude mice (see, e.g., 6,17,18), attempts to detect class II-specific nude mouse T cells have been entirely unsuccessful (6,19). It should be noted, however, that the defect in nude mice is complex: apart from a failure to express Ia antigens on epithelial and dendritic cells in the thymic rudiment, they also are defective in expressing

other epithelial markers (15,16) and the dendritic cell
marker TR6 (16). Secondly, thymic lymphocytes do not
express their genotypically determined class II-antigens
but, as was concluded from studies with radiation bone
marrow chimeras (20), class II-antigens passively acquired
from radiation-resistant thymic stromal cells. Electron
microscopy studies revealed (12) that expression of class
II-antigens by thymocytes was restricted to the membrane in
contact with the Ia-positive stromal cells. Thymocytes
exhibited this feature with all types of stromal cells,
i.e., both epithelial and dendritic. The demonstration of
Ia-antigens associated with thymocytes only at points of
intercellular contact with stromal cells may reflect specific
Ia-antigen recognition and receptor-mediated binding of Ia
molecules by thymocytes.

CLASS II-BEARING DENDRITIC CELLS

Mononuclear phagocytes and interdigitating (dendritic)
cells in the thymus also express Ia antigens (13,16,21).
These cells occur mainly in the perivascular area of the
corticomedullary junction and of the medulla. Morphological
studies on thymuses from radiation bone marrow chimeras indicate that, while epithelial cells are of recipient origin,
class II-bearing medullary dendritic cells are of bone
marrow origin (21). Because functional Ia-bearing antigen
presenting cells (APC), isolated from the thymus, also are
of bone marrow origin (22,23), one could hypothesize that
medullary dendritic cells and thymic antigen presenting
cells are the same. As a monoclonal antibody, TR6, specific
for medullary dendritic cells has recently been identified
(on the basis of immunohistochemical studies) (24), this
notion can now be tested.

The role of these Ia-bearing dendritic cells in T cell
differentiation is not entirely clear. They might be involved in providing a stimulatory signal to self-class
II-specific thymocytes (25). Furthermore, the self-class
II restriction specificity of T cells developing in radiation bone marrow chimeras correlates with the class II-
phenotype of thymic APC (22,23). When nude mice were
grafted with thymuses whose APC class II-genotype differed
from that of the epithelial stromal element (26), developing
class II-restricted T cells again recognized the thymic
APC-class II antigens as self and made Ir-gene controlled
responses for which the APC-genotype is a responder. Therefore, the critical thymic stromal cell responsible for determining class II-restriction specificities appears to be

a bone marrow-derived APC, which might be identical to the medullary dendritic cell (21).

Another approach to exploring the role of thymic APC was to treat newborn mice with monoclonal anti-Ia antibodies (27-29), leading to reduced expression of class II-antigens in the thymus. In addition, this manipulation results in abrogation of thymic APC function (28) and complete lack of development of the class II-specific lineage of Lyt $2^- $ L3T4$^+$ T cells, as defined both functionally and phenotypically (28, 29). The class I-specific T cell lineage (Lyt2^+L3T4$^-$) develops normally in such anti-Ia-treated mice (28). Thus, expression of intrathymic class II-antigens is required for development of class II-specific T cells. In addition, these findings indicate that generation of the two major subsets of T cells occurs through separate events, involving unique sites of interaction between precursor T cells and thymic stromal cells. It should be stressed that these studies in anti-Ia treated mice do not argue that, because normal levels of class I-specific T cells are present, thymic APC do not play a role in development of class I-specific T cells. It is conceivable that thymic APC are present but non-functional as APC for class II-specific T cells, through loss of Ia-antigens (28,30). Thus, they might no longer be capable of providing activation signals for self-class II-specific thymocytes, but could still be delivering class I-specific signals and other nonspecific signals. Future studies will address these questions, as well as examine the effect of anti-Ia antibody treatment on the class II-bearing epithelial compartment.

A last type of experiment indirectly determining the role of class II-bearing dendritic cells involves organ culture of thymic rudiments in the presence of deoxyguanosine (dGuo) (31,32). Explants from thymuses from 14 day old embryos become completely devoid of lymphoid cells after 5 days of culture in dGuo (31), while maintaining normal organization and Ia-expression of epithelial cells (16,31). In addition, morphological studies indicate a substantial reduction or elimination of dendritic cells (31). A similar depletion of cells of haemotopoietic origin can be achieved by low temperature organ culture (LTOC) (33,34). When dGuo-treated or LTOC-grafts are transplanted into allogenic intact recipients, the host-derived intrathymic lymphocytes are not tolerized to thymic-class II antigens (32,35). Thus, it was concluded that class II-bearing epithelial cells are not involved in tolerization of developing thymocytes, but that, instead, only class

II-bearing dendritic cells can induce tolerance. Also tolerance to class I-antigens cannot be induced by dGuo grafts (36). Others, however, considered it premature to exclude thymic epithelial cells from having a role in tolerance induction, because LTOC-thymuses grafted into allogeneic nude, instead of intact recipients, did induce class II-tolerance (35). The explanation for this apparent paradox may be that in intact recipients, tolerance is marked by host T cells which matured in the host thymus and migrated into the allogeneic thymic graft. The crucial issue in these studies remains to determine whether the alleged epithelial grafts are indeed devoid of thymic APC, i.e., whether morphological evidence of absence of dendritic cells correlates with absence of functional APC.

CLASS I-BEARING THYMIC STROMAL CELLS

Staining patterns observed with anti-classI-antibodies are somewhat confusing: in the human thymus, some antibodies only react with medullary epithelial cells, while others react with both medullary and cortical epithelial cells (14). In the mouse thymus, only medullary epithelial cells were reported to react with anti-class I-antibodies (13), but a limited number of monoclonal antibodies was studied and after overnight culture, all epithelial cells become positive for class I antigens (15). These results suggest that in situ, all antigenic determinants of class I-molecules can be detected on medullary epithelial cells, while only a subset can be detected on cortical epithelial cells. All epithelial cells that express class I antigens probably also express class II antigens (15,31). Also dendritic cells express class I antigens (31).

An understanding of how class I-molecules on epithelial cells determine restriction specificities is not yet available. It is clear from studies in radiation bone marrow chimeras that developing class I-specific cytotoxic T cells acquire specificity for the class I-antigens on thymic stromal cells (1,2,5). Most likely, the restricting element for class I-specific T cells is a thymic epithelial cell (37), while the stromal cells imparting specificity to class II-specific T cells are bone marrow derived (see above) (22, 23). One study, however, contends that thymic epithelial cells are not involved in tolerization for class I-antigens (36). Direct evidence of recognition of class I-antigens on epithelial cells by thymocytes is not available to date, but thymocytes can passively acquire class I-antigens from radiation resistant thymic cells (20). The nature of the "donating" cells has not been determined.

OTHER STROMAL CELL MARKERS

Another level of heterogeneity in thymic epithelial cells was recently revealed, as monoclonal antibodies raised against thymic stromal cells became available. Both human (38) and mouse (24) cortical thymic epithelium is antigenically different from medullary epithelium. In addition, monoclonal antibody A2B5 which binds to human and mouse neuroendocrine cells, appears to define a subpopulation of stromal cells distinct from the bulk of class II-antigen expressing epithelial cells (31). In the mouse, also medullary dendritic cells are identified by a specific monoclonal antibody, not reactive with cortical and medullary epithelial cells (24). Thus, monoclonal antibodies have now confirmed the heterogeneity of thymic stromal cells previously reported on the basis of morphological studies. Whether the antigens defined by these stromal-cell specific antibodies are themselves involved in T cell differentiation has not yet been studied. We have used the approach of treating neonatal mice with anti-class II-antibodies to analyze the functional significance of thymic class II antigen in T cell development (see above) (27-29). In analogy, future work will focus on gaining better insight in the role of other stromal cell markers through treatment of neonatal mice with TR6 (the medullary dendritic cell marker) and TR4 and TR5 (the cortical and medullary epithelial cell markers) (Kruisbeek and Van Ewijk, in preparation).

THYMIC STROMAL CELLS IN ONTOGENY

Analysis of the thymic microenvironment during ontogeny should also facilitate a better understanding of the thymic stroma-T cell development relationship. One of the main questions to be answered is when developing thymocytes could first be capable of recognizing MHC (and other) antigens on thymic stromal cells, and thus become susceptible to repertoire selection and acquisition of tolerance. T cell-receptor-like molecules were reported to be detectable at day 17 of gestation (39,40), shortly after the β-chain genes have become rearranged (day 15-16) (39-41) and have become transcriptionally active. Because messenger RNA (mRNA) for the α-chain is not detected until day 19 (39), it has been postulated that early thymocytes express receptors formed by a combination of γ and β chains. The γ-chain genes are already transcribed at day 15, and transcription rapidly declines thereafter (39,41). What, then, can developing thymocytes recognize? Class II-antigen expression is present first on day 13 in the medulla and expands throughout the thymus lobe by day 16 (15,31). Also thymic APC function is first detectable on day 13 (42). Class I-antigen is first expressed by day 16 (31) but appears to be difficult to detect; when thymic explants from day 14-old embryos are cultured overnight, strong class I-antigen expression is obtained (31). The complex mixture of cell types which make up the thymic stroma appears complete by day 13 of gestation, as all three types of stromal cells can be identified by monoclonal antibodies (16) (i.e., cortical and medullary epithelial cells, and medullary dendutic cells). In summary, expression of MHC-antigens on stromal cells occurs long before expression of T cell receptors. If surface expression of the T cell antigen receptor complex is required for repertoire selection, this event could not occur until day 17 in embryonic development, as this is the earliest possible time at which a receptor might be present (39-41).

REFERENCES
1. Fink PJ, MJ Bevan (1978). J Exp Med 48:766.
2. Zinkernagel RM, Callahan GN, Klein J, Dennert G (1978). Nature 271:251.
3. Singer A, Hathcock KS, Hodes RJ (1982). J Exp Med 155:339.
4. Hedrick SM, Watson J (1979). J Exp Med 150:646.
5. Bradley SM, Kruisbeek AM, Singer A (1982). J Exp Med 156:1650.
6. Kruisbeek AM, Davis ML, Matis LA, Longo DL (1984). J Exp Med 160:839.
7. Kyewski BA, Rouse RV, Kaplan HS (1982). Proc Natl Acad Sci USA 79:5646.
8. Kyewski BA, Kaplan HS (1982). J Immunol 128:2287.
9. Cardier AC, Haumont SM (1980). Am J Anat 157:227.
10. Cordier AC, Heremans JF (1975). Scan J Immunol 4:193
11. Bockman DE, Kirby ML (1984). Science 223:498.
12. Farr A, Nakane P (1983). Am J Path 111:88.
13. Rouse RV, Van Ewijk W, Jones PP, Weissman IL (1979). J Immunol 122:2508.
14. Rouse RV, Parham P, Grumet FC, Weissman IL (1982). Scan J Immunol 5:21.

15. Jenkinson EJ, Van Ewijk W, Owen JJT (1981). J Exp Med 153:280.
16. Van Vliet E, Jenkinson EJ, Kingston R, Owen JJT, Van Ewijk W (1985). Eur J Immunol 15:645.
17. Hunig T, Bevan MJ (1980). J Exp Med 152:688.
18. Maryanski JL, MacDonald HR, Sordat B, Cerottini JC (1981). J Immunol 126:871.
19. Kast WM, deWaal LP, Melief CJM (1984). J Exp Med 160:1752.
20. Sharrow SO, Mathieson BJ, Singer A (1981). J Immunol 126:1327.
21. Barclay AN, Maythofer G (1981). J Exp Med 153:1666.
22. Longo DL, Schwartz RH (1980). Nature 287:44.
23. Longo DL, Davis ML (1983). J Immunol 130: 2525.
24. Van Vliet E, Melis M, Van Ewijk W (1984). Eur J Immunol 14:524.
25. Rock KL, Benacerraf B (1984). Proc Natl Acad Sci USA 81:1221.
26. Longo DL, Kruisbeek AM, Davis ML, Matis LA (1985). Proc Natl Acad Sci USA (in press).
27. Kruisbeek AM, Fultz MJ, Sharrow SO, Singer A, Mond JJ (1983). J Exp Med 157:1932.
28. Kruisbeek AM, Moud JJ, Fowlkes BJ, Carmen JA, Bridges, S, Longo DL (1985). J Exp Med 161: 1029.
29. Kruisbeek AM, Bridges S, Carmen J, Longo DL, Mond JJ (1985). J Immunol 134:3597.
30. Kruisbeek AM, Titus JA, Stephany DA, Gause BL, Longo DL (1985). J Immunol 134:3605.
31. Owen JJT, Jenkinson EJ (1984). Am J Anat 170:301.
32. Ready AR, Jenkinson EJ, Kingston R, Owen JJT (1984). Nature 310:231.
33. Robinson J, Jordan RK (1983). Immunol Today 4:41.
34. Jordan RK, Bentley AL, Perry GA, Crouse DA (1985). J Immunol 134:2155.
35. Jordan RK, Robinson JH, Hopkinson NA, House KC, Bentley AL (1985). Nature 314:454.
36. von Boehmer H, Schubiger K (1984). Eur J Immunol 14:1408.
37. Zinkernagel RM (1982). J Exp Med 156:1842.
38. Mc. Farland RM, Scearce, Haynes BF (1984). J Immunol 133:1241.
39. Snodgrass HR, Kisielow P, Kiefer M, Steinmetz M, von Boehmer H (1985). Nature 313:592.
40. Born W, Yague J, Palmer E, Kappler J, Marrack P (1985). Proc Natl Acad Sci 85:2925.

DEVELOPMENT OF T CELL RECEPTOR EXPRESSION IN FETAL THYMUS ORGAN CULTURES

Willi Born, Neal Roehm, Janice White, Ella Kushnir, Edward Palmer, John Kappler and Philippa Marrack

Department of Medicine, (W.B.,N.R.,J.W.,E.K., P.M.), National Jewish Center, and Departments of Medicine, of Microbiology and Immunology, and of Biochemistry, Biophysics and Genetics, (E.P., J.K., P.M.) University of Colorado Health Sciences Center, Denver, Colorado 80206

INTRODUCTION

In a series of elegant experiments with bone marrow and thymus chimeras it has been demonstrated that the major histocompatibility complex (MHC) type of the thymus determines to a large extent the repertoire of specificities in peripheral T cells (Bevan, 1977; Zinkernagel et al., 1978; Kruisbeek et al., 1981). While this linkage is well established, we still know little about the actual mechanisms by which repertoire is selected to yield self MHC-restricted specificities, and what role this selection plays in maintaining immunological self tolerance.

Most likely the selection process involves expression of T cell receptors for antigen/MHC on the surface of thymocytes. Therefore, we and others have analyzed the expression of T cell receptors in adult thymus populations and during thymocyte development in ontogeny (Acuto et al., 1985; Roehm et al., 1984; Snodgrass et al., 1985a, 1985b; Raulet et al., 1985; Born et al., 1985). It was found that, shortly after β and α gene rearrangements during early stages of development, the α/β heterodimeric receptor molecules appear, initially at low levels, on the surface of the cells. With further maturation of the cells receptor expression seems to increase gradually because we observed a wide spectrum of low, intermediate and high receptor densities on adult thymocytes, and uniformly high expression levels on peripheral T lymphocytes (Roehm et al., 1984).

Wondering whether T cell receptor expression would also initiate in vitro, i.e. under experimentally better controlled conditions, we have studied early events (β chain gene rearrangements) and late events (cell surface expression of the receptor molecules) in fetal thymus organ cultures[†]. Here we report that in these cultures, in the absence of immigrating precursor cells, antigen/MHC receptor expression develops in an apparently normal fashion over a period of several days.

MATERIALS AND METHODS

Timed pregnant BALB/cBy mice were generated in our own vivarium or purchased from The Jackson Laboratory. The day of finding a vaginal plug was designated as day 0 of embryonic development.

Organ cultures were set up as previously described by others (Mandel et al., 1978). Briefly, individual thymus lobes were incubated at the interface of 90% air/10% CO_2 and standard culture medium, supported by millipore filter strips (0.22μm) and gelatine rafts, at 37°C.

Hybridomas were prepared as previously described (Born et al., 1985), by fusion to the azaguanine-resistant AKR thymoma, BW5147.G.1.4 Oua^r.1.

Southern hybridizations were carried out by standard methods as previously described (Born et al., 1985). The probe used in these experiments (pDOβ2) hybridizes to $J\beta2_6$ and both $C\beta_1$ and $C\beta_2$. To map rearrangements within the β gene complex we prepared genomic restriction enzyme digests with the enzymes HindIII, PvuII and HpaI. A simultaneous analysis with all three enzymes allows the indentification of $D\beta_1$-to-$J\beta_1$, $D\beta_1$-to-$J\beta_2$ and $D\beta_2$-to-$J\beta_2$ rearrangements and detects VβDβJβ joining events as well as aberrant rearrangements involving the β gene complex (Born et al., 1985).

[†]We thank Dr. Thomas H. Mandel for familiarizing us with the fetal thymus organ culture system.

The properties and initial characterization of monoclonal antibody KJ16-133 have been previously described (Haskins et al., 1984). This antibody detects an allotypic determinant encoded by at least 3 Vβ genes (Behlke et al., 1985; Sim et al., 1985), present in the genome of most mouse strains but absent in SJL, SWR, C57BR and C57L animals, and expressed on approximately one fifth of all peripheral T cell receptors in adult BALB/cBy mice. For immunofluorescence studies, cells were incubated with KJ16-133 at 37°C for 20 minutes, washed and reincubated on ice with fluorescein-conjugated mouse anti-rat kappa chain antibody (RG7/9.1), and analyzed using an ORTHO Cytofluorograf System 50H, as previously described in detail (Roehm et al., 1984).

RESULTS AND DISCUSSION

TABLE 1. β chain gene rearrangements during fetal thymus organ culture

Normal cell origin	Number of hybrids with at least one rearranged β complex (%)[*]	Total β complex rearrangements	Ratio of Jβ2 to Jβ1 rearrangements
d14 fetal thymus	3(15)	4	1.0
d17 fetal thymus	19(90)	28	1.0
d14 fetal thymus + 5 day organ culture	6(100)	8	1.5
adult thymus	23(100)	37	2.2

[*]Only hybridomas with at least one normal cell-derived β complex were included in the analysis.

Table 1 shows an analysis of β chain gene rearrangements in controls and in 6 thymocyte hybridomas which were generated with d14 fetal thymus cells after five additional days of organ culture.

Previously we have found that d14 fetal thymus hybridomas only rarely contain β complex rearrangements. All that were found were of the partial, D-to-J joining type. After 5 days of organ culture, all thymocyte hybridomas carried β complex rearrangements. Five of these rearrangements were compatible with the predicted pattern of D-to-J joinings, whereas the pattern of the remaining 3 rearrangements was indicative of VDJ joins or aberrant rearrangements.

Although the number of hybrids studied so far is too small for a detailed statistical analysis, the data suggest that β chain gene rearrangements progress <u>in vitro</u>. This apparently normal progression occurs within the isolated thymus environment, separated from any immigrating precursor cells. Therefore, even at this early stage of development, and similarly to the adult thymus, thymus immigrants seem no longer to play a significant role in the generation of the diverse thymocyte populations. Furthermore, although not formally proving this fact, our data suggest that the diverse repertoire of T cell receptors, at least with respect to the β chains, is normally generated within the thymus.

In a second series of experiments (Table 2), we have followed the cell surface appearance of T cell receptors during thymocyte development in fetal thymus organ cultures, using monoclonal antibody KJ16-133 and automated immunofluorescence analysis.

TABLE 2. Appearance of KJ16-133-reactive thymocytes during fetal thymus organ culture

Source of thymocytes*	Fraction (%) of KJ16+ cells	Relative levels of staining
d16 fetal thymus**	0.0	
d17 fetal thymus	1.3	low
d14 fetal thymus + 5 day organ culture	2.4	low
d17 fetal thymus + 3 day organ culture	7.8	low
d17 fetal thymus + 4 day organ culture	11.0	low
newborn thymus	10.4	low
adult thymus	14.6	low intermediate high
adult lymph node***	18.2	high
adult lymph node (SJL)	0.0	
d18 fetal thymus (SWR) + 3 day organ culture	0.1	

*Thymocytes were derived from BALB/cBy mice unless otherwise indicated.

Data are pooled from 5 different experiments. For standardization, adult nylon wool-nonadherent lymph node cells* were analyzed in every experiment, with very little variation in numbers of KJ16-133-reactive cells found (19 ± 1.5%).

KJ16-133 reacts with a large fraction of peripheral T lymphocytes (approx. 20%) of most mouse strains and was used here in lieu of a monoclonal antibody against constant portions of T cell receptors which has yet to be described in mice. Therefore, in a strict sense, our analysis is confined to the Vβ segments which encode the KJ16 determinant, and may depend on the possible developmentally controlled expression of these Vβ genes.

We found that during short periods of organ culture, T cell receptor surface expression develops similarly to the normal counterparts, both with respect to numbers of KJ16-133-reactive cells and with regard to levels of cell surface staining. Until the stage of newborn thymus, cell surface receptor densities appear to be uniformly low, much in contrast to the adult thymus and peripheral T lymphocytes. The low levels of surface receptors seem to be a property of cortical subsets (Roehm et al., 1984) and may be influenced by lymphostromal interactions with cortical epithelium (Farr et al., 1985).

Clearly, KJ16 staining of organ cultured thymocytes is not nonspecific, since organ cultured thymi of KJ16⁻ mouse strains (SJL,SWR) do not acquire staining in vitro, and because the time course of staining is related to the corresponding stages of development rather than to the length of organ culture.

Taken together, our data show that both early and late events of T cell receptor gene expression can occur in vitro, in isolated thymus fragments. This then suggests that the thymus is sufficient a microenvironment not only for phenotypic T cell differentiation (Kisielow et al., 1984), but also for antigen/MHC receptor diversification and surface expression, which most likely are the prerequisites for subsequent selection processes. This behavior recommends thymus organ cultures as a suitable model for experimental manipulations aimed at the selection mechanism itself.

REFERENCES

Acuto, O, Hussey, RW, Fitzgerald, KA, Protentis, HP, Meuer, SC, Schlossman, SF, Reinherz, EL (1983). The human T cell receptor: appearance in ontogeny and biochemical relationship of α and β subunits on IL-2 dependant clones and T cell tumor. Cell 34:717-726.

Behlke, MA, Spinella, DG, Chou, HS, Sha, W, Hartl, DL, Loh, DY (1985). T-cell receptor β-chain expression: dependence on relatively few variable region genes. Science 229:566-570.

Bevan, MJ (1977). In a radiation chimera hosts H-2 antigens determine the immune responsiveness of donor cytotoxic cells. Nature 269:417-419.

Born, W, Yagüe, J, Palmer, E, Kappler, J, Marrack, P (1985). Rearrangement of T-cell receptor β chain genes during T cell development. Proc Natl Acad Sci USA 82:2925-2929.

Farr, A, Anderson, S, Marrack, P, Kappler, J (1985). Expression of antigen receptor molecules by cortical and medullary thymocytes in situ. Cell in the press.

Haskins, K, Hannum, C, White, J, Roehm, N, Kubo, R, Kappler, J, Marrack, P (1984). The major histocompatibility complex-restricted antigen receptor on T cells. VI. An antibody to a receptor allotype. J Exp Med 160:452-471.

Kisielow, P, Lieserson, W, von Boehmer, H (1984). Differentiation of thymocytes in fetal organ culture: analysis of phenotypic changes accompanying the appearance of cytolytic and interleukin 2-producing cells. J Immunol 133:1117-1123.

Kruisbeek, AM, Hodes, RJ, Singer A (1981). Cytotoxic T lymphocyte responses by chimeric thymocytes: self-recogniton is determined early in T cell development. J Exp Med 153:13-29.

Mandel, TH, Kennedy, MM (1978). The differentiation of murine thymocytes in vivo and in vitro. Immunology 35:317-327.

Roehm, N, Herron, L, Cambier, J, DiGuisto, D, Haskins, K, Kappler, J, Marrack, P (1984). The major histocompatibility complex-restricted antigen receptor on T cell: distribution on thymus and peripheral T cells. Cell 38:577-584.

Raulet, DH, Gasman, RD, Saito, H, Tonegawa, S (1985). Developmental regulation of T cell receptor gene expression. Nature 314:103-107.

Sim, GK, Augustin, A (1985). Cell in the press.

Snodgrass, HR, Kisielow, P, Kiefer, M, Steinmetz, M, von Boehmer, H (1985). Ontogeny of the T cell antigen receptor within the thymus. Nature 313:592-595.

Snodgrass, HR, Dembic, Z, Steinmetz, M, von Boehmer, H (1985). Expression of T cell antigen receptor genes during fetal development in the thymus. Nature 315:232-283.

Zinkernagel, RM, Callahan, GN, Althage, A, Cooper, S Klein, PA, Klein, J (1978). On the thymus in the differentiation of H-2 self-recognition by T cells: evidence for clonal recognition? J Exp Med 147:882-896.

The Components of the Murine T Cell Antigen Receptor Complex

Lawrence E. Samelson, Joe B. Harford and Richard D. Klausner
Cell Biology and Metabolism Branch
National Institute of Child Health and Human Development, National Institutes of Health
Bethesda, Maryland 20892

INTRODUCTION

The antigen receptors of several murine and human MHC-restricted T cell clones have been isolated and characterized with clone specific monoclonal antibodies (Allison et al., 1982; Meuer et al., 1983a; Haskins et al., 1983; Samelson et al., 1983). In all cases, this receptor is a disulfide-linked heterodimeric glycoprotein containing an alpha and beta chain, each of approximately 43kd. Recent evidence suggests that the human T cell antigen receptor is noncovalently associated with additional proteins termed the T3 complex. This polypeptide complex is T cell specific and is comprised of three peptides, two glycoproteins of 20kd and 25kd and a non-glycosylated protein of 20kd (Borst et al., 1983; Kanellopoulos et al., 1983). Under certain circumstances, monoclonal antibodies that immunoprecipitate the human 20kd T3 glycoprotein co-precipitate the clonotypic alpha and beta chains as well as the other two polypeptides of the T3 complex providing evidence that these polypeptides are associated in a receptor complex on the cell surface (Reinherz et al., 1983; Oettgen et al., 1984).

Reports indicating that analogous proteins may be associated with murine T cell antigen receptors have recently appeared. Structures with molecular weights similar to those seen in human T cells have been cross-linked to the murine clonotypic receptors (Allison and Lanier, 1984; Samelson and Schwartz, 1984). We have shown that antigen- or lectin-induced activation of T cell hybridomas results in phosphorylation of a 21kd polypeptide that is co-precipitated with the T cell antigen receptor (Samelson et al., 1985). The current report extends our description of a proposed murine T cell antigen receptor complex. We have observed that four polypeptides are specifically co precipitated with monoclonal antibodies that bind T cell antigen receptors. There are two glycoproteins of molecular weights 21,000 and 25,000, and two non glycosylated proteins of molecular weights 26,000 and 16,000. The latter polypeptide appears to exist in the receptor complex as a disulfide-linked homodimer of 32,000. The 21kd glycoprotein is the 20-22kd polypeptide previously reported to be phosphorylated in response to T cell activation (Samelson et al., 1985). This chain and a 26kd protein are both phosphorylated when the T cells are treated with phorbol 12 myristate 13-acetate (PMA).

RESULTS

The T cell hybridoma 2B4 is specific for the carboxy terminal portion of pigeon cytochrome c (Hedrick et al., 1982). The antigen receptor on this cell can be precipitated with A2B4-2, a monoclonal antibody recognizing the clonotypic receptor structure (Samelson et al., 1983). In addition this monoclonal antibody specifically co-immunoprecipitates four additional molecules. To further characterize these components, two dimensional diagonal electrophoresis was employed. Material immunoprecipitated with A2B4-2 from surface labeled 2B4 cells was electrophoresed under nonreducing conditions in an SDS-polyacrylamide tube gel for the first dimension. After reduction of the material in the tube, SDS-PAGE was run under reducing conditions for the second dimension. In such a gel system the T cell antigen receptor α and β subunits fall below the diagonal (Figure 1) running at 84-88kd in the first dimension and 42-48kd in the second. The antigen receptor pattern is complex because there are both α-β and α-β' heterodimers on the 2B4 cell (Samelson, 1985). In the lower molecular weight region of the gel four polypeptides were clearly resolved. Two of these ran on the diagonal at 25kd (γ) and 21kd (δ) respectively, and the third chain (ε) ran above the diagonal with apparent molecular weights of 22kd nonreduced and 26kd reduced. Structures that run above the diagonal in this fashion are likely to have intrachain disulfide bonds. Material that migrated at 32kd under non-reducing conditions fell below the diagonal to 16kd (ζ) after reduction. This is consistent with the interpretation that this 32kd molecule is a dimeric structure composed of two 16kd subunits. For convenience we have assigned Greek letter names to the four polypeptides associated with the murine antigen receptor complex.

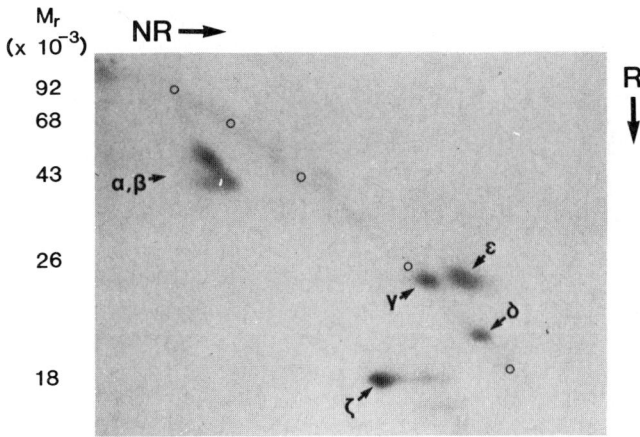

Figure 1. Two Dimensional Diagonal SDS-PAGE Analysis of the T Cell Antigen Receptor Complex of the 2B4 Hybridoma.

The presence of N-linked carbohydrates on the receptor-associated chains was evaluated by eluting the bands from a non-reducing gel, reducing the eluent, and treating with endoglycosaminidase F (endo F) (Elder and Alexander, 1982). The samples were then subjected to a second SDS-PAGE under reducing conditions (data not shown). The 32kd ζ dimer migrated upon reduction at 16kd and was unaltered by enzyme treatment. The 25kd γ chain that had run on the diagonal in the experiment shown in figure 1 contains N-linked carbohydrates and after endo F treatment yields a polypeptide that migrated at 14-15kd under reducing conditions. The ε chain that displayed an apparent molecular weight of 22kd nonreduced was increased to 26kd upon reduction and was not altered by treatment with endo F. The 21kd δ polypeptide has

N-linked carbohydrates and migrates at 16kd after endo F treatment. Thus, of the four associated chains, two (γ and δ) contain N-linked carbohydrate, one is a dimer (ζ) and one may have intrachain disulfide bonds (ϵ).

Phosphorylation of the Complex

Antigen or concanavalin A activation of the 2B4 cell results in the phosphorylation of a 20-22kd polypeptide that is associated with the T cell antigen receptor (Samelson et al, 1985). In addition, a 26kd polypeptide, which is also associated with the T cell antigen receptor, as well as the 21kd polypeptide, is phosphorylated in response to phorbol 12 myristate 13-acetate. The near comigration of ϵ and γ under reducing conditions and of ϵ and δ under nonreducing conditions made it difficult to unambiguiously identify the phosphoproteins. To accomplish this identification, we examined the structural features of the ^{32}P labeled species from stimulated cells in the light of our knowledge of the properties of the components of the antigen receptor complex gained from ^{125}I labeling experiments.

The 2B4 cells were loaded with [^{32}P] orthophosphate and were activated with antigen in the presence of B cell tumors added as antigen presenting cells or treated with 100 ng/ml PMA in the absence of B cells. After detergent solubilization of the cell pellet in the presence of phosphatase inhibitors, immunoprecipitation was performed with either the A2B4-2 monoclonal antibody or with culture supernatant without antibody (Figure 2). After stimulation with antigen, a phosphorylated protein of 21kd was observed. A 26kd phosphorylated protein was also specifically precipitated, but the degree of phosphorylation of this band in response to antigen was consistently very low. In contrast, the phosphorylation pattern in PMA treated cells was characterized by labeling of the 21kd and 26kd polypeptides to approximately equal degrees. The 21kd phosphoprotein comigrated under reducing or nonreducing conditions with the iodinated δ chain of the same apparent molecular weight (Figure 1). The 26kd [^{32}P] protein isolated from PMA treated 2B4 cells migrated with an apparently smaller molecular weight in the absence of reducing agents. This difference in migration on SDS PAGE as a result of disulfide reduction was also observed in the 26kd iodinated ε chain analyzed in Figure 1.

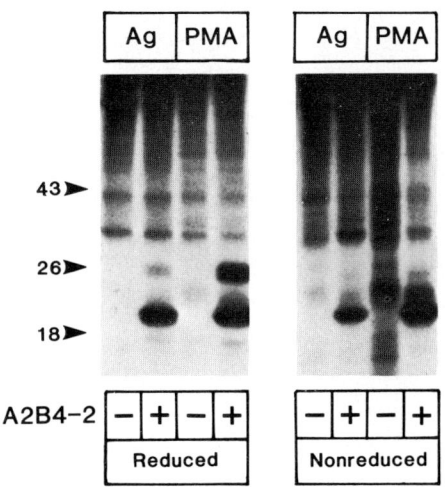

Figure 2. Biochemical Characterization of Phosphoproteins Precipitated with the Murine T Cell Antigen Receptor.

We determined which amino acid of the δ chain was phosphorylated upon activation with antigen plus B cells or in response to treatment with PMA. In both cases the residue proved to be phosphoserine (data not shown).

DISCUSSION

Monoclonal antibodies that bind the antigen receptor on murine T cells can immunoprecipitate four polypeptides in addition to the heterodimeric clonotypic receptor. The immunoprecipitation is specific and only monoclonal antibodies that bind the T cell antigen receptor co precipitate these proteins; the polypeptides are not precipitated with antibodies directed against other T cell surface molecules. Our working hypothesis is that the α-β heterodimer and these four additional polypeptides are noncovalently associated as the T cell antigen receptor complex. The four co-precipitated structures each have been defined in terms of certain characteristic biochemical properties (Table 1).

TABLE I
Biochemical Properties of Components of
the Murine T Cell Antigen Receptor Complex

Chain	Molecular Weight		CHO^a	pH^b	PO_4
	Reduced	Non Reduced			
α	43		30	5.0-5.5	
		> 84			
β	43		30	6.5-8.0	
γ	25	25	14	6.0-7.5	
δ	21	21	16	8.2-8.5	[c]
ε	26	22	26	6.0-7.5	[d]
ζ	16	32	16	8.6	

a   The apparent molecular weight after removal of N-linked carbohydrates by endo F is indicated.
b   The charge of the α and β of the 2B4 antigen receptor were determined by isoelectric focusing (Samelson, 1985). The charge of the other subunits was determined on NEPHGE gels as described.
c   Activation of the 2B4 T cell with antigen resulted in phosphorylation of the δ chain. Similarly, the δ chain is phosphorylated after treatment of the T cells with PMA. Phosphate groups constituitively present on the δ chain can be removed with alkaline phosphatase (data not shown).
d   The ε chain is phosphorylated after treatment of the T cells with the PMA.

We do not know the stoichiometry of these subunits in the T cell antigen receptor complex. Furthermore, we do not know whether all α β heterodimers are associated with this set of proteins or whether the entire cellular complement of each of the smaller subunits are found in the complex. Based on the data presented above, a minimal model for the structure of the T cell antigen receptor contains seven chains (α, β, γ, δ, ϵ, ζ_2). The nature of the association of these structures is not yet fully understood. Non-covalent interactions seem to be critical because ionic detergents such as SDS prevents the coprecipitation of these additional polypeptides with the antigen receptor. The ability to stimulate the phosphorylation of the δ and ϵ chains in intact cells supports the contention that these two chains span the plasma membrane. Our analysis of the structure of the murine T cell receptor complex suggests an analogy between this complex and the T3 complex associated with the human T cell antigen receptor.

In summary, we have detected and partially characterized four polypeptides that are associated with the murine T cell antigen receptor in a cloned T cell hybrid. All four appear to be transmembrane proteins and two (γ, δ) contain N-linked carbohydrate chains. Two of the chains (δ, ϵ) can exist as phosphoproteins. Information is provided regarding disulfide linkages in two of the chains; the ϵ chain appears to have an intrachain disulphide bridge and the ζ chain appears to self associate as a disulfide linked dimer. The possibility exists that some or all of these polypeptides are involved in the transduction to the cell interior of the signal arising from antigen binding or mitogen stimulation. In this regard, we have shown that the δ chain is phosphorylated concomitant with T cell activation _via_ antigen or mitogen (Samelson et al., 1985). The exact role, if any, of this phosphorylation in the process of T cell activation remains obscure as does the function of the other components of the complex. It is our hope that this partial characterization will aid in further studies to elucidate this complex and its mechanism of action.

REFERENCES

Allison JP, McIntyre BW, Bloch D (1982). Tumor specific antigen of murine T lymphoma defined with monoclonal antibody. J Immunol 129:2293 2300.

Allison JP, Lanier LL (1985). Identification of antigen receptor associated structures on murine T cells. Nature 314:107 109.

Borst J, Prendiville MA, Terhorst C (1983). The T3 complex on human thymus derived lymphocytes contains two different subunits of 20 kDa. Eur J Immunol 13:576 580.

Elder JH, Alexander S (1982). Endo β N Acetyl glucosaminidase F: Endoglycosidase from Flavobacterium meningosepticum that cleaves both high mannose and complex glycoproteins. Proc Natl Acad Sci USA 79:4540 4544.

Haskins K, Kubo R, White J, Pigeon M, Kappler J, Marrack P (1983). The major histocompatibility complex restricted antigen receptor on T cells. I. Isolation with a monoclonal antibody. J Exp Med 157:1149 1169.

Hedrick SM, Matis LA, Hecht TT, Samelson LE, Longo DL, Heber-Katz E, Schwartz RH (1982). The fine specificity of antigen and Ia determinant recognition by T cell hybridoma clones specific for pigeon cytochrome c. Cell 30:141 152.

Kanellopoulos JM, Wigglesworth NM, Owen MJ, Crumpton MJ (1983). Biosynthesis and molecular nature of the T3 antigen of human T lymphocytes. EMBO Journal 2:1807 1814.

Meuer SC, Fitzgerald KA, Hussey RE, Hodgdon JC, Schlossman SF, Reinherz EL (1983a). Clonotypic structures involved in antigen specific human T cell function. Relationship to the T3 molecular complex. J Exp Med 157:705 719.

Oettgen HC, Kappler J, Tax WJM, Terhorst C (1984). Characterization of the two heavy chains of the T3 complex on the surface of human T lymphocytes. J Biol Chem 259:12039 12048.

Reinherz EL, Meuer SC, Fitzgerald KA, Hussey RE, Hodgdon JC, Acuto O, Schlossman SF (1983). Comparison of T3 associated 49 and 43 kilodalton cell surface molecules on individual human T cell clones: Evidence for peptide variability in T cell receptor structures. Proc Natl Acad Sci USA 80:4104 4108.

Samelson LE, Germain RN, Schwartz RH (1983). Monoclonal antibodies against the antigen receptor on a cloned T cell hybrid. Proc Natl Acad Sci USA 80:6972 6976.

Samelson LE, Schwartz RH (1984). Characterization of the antigen specific T cell receptor from a pigeon cytochrome c specific T cell hybrid. Immunol Rev 81:131 144.

Samelson LE (1985). An analysis of the structure of the antigen receptor on a pigeon cytochrome c specific T cell hybrid. J Immunol 134:2529 2535.

Samelson LE, Harford J, Schwartz RH, Klausner RD (1985). A 20 kDa protein associated with the murine T cell antigen receptor is phosphorylated in response to activation by antigen or concanavalin A. Proc Natl Acad Sci USA 82:1969- 1973.

# T CELL MARKERS AND SUBSETS INVOLVED IN T CELL DIFFERENTIATION

Bonnie J. Mathieson and Charles A. Janeway, Jr.

Monoclonal Antibody/Hybridoma Section, Biological Therapeutics Branch, BRMP, DCT, NCI, Frederick Cancer Research Facility, Frederick, MD 21701 and Dept. of Pathology, Yale University School of Medicine, New Haven, CT 06510

Discrete steps in the sequence and pathways for T cell differentiation from an uncommitted bone marrow-derived precursor to functionally mature T cells appear to be expressed at the cell surface of differentiating T cells by unique patterns of cell surface markers. We have focused this review of the posters and workshop on this topic at the RES/LCC conference on a series of questions that were posed for the workshop discussion and on the data and ideas presented and discussed there.

<u>What markers are available that identify subsets of thymocytes and T cells? And, how are the subsets distinct?</u>
A number of cell surface markers have been successfully used to subset T cells in the mouse, in man and in rats. These markers include the following: Ly1 (65-67 KD) antigen of the mouse, which is comparable to the CD5 antigens (e.g. T101 or Leu1) on human lymphocytes and OX19 in the rat; Lyt2/3 (28-35 KD) in the mouse, which is homologous with the CD8 antigens (T8, Leu2 or RF8) on human cells or OX8 in the rat; and L3T4 (55 KD), only recently defined in the mouse, which is similar to the antigen first defined in the rat as W325 and is homologous to the CD4 markers detected by T4 or Leu 3 on human lymphocytes. See Mathieson and Fowlkes (1984) for details of the thymocyte subsets defined by these mouse antigens; Bernard et al. (1984) for details of the clusters of differentiation (CD) antigens defined at the first IUIS/WHO Workshop on Leucocyte Differentiation; and Williams et al. (1977) for a review of the rat antigens.

Within the normal adult mouse thymus, the most immature precursor cells that have been demonstrated to have a committment to T cell differentiation are the dull Lyl (dLyl) cells (Fowlkes et al., 1985). The dLyl, high Thyl cells are a subset of the "double negative" cells which lack both the Lyt2/3 and L3T4 marker. The dLyl subset can be further divided into 2 subsets by the presence of the IL2 receptor as detected by monoclonal antibodies (MoAbs) 7D4, 3C7 (Malek et al., 1984) and PC-61 (Ceredig et al., 1985) and by several other markers (Fowlkes, 1984; Ceredig and MacDonald, 1985). However, there is evidence that the IL2 receptor positive cells do not respond to exogenous IL2 (Ceredig et al., 1985, Raulet, 1985, and Hardt et al., 1985).

The majority of thymocytes are Lyt2+,L3T4+ ("double positive") cells. Both Shortman and Ceredig presented models in the plenary session which proposed that the mature subsets were derived directly from "double negative" cells and that "double positive" cells may be non-functional or dead-end cells. There are also two minor subsets, the Lyt2+ and L3T4+ cells, which are mature functional cells within the thymus. (Both of these populations express high levels of Lyl.) But, neither of these subsets are observed, either in the kinetics of repopulation after irradiation or in fetal ontogeny, without the previous transitional appearance of the "double positive" subset. Furthermore the dLyl to "double positive" is the one transition which can be generated in vitro (Fowlkes et al., 1984). Thus thymocytes undergo the following developmental sequence:

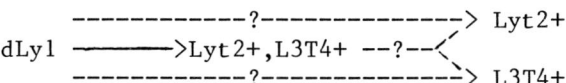

Data for several additional markers were presented which further subset T cells. 9F3 (Dumont et al. Abstract 131), I-J (Nanda and Mitchison, Abstract 141), PNL in bovine cells (Hurley and Mastro, Abstract 135) and Lyml0 (Chan et al., Abstract 128).

The 9F3 marker defines a heterogeneity within the Lyt2+ cells. This marker appears to be absent on the functional Lyt2+ cells that can be generated by antigen or mitogen stimulation but present on Lyt2+ cells that are not responsive to antigen stimulation. The 9F3 marker does not subdivide the functional and nonfunctional L3T4+ subsets.

The data from Nanda and Mitchison indicated that lysis with anti-I-J reagents could abrogate all of the transferable T cell suppressive activity. Furthermore the suppressive activity was eliminated with anti-Lyt2 but not anti-L3T4 (GK1.5), thus indicating that these reagents could also subset the Lyt2+ cells. Although the absence of comparable markers for bovine cells makes the comparison difficult, it would appear that the peanut lectin binding molecule on T cells can similarly separate the active functional suppressor cells from the precursors for this activity (Hurley and Mastro). The Lym10 marker which was assessed by MoAb + complement (C) lysis, is present on cytotoxic T lymphocytes (CTL) and T helper (Th) (IL 2-producing) subsets activated by MLR or antigen stimulation. By this same methodology, Lym10 is not detected on any of the precursor populations to functional, peripheral T cell subsets that were tested. Thus Lym10 appears to be a marker for T cell activation on cells with different functions and is not correlated with other T cell subset markers.

Two posters dealing with gut-associated lymphocytes (Dillon and MacDonald, Abstract 130 and Roy et al., Abstract 144) indicated that such lymphocytes presumed to be T cells by phenotype may not be typical T cells. Dillon presented evidence that Lyt2+ intraepithelial lymphocytes (IEL) from the small intestine of mice constitute up to 70% of IEL and have a very low ConA + IL 2 response relative to spleen-derived splenic Lyt2+ cells. Roy et al. indicated that gut-associated lymphocytes with a T cell marker (L11/135) infiltrated rabbit appendices as early as 2 days after birth. The phenotype of these cells and the very early architectural association within gut tissue might indicate a higher degree of maturity than could be attained through an intrathymic maturation pathway.

Do these markers identify: Function, Activation or Differentiated State?

Cantor and Boyse (1975) initially proposed that the presence or absence of the Lyt2 phenotype was predictive of both the MHC class restriction and the cell's functional capacity. As the generation of T cell lines with IL 2 became more reproducible, a number of T cell clones became available that clearly did not fit this pattern. At this meeting, Macphail and Stutman (Abstract 139) presented evidence that cells initially selected for the L3T4 marker generated highly effective CTL against allogeneic stimulators with high Ia expression. This extends the earlier predictions of Swain and Panfili (1979), that proposed that the Lyt2 phenotype of peripheral T cells was not predictive of the function of the cells but rather predictive of the MHC class restriction. However, Macphail indicated in the discussion that although these L3T4+ CTL effectors can be blocked by anti-L3T4 MoAb, anti-Ia (class II) MoAb may not be effective for blocking these effectors.

In general, a current consensus appears to be that L3T4+ peripheral T cells are class II MHC-restricted, and more likely to be helpers than killers. However some L3T4+ T cell lines or clones respond to non-self or autologous class I products. Lyt2+ peripheral T cells are class I MHC-restricted, and much more likely to be killers than helpers. But again, Lyt2+ cells can be specific for non-self class II products. Thus Lyt2 and L3T4 molecules appear to be more important for, and thus more closely associated with, restricted recognition of antigens plus self MHC, and relatively less critical in responses to non-self MHC.

In addition to this imprecise association of phenotype and function, the sequence of appearance of the different subsets in vivo during an immune response, as indicated by Tuohy et al. (Abstract 148), leads us to predict specific controls exist for the different subsets that as yet are undefined.

<u>What is the function of the marker itself?</u>
Shimonkevitz et al. (Abstract 147) presented evidence that the Lyt2/3 molecule on the more commonly generated Lyt2/3+, KD-restricted, CTL acts as an accessory molecule to increase the avidity of the effector-target interaction. This was determined by the relative ability of anti-Lyt2/3 to block targets with different levels of class I MHC expression. They observed that CTL clones, which could only lyse targets with high alloantigen expression, could be blocked by anti-Lyt2/3 MoAb. Whereas, CTL clones that could lyse targets with either high or low levels of class I MHC expression could not be blocked by anti-Lyt2/3.

An alternative view, presented in the workshop (CAJ) (Tite, Sloan and Janeway, JNCI, in press) is that Lyt2 and L3T4 are required for initial contact, allowing time for the T cell receptor to bind antigen:MHC complexes. If the cell does not bear foreign antigen, then L3T4 or Lyt2 transduces a net negative signal, leading to cell separation.

Weber et al. (Abstract 149) indicated that the T3 marker for human cells can be used as a target for anti-T3 (MoAb WT23) functional stimulation for all of the T cells. Clonal analysis of these cells indicated that both CTL and IL 2 producing clones could be observed with up to 20% of the clones expressing NK function. Since the T3 marker has been shown by a number of other laboratories to be highly mitogenic for T cells, it is now clear that this marker is directly involved with the activation of T cells in specific immune responses.

Two posters (Lee and Repasky, Abstract 138 and Repasky and Bankert, 142) indicated that a "submembrane" marker, capped spectrin, may also be a useful marker for distinguishing T cells with either a more mature or more functionally active state of differentiation. Since spectrin is detected in all lymphocytes, the movement of the molecules to an aggregated cap rather than presence or absence of the molecules is indicative of the state of activation. The association of this protein with other cytoskeletal proteins within the membrane may be important in membrane fluidity and other functions.

Konigsberg and Podack (Abstract 136) presented evidence in their poster that indicated that the cytolytic granules isolated from CTLL2 shows all of the activity of the functional CTLs thus being one of the most definitive "markers" for differentiation. (This topic was more extensively considered in another session.)

What precursors of mature T cells have been identified?
In 2 posters (Abstracts 134 and 140) Goube de Laforest claimed to have produced extrathymic differentiation of T cell precursors from bone marrow. This system depended on a culture supernatant with "prothymocyte differentiating activity" (PTDA) that was generated from presumably T depleted bone marrow and which was in turn used on similarly T-depleted bone marrow to produce T3+,T4+ or T3+,T8+ cells. This work contrasted with work from Globerson et al. (Abstract 133) where Thy-1+ cell lines were derived from fetal liver cells where there was no likelihood of adult peripheral T cell contamination. Furthermore she observed that only a rare cell line could be obtained with the more

differentiated Lyt2+ phenotype. Because Thy-1 was found on a higher proportion of the lymphocyte lines, it was suggested that these cells that might still have further potential for differentiation if given the appropriate signals.

What are the sources of problems involved in mapping lineages? Lugo claimed in the workshop discussion that the "double negative" cells could be differentiated in vitro into Lyt2+ cells with phorbol ester (PMA) + Ionomycin + IL 2. However, it was noted by Ceredig in the plenary session and raised again in the discussion that contamination of the "double negative" population with as little as 0.5% of the "mature" Lyt2+ subset can lead to selective overgrowth of the Lyt2+ subset in the presence of IL 2 + PMA and lead to erroneous interpretation of the in vitro stimulation data. These experiments require either limiting dilution or "add-back" experiments as controls. Personal experience (Mathieson and Matsushima) has shown that PMA + IL 2 will not differentiate the highly selected dLy1 subset which contains nearly all of the IL 2 receptor positive cells within the thymus, but selectively expands the Lyt2+ subset of thymocytes. Further, suitable combinations of IL 1 + IL 2 will provide stimulation for extensive proliferation without differentiation to mature subsets. Likewise, the problem of complete depletion of contaminating T cells from bone marrow or peripheral blood cells was discussed. Such depletions often require 2 to 3 cycles of antibody plus complement treatment with reagents detecting different antigens on the same cells to remove all of the antigen positive cells.

What does the thymus "really" do to/for T cells?
In regard to this question, two pieces of work presented in the poster and workshop sessions and the work of Kruisbeek (See this book) speak to this problem. Latime and Stutman (Abstract 137) indicated that the minor self Ia-restricted response seen for IL 2 production may be a particularly relevant response for the initial stimulation of thymic progenitor cells. In line with this, Fleming and Wood (Abstract 132) presented evidence that showed specific thymocyte macrophage interactions resulting in rosette formation. These several pieces of evidence, as well as a large body of other evidence, suggest that the unique environment of the thymus, at the very least, enhances the development of the T cell receptor and the appropriate subset differentiation for class restricted responses.

REFERENCES

Bernard A, Boumsell L, Dausset J, Milstein C, Schlossman SF (1984). Clusters of differentiation defined by the first international workshop on human leucocyte differentiation antigens. In "Leucocyte Typing: Human Leucocyte Differentiation Antigens Detected by Monoclonal Antibodies," New York: Springer-Verlag, Poster.

Ceredig R, MacDonald HR (1985). Intrathymic differentiation: Some unanswered questions. Surv Immunol Res 4:87-95.

Ceredig R, Lowenthal JW, Nabholz M, MacDonald HR (1985). Expression of interleukin-2 receptors as a differentiation marker on intrathymic stem cells. Nature 314:98-100.

Fowlkes BJ (1984). Characterization and differentiation of thymic lymphocytes in the mouse. Thesis. George Washington University Graduate School of Arts and Sciences, Washington, D.C.

Fowlkes BJ, Edison L, Mathieson B, Chused TM (1984). Differentiation in vitro of an adult precursor thymocyte. In Sercarz E, Cantor H, Chess L (eds) "Regulation of the Immune system. UCLA Symposia on Molecular and Cellular Biology, New Series, vol. 18, pp 275-293.

Fowlkes BJ, Edison L, Mathieson BJ, Chused TM (1985). Early T lymphocytes: Differentiation in vivo of adult intrathymic precursor cells. J Exp Med 162:802-822.

Hardt C, Diamanstein T, Wagner H (1985). Developmentally controlled expression of IL 2 receptors and of sensitivity to IL 2 in a subset of embryonic thymocytes. J Immunol 134:3891-3900.

Malek TR, Ortega-R G, Jakway JP, Chan C, Shevach EM (1984). The murine IL 2 receptor: II. Monoclonal anti-IL 2 receptor antibodies as specific inhibitors of T cell function in vitro. J Immunol 133:1976-1982.

Mathieson BJ, Fowlkes BJ (1984). Cell surface antigen expression on thymocytes: Development and phenotypic differentiation of intrathymic subsets. Immunol Rev 82: 141-173.

Raulet DH (1985). Expression and function of interleukin-2 receptors on immature thymocytes. Nature 314:101-103.

Swain SL and Panfili PR (1979). Helper cells activated by allogeneic H-2K or H-2D differences have an Ly phenotype distinct from those responsive to I differences. J Immunol 122:383-391.

Williams AF, Galfre G, Milstein C (1977). Analysis of cell surfaces by xenogeneic myeloma-hybrid antibodies: Differentiation antigens of rat lymphocytes. Cell 12: 663-673.

Section II. Effect of Interleukins on T and B Lymphocytes

REGULATION OF HUMAN INTERLEUKIN-2 GENE EXPRESSION

Raymond Kaempfer and Shimon Efrat

Department of Molecular Virology, The Hebrew University-Hadassah Medical School, 91010 Jerusalem, Israel

INTRODUCTION

Interleukin-2 (IL-2), or T-cell growth factor, is an inducible lymphokine produced by T cells upon antigenic or mitogenic stimulation. This key immunoregulatory protein is absolutely required for the proliferation of activated T cells of various types. It is thought that the strength of the immune response is determined to a large extent by the amount of IL-2 made available for T cell growth in response to a stimulus (Gillis and Smith, 1977; Andersson et al., 1979; Smith, 1981). Study of the control of IL-2 gene expression is, therefore, of direct relevance to understanding the molecular basis for the regulation of the strength of the immune response.

We show here that induction of the human gene encoding interleukin-2 (IL-2) leads to the appearance of a brief wave of IL-2 mRNA. De novo synthesis of IL-2 mRNA molecules is followed promptly by cessation of transcription and decay of mRNA sequences (halflife, about 15 h). IL-2 mRNA activity, quantitated by microinjection analysis, appears coordinately with IL-2 mRNA sequences, quantitated by Northern blotting, and IL-2 synthesis by the lymphocytes; thus, translational control does not determine the observed wave of IL-2 mRNA. Formation of IL-2 mRNA is tightly controlled by the early appearance of a labile protein repressor whose neutralization, by any one of a series of translation inhibitors, causes extensive (up to 60-fold) superinduction of IL-2 mRNA in tonsil cells and of IL-2 in the culture medium. Superinduction of the human IL-2 gene is not accompanied by any increase in primary transcription, nor in the stability of IL-2 mRNA. Instead, superinduction conditions cause a greatly increased flow of large IL-2 RNA precursors into mature IL-2 mRNA molecules. Our data support the concept that IL-2 gene expression in human T cells is controlled at transcription and, in addition, by a labile repressor that acts posttranscriptionally to reduce, by up to 98%, the processing of IL-2 mRNA precursors. This labile repressor mechanism determines the magnitude of the IL-2 mRNA wave over an approx. 50-fold range, and thereby, the strength of the eventual IL-2 signal in the immune response. Normally, the human IL-2 gene is, therefore, expressed to only about 2% of its potential. This mode of regulation by a labile repressor allows for dramatic up-regulation of the gene within a short time-span.

We present evidence that this regulatory mechanism is elicited by the action of a distinct class of T lymphocytes that is OKT8$^+$ and sensitive to γ-irradiation.

RESULTS AND DISCUSSION

A. Induction and Shutoff of Biologically Active IL-2 mRNA Formation

Figure 1A depicts the kinetics of accumulation of mRNA encoding IL-2 in human tonsil lymphocytes cultured in the presence of the mitogen PHA. In this experiment, total mRNA was isolated from the cells at time intervals and was microinjected at a constant concentration into oocytes of Xenopus laevis (Efrat et al., 1982; Efrat and Kaempfer, 1984a, b). It is evident that the appearance of IL-2 mRNA during induction is followed by a prompt shutoff, giving rise to a wave of IL-2 mRNA activity in the induced lymphocytes.

When DRB (5,6-dichloro-1-β-D-ribofuranosyl benzimidazole), a reversible inhibitor of primary transcription, was present from 4 hr of induction, little, if any, IL-2 mRNA activity appeared up to 22 hr of induction (Fig. 1A). Induction of IL-2 mRNA activity thus involves synthesis of new mRNA molecules. DRB, when added at 20 hr, did not significantly affect the rate of decline of IL-2 mRNA activity (Fig. 1A), showing that little, if any, synthesis of additional active IL-2 mRNA takes place during the decline

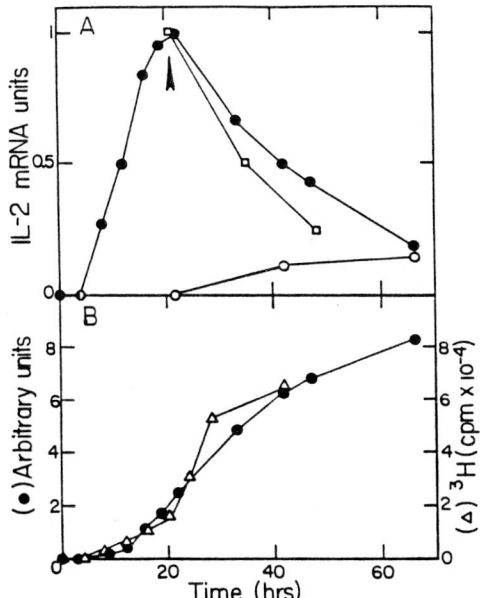

Fig. 1. Kinetics of accumulation of IL-2 mRNA during induction of human tonsil lymphocytes (oocyte microinjection analysis). (A) ●, normal induction; o, induction with DRB (40 µM) added at 4 hr; ☐, induction with DRB added at 21 hr (arrow). (B) Comparison between expected accumulation curve of IL-2 activity, calculated from the mRNA values in A (●), and actual IL-2 activity in conditioned medium (Δ). From Efrat and Kaempfer (1984a).

period. Therefore, this decline is the result of an inactivation or breakdown process only. The functional half-life of human IL-2 mRNA may be estimated from the upper curve of Fig. 1A at about 15-20 hr.

In Fig. 1B, the expected accumulation of IL-2 activity during induction, predicted from the amount of active IL-2 mRNA present in the cell during successive time intervals in Fig. 1A, is compared with the accumulation of IL-2 activity actually observed in the medium. The extremely close correspondence between predicted and observed values shows that the mRNA levels quantitated by the method used in Fig. 1A accurately reflect intracellular concentrations of active

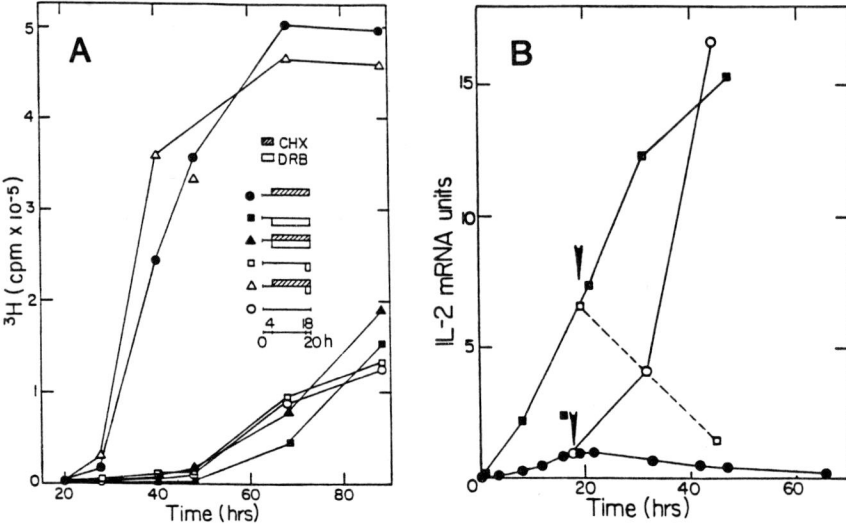

Fig. 2. (A) Superinduction of IL-2. CHX (20 µg/ml) or DRB was added to lymphocyte cultures at 4 or 18 hr after induction as indicated. At 20 hr, all cultures were washed and the cells were resuspended in fresh PHA-free medium. At the indicated times, IL-2 activity in the medium was assayed. From Efrat and Kaempfer (1984a).

(B) Superinduction of active IL-2 mRNA. IL-2 mRNA activity was assayed by microinjection as for Fig. 1. CHX was added at 4 hr (■), at 18 hr (o) (arrow), or at 4 hr and removed at 19 hr (□) (arrow). For comparison, mRNA values for normal induction (from Fig. 1A) are plotted on the same scale (●). Note the scale change between Figs. 1A and 2B. From Efrat and Kaempfer (1984a).

IL-2 mRNA. Since IL-2 synthesis by lymphocytes is precisely that predicted from active mRNA levels, translational control does not determine the observed wave of IL-2 mRNA.

B. Superinduction of IL-2 and IL-2 mRNA

   To examine the nature of the mechanisms that regulate the level of IL-2 mRNA activity, induction was studied in the presence of reversible inhibitors of macromolecule synthesis. Accumulation of IL-2 activity was followed in cell cultures that had been preincubated for 20 hr in the presence of PHA and then transferred to fresh medium lacking PHA. CHX and/or DRB were included during part of the preincubation period, and their effect on the accumulation of IL-2-encoding capacity was assessed upon their removal at the end of the preincubation period, when expression of this capacity was allowed in fresh medium.

Fig. 2A depicts the kinetics of accumulation of IL-2 activity under various conditions of induction. The presence of CHX during the 4- to 20-hr time interval led to extensive superinduciton of IL-2, relative to the control incubated only with PHA. Superinduction by CHX was manifested both by a far earlier appearance of IL-2 and by greatly increased levels: by 48 hr, the extent of superinduction was about 15-fold. In spite of this great increase in IL-2 synthesis, the rate of accumulation of IL-2 in the CHX-treated culture began to decline with roughly the same kinetics as during normal induction (Fig. 1B).

When DRB was present during the 4- to 20-hr time interval, the subsequent appearance of IL-2 was delayed relative to the control. This delay might be expected, because IL-2 mRNA synthesis is inhibited in the presence of DRB (Fig. 1A). Even at later times, however, there was no indication of superinduction subsequent to the removal of DRB. Indeed, the presence of DRB from 4 to 20 hr prevented almost totally the CHX-mediated superinduction, implying that superinduction depends on de novo transcription. When DRB was added after 18 hr of induction, it no longer affected the subsequent formation of IL-2 in normal or superinduced cell cultures.

The results of Fig. 2B show that the superinduction of IL-2 seen in the presence of CHX involves changes in the level of active IL-2 mRNA. In the presence of CHX, the amount of biologically active IL-2 mRNA increased dramatically, reaching 7.5-fold higher levels by 20 hr and 30-fold higher levels by 48 hr of induction. Note that by 8 hr, only 4 hr after addition of CHX, superinduction of IL-2 mRNA is already at least 6-fold. This implies that the CHX-sensitive mechanism starts to act early during induction.

In view of the relatively long half-life of IL-2 mRNA observed both in the presence or absence of DRB (Fig. 1A), about 15 hr, stabilization of mRNA by CHX cannot account for

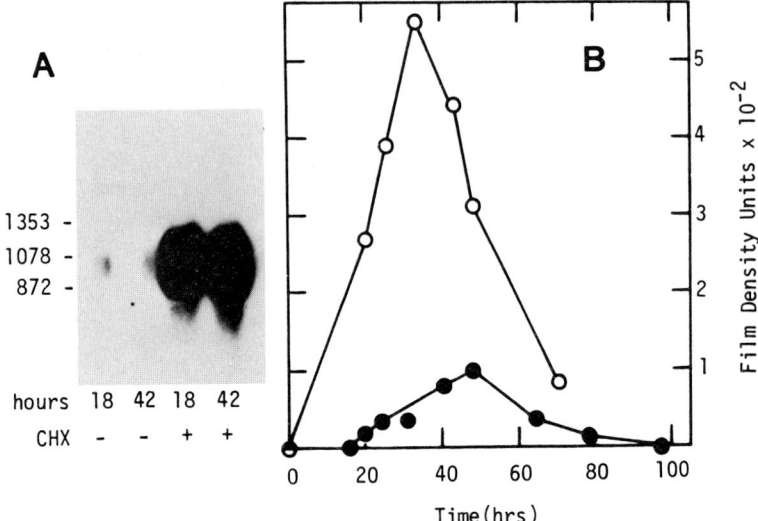

Fig. 3. Superinduction of IL-2 mRNA sequences. Human lymphocytes were induced with PHA. Where indicated, CHX (20 μg/ml) was included from 4 hr onwards. At the indicated times, total RNA was extracted, subjected to formaldehyde/ agarose gel electrophoresis and blot-hybridized with nick-translated, ^{32}P-labeled p3-16 DNA carrying an insert of human IL-2 cDNA (Taniguchi et al., 1983). (A), autoradiograph. (B), microdensitometric quantitation of similar RNA blots sampled at the indicated times from cultures incubated with (o) or without (●) CHX. Size markers are on left.

the observed superinduction. Even if CHX were to stabilize IL-2 mRNA completely, this would yield at most a twofold superinduction at late times.

In Fig. 2B, the IL-2-encoding capacity of equal amounts of microinjected mRNA is measured. Clearly, CHX does not act merely by inhibiting the accumulation of non-IL-2 mRNA, for its presence led to an absolute increase in IL-2 produced in culture (Fig. 2A).

When CHX was added at 18 hr, a time when shutoff of active IL-2 mRNA formation normally follows (Fig. 1A), there was an immediate and dramatic rise in IL-2 mRNA activity, and neither shutoff nor decrease in mRNA level was observed

(Fig. 2B). Furthermore, removal of CHX at 20 hr resulted in immediate cessation of active IL-2 mRNA accumulation and a decline in mRNA level at a practically normal rate (Fig. 2B).

The superinduction of active IL-2 mRNA formation in the presence of CHX represents a true increase in active mRNA encoding IL-2, as judged by the sensitivity to anti-Tac antibody of IL-2 activity elicited by this mRNA in microinjected oocytes (Efrat and Kaempfer, 1984a).

C. Superinduction of IL-2 mRNA Sequences: Demonstration of Two Distinct Repression Mechanisms

Apparently, IL-2 gene expression is tightly controlled by a labile protein repressor. In Fig. 3, a cloned IL-2 cDNA probe (Taniguchi et al., 1983) was used to quantitate IL-2 mRNA sequences in total RNA prepared at time intervals after induction. This probe detects an RNA species migrating at about 1,000 nucleotides, the expected size of IL-2 mRNA (Taniguchi et al., 1983). As seen in Fig. 3A, the presence of CHX results in an equally striking superinduction of IL-2 mRNA sequences, by a factor of at least 25- to 35-fold. Other translation inhibitors with distinct modes of action (sparsomycin, T-2 toxin, or pactamycin) yielded similar results (Efrat et al., 1984). The extensive increase in mature IL-2 mRNA cannot be due to a pool effect, since IL-2 mRNA sequences (Fig. 3) and IL-2 mRNA activity (Fig. 2B) rise commensurately with IL-2 production by the lymphocytes in culture (Fig. 2A).

Fig. 3B depicts a kinetic analysis of IL-2 mRNA sequences present in a culture that was normally induced, as compared to a culture that also received CHX. In spite of the fact that the presence of CHX results in a pronounced superinduction of IL-2 mRNA sequences at every time tested, it is clear that the shutoff and decline observed during normal induction (Figs. 1 and 3B) also occur during superinduction (Fig. 3B).

Whether IL-2 gene expression is induced normally or is superinduced, shutoff is followed by decay of mRNA. Although cell viability does decrease after long incubations with CHX, the rate is too slow to account for the observed decay of IL-2 mRNA (Efrat and Kaempfer, 1984a); in addition, equal

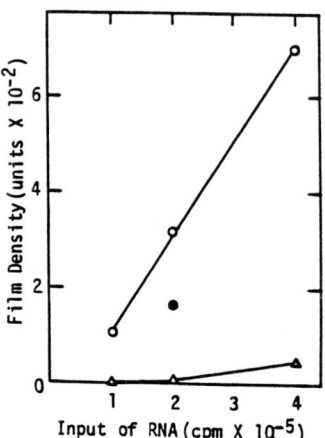

Fig. 4. Quantitation of nascent IL-2 transcripts during normal induction and superinduction. RNA labeled with [α-^{32}P]UTP in nuclei (Schibler et al., 1983) from normally induced (o) or superinduced cells (●) was hybridized with IL-2 cDNA or pBR322 DNA (Δ). Microdensitometric analysis of hybridized IL-2 RNA in dot blots is plotted vs. total input RNA.

amounts of RNA were compared in Fig. 3. The half-life of IL-2 mRNA in this experiment is 12 to 15 hr, again showing that CHX does not stabilize IL-2 mRNA.

These results demonstrate the existence of two distinct repression mechanisms that regulate the accumulation of IL-2 mRNA sequences. One is sensitive to CHX, and its neutralization causes extensive superinduction. The other, apparently insensitive to CHX, is responsible for the shutoff observed both during normal induction and during superinduction. Since induction of IL-2 mRNA depends on de novo transcription, as shown by the inhibitory effect of DRB (Fig. 1), and since decay of translatable IL-2 mRNA after shutoff is not noticeably affected by DRB (Fig. 1), transcription apparently ceases upon shutoff. Hence, the most plausible interpretation of our findings is that the CHX-insensitive repressor mechanism acts to shut off transcription.

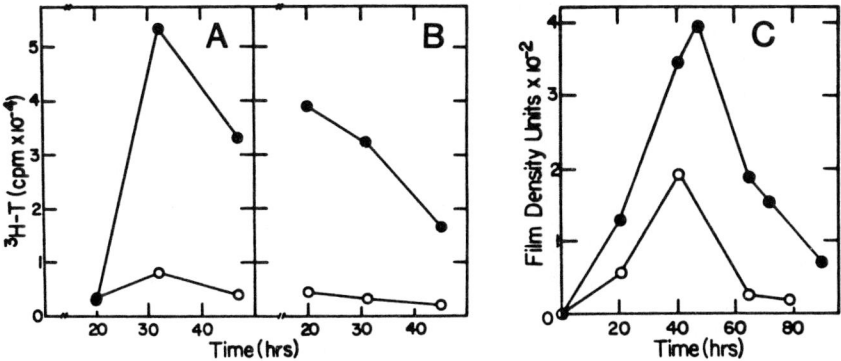

Fig. 5. Superinduction of active IL-2 mRNA and IL-2 mRNA sequences by γ-irradiation. Tonsillar cells were γ-irradiated with 1,500 Rads before induction with PHA. At the indicated times, RNA was extracted. Purified mRNA was microinjected into oocytes and the oocyte medium was assayed for IL-2 activity (A, B). Total RNA was subjected to agarose gel electrophoresis and blot hybridization with a cloned IL-2 cDNA probe (C); the film density of the 1000-nucleotide band is depicted. (●), γ-irradiated cultures; (o) non-irradiated controls.

D. The Labile Repressor Acts Posttranscriptionally

In Fig. 3A, the striking superinduction of IL-2 mRNA sequences in the presence of CHX is not accompanied by a detectable rise in RNA sequences migrating as larger IL-2 mRNA precursors, as might have been expected if transcription were increased. Fig. 4 presents direct evidence that primary transcription of the IL-2 gene in superinduced cells does not exceed that observed in normally induced cells. In this experiment, nuclear run-on transcription is quantitated in nuclei from cells induced in the presence or absence of CHX. It is seen that the extent of hybridization of IL-2 RNA molecules, labeled in nuclei from normally induced cells, to the IL-2 cDNA probe increases linearly with input radioactivity. IL-2 RNA sequences labeled in nuclei from superinduced cells hybridize within this linear range. It is clear from Fig. 4 that their amount is not increased over that observed for nuclei from normally induced cells and, indeed, is actually somewhat less.

To further analyze the mode of action of CHX-sensitive repressor, we studied IL-2 gene induction in the presence of cordycepin (3'-deoxyadenosine). This agent inhibits the polyadenylation of nuclear mRNA precursors and hence, their subsequent processing, but is thought not to affect primary transcription. Superinduction was found to cause a greater increase in IL-2 RNA sequences as they approach the size of mature IL-2 mRNA. Superinduction of the human IL-2 gene by CHX, as expressed by a very pronounced increase in IL-2 mRNA sequences and IL-2 mRNA activity, thus appears to be correlated with a strongly increased flow of precursor RNA molecules into mature IL-2 mRNA.

E. Requirement for an OKT8$^+$, γ-Irradiation-Sensitive T Cell Class in Regulation of IL-2 Gene Expression

Exposure of human lymphocyte cultures to low doses of γ-irradiation (500-1,500 Rads) leads to strongly increased production of IL-2 upon subsequent stimulation by PHA and, as shown in Fig. 5, to greatly increased levels of IL-2 mRNA. γ-Irradiation results in a pronounced superinduction of IL-2 mRNA activity, as determined by oocyte microinjection analysis (Figs. 5A and B). Panels A-C show data obtained with lymphocyte cultures from different donors. While a wave-shaped induction curve is always observed, the kinetics of appearance of IL-2 mRNA and actual timing of shutoff can vary between cultures (cf. Figs. 1 and 3). This variation is also seen in Fig. 5: maximal IL-2 mRNA activity is reached between 30 and 40 hr in A and by 20 hr in B. Yet, it is clear that, as in the presence of CHX, superinduction by γ-irradiation does not prevent shutoff of active IL-2 mRNA formation, nor subsequent decay of mRNA activity. The blot analysis of Fig. 5C further demonstrates that γ-irradiation acts to increase the magnitude of the wave of IL-2 mRNA sequences, but does not affect the shape of this wave.

These results reveal a remarkably parallel response by lymphocyte cultures to γ-irradiation on one hand, and to treatment with CHX on the other. They suggest that γ-irradiation affects the regulatory mechanism that is sensitive to CHX, i.e., the labile posttranscriptional repressor mechanism.

By incubating tonsil lymphocyte cultures with OKT8 monoclonal antibodies and then lysing the OKT8$^+$ cells with complement, or by labeling OKT8$^+$ cells with fluorescent antibody and fractionating the lymphocyte population in a fluorescence-activated cell sorter, we have found that normal human tonsil lymphocyte populations depleted of OKT8$^+$ cells by either method produce up to 10-fold more IL-2 upon mitogenic stimulation. This finding supports the concept that an OKT8-positive,γ-irradiation-sensitive class of T lymphocytes is required in order to elicit posttranscriptional control of human IL-2 gene expression.

These properties are consistent with the involvement of activated suppressor T cells in this process of control. γ-Irradiation would then act to prevent the activation of suppressor T cells, while depletion of OKT8$^+$ cells would remove them from the population. Additional evidence, to be reported elsewhere, strongly supports this view.

ACKNOWLEDGMENTS

We thank Dr. T. Taniguchi for the IL-2 cDNA probe and Susan Marsh and Avivah Yeheskel for excellent assistance. Supported by grants from the National Council for Research and Development (NCRD) of Israel, from NCRD and DKFZ (Heidelberg), from the Israel Academy of Sciences and Humanities, and from the Cancer Research Institute (New York).

REFERENCES

Andersson J, Grönvik K-O, Larsson E-L, Coutinho A (1979). Studies on T lymphocyte activation. I Requirements for the mitogen-dependent production of T cell growth factors. Eur J Immunol 9:581-587.

Efrat S, Pilo S, Kaempfer R (1982). Kinetics of induction and molecular size of mRNA species encoding human interleukin-2 and γ-interferon. Nature 297:236-239.

Efrat S, Kaempfer R (1984a). Control of biologically active interleukin-2 messenger RNA formation in induced human lymphocytes. Proc Natl Acad Sci USA 81:2601-2605.

Efrat S, Kaempfer R (1984b). A qualitative difference in the interleukin-2 requirement of helper and cytotoxic T lymphocytes. Cell Immunol 88:207-212.

Efrat S, Zelig S, Yagen B, Kaempfer R (1984). Superinduction of human interleukin-2 messenger RNA by inhibitors of translation. Biochem Biophys Res Commun 123:842-848.

Gillis S, Smith KA (1977). Long term culture of tumor-specific cytotoxic T cells. Nature 268:154-156.

Gillis S, Ferm MM, Ou W, Smith KA (1978). T cell growth factor: Parameters of production and a quantitative microassay for activity. J Immunol 120:2027-2032.

Schibler U, Hagenbüchle O, Wellauer PK, Pittet AC (1983). Two promoters of different strength control the transcription of the mouse alpha-amylase gene $Amy-1^a$ in the parotid gland and the liver. Cell 33:501-508.

Smith KA (1981). T-cell growth factor: Present status and future implications. In Pick E (ed): "Lymphokines", Vol. 2, New York: Academic Press, pp 21-30.

Taniguchi T, Matsui H, Fujita T, Takaoka C, Kashima N, Yoshimoto R, Hamuro J (1983). Structure and expression of a cloned cDNA for human interleukin-2. Nature 302:305-310.

IL 2 AND AUTOIMMUNITY. HYPERPRODUCTION OF IL 2 IN OBESE
STRAIN CHICKENS WITH SPONTANEOUS AUTOIMMUNE THYROIDITIS
IS DUE TO A DEFECT IN NON SPECIFIC SUPPRESSOR MECHANISMS.

Konrad Schauenstein, Guido Krömer and Georg Wick

Institute of General and Experimental Pathology,
University of Innsbruck, School of Medicine,
A-6020 Innsbruck, Austria

INTRODUCTION

One essential feature of autoimmune reactions appears to be a disturbed immunoregulation. In previous studies we and others have found the spontaneous autoimmune thyroiditis (SAT) of Obese Strain (OS) chickens (Wick et al., 1982) to be associated with a marked hyperreactivity of the T cell system (Kite et al., 1979; Schauenstein et al., 1985) as expressed in various T cell specific proliferative responses and the production of interleukin 2 (IL 2). More recently, signs of T cell activation have been observed at the site of the autoimmune process, i.e. the thyroid gland (Krömer et al.,1985a). Hence we assume that this dysregulation is involved in the pathogenesis of the disease.

In the present experiments we aimed to explore the mechanisms leading to the enhanced T cell response and IL 2 activity in the OS.

RESULTS AND DISCUSSION

Cocultivation experiments in communicating culture chambers

The first question to be addressed was whether the differences observed between OS and control (Normal White Leghorn, NWL) chickens in responding to T cell mitogens (Con A) were due to soluble regulatory factors. To this end we performed coculture experiments with Con A activated OS and NWL chicken spleen cells. Pairs of communicating culture chambers were manufactured in flat bottomed Microtiter plates allowing

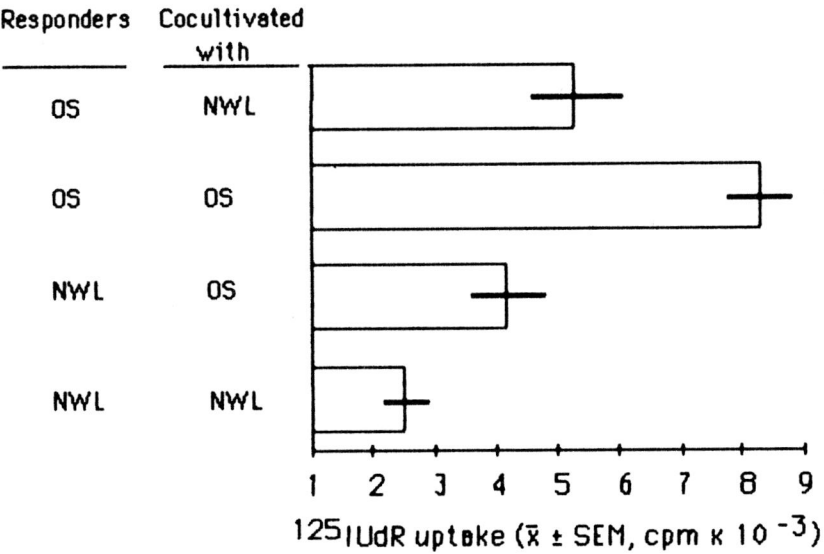

Figure 1. Cocultivation of NWL and OS lymphocytes in communicating culture chambers results in abrogation of the originally observed difference in the response to Con A.

for the mutual exchange of conditioned medium (CM) between two cell cultures. Cocultivation of Con A stimulated OS and NWL splenocytes for 48 hrs in this system led to the abrogation of the originally observed difference in Con A responses (Fig. 1): CM of OS cells had a helper effect on the low NWL response, and the high response of OS cells was suppressed by about 40% by the CM of NWL lymphocytes.

<u>Low molecular weight inhibitory factor(s) in CM from NWL cells suppress the enhanced IL 2 production by OS lymphocytes</u>

Previous data (Schauenstein et al., 1985) have indicated the suppressive activity of CM from NWL cells to be due to low m.w. factors that are removed by dialysis. Hence, addition of the dialysate (m.w. <10.000 daltons) of CM from NWL cells was found to suppress the Con A induced proliferation of OS cells in a dose dependent manner to the level of the NWL response. CM from Con A stimulated OS lymphocytes did not exhibit this suppressive effect. From data shown in Fig.2 it can be concluded that the suppression by NWL-CM is mediated by an inhibition of the IL 2 hyperproduction of OS cells: The IL 2 activity of CM from Mitomycin C treated and Con A

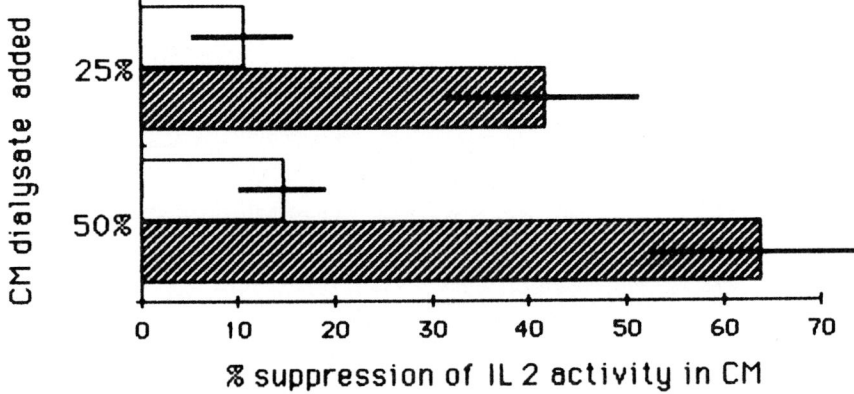

Figure 2. Suppression of IL 2 production of Mitomycin C treated and Con A stimulated splenocytes of NWL (☐, original IL 2 activity 1.5 U/ml) and OS (▧, original IL 2 activity 8.3 U/ml) chickens by the dialysate (m.w. <10.000) of CM from Con A activated NWL spleen cells.

pulsed OS cells was reduced in the presence of 50% dialysate of NWL-CM by about 60% of the untreated controls. The IL 2 production of NWL cells was only marginally affected by this treatment, probably due to saturation by endogenous production of this low m.w. suppressor factor.

To determine if the low suppressor activity in OS-CM was due secondarily to an excess production of IL 2, exogenous IL 2 was added to NWL cells (Fig. 3). This appeared unlikely since the addition of dialysed (i.e. suppressor free) CM to Con A stimulated NWL cells did not influence the suppressive activity of their crude CM in IL 2 assays.

The serum of OS animals is deficient in a non specific suppressor activity

Similarly to CM, sera of young adult NWL chickens exhibited a non specific suppressive activity in IL 2 assays, that is removable by dialysis. OS chickens exhibiting T cell hyperresponses were found to be consistently deficient in this serum suppressor (Fig. 4). This was also found in F_1 animals derived from matings of OS with normal chickens, which exhibit enhanced T cell responses to the same degree as do the OS parental animals.

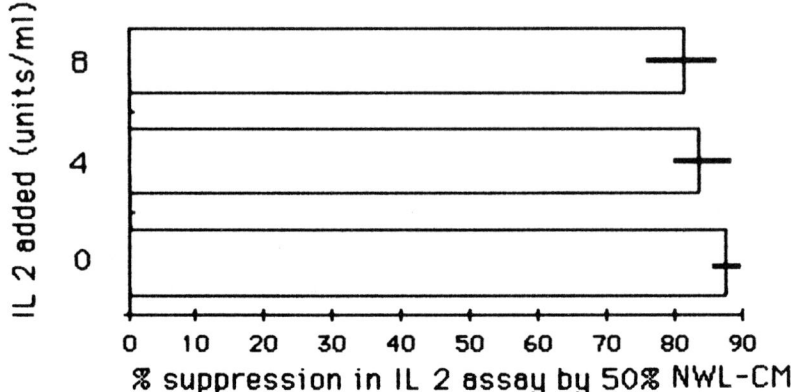

Figure 3. Addition of IL 2 (dialysed CM) does not affect the inhibitory activity in CM of Con A stimulated NWL splenocytes

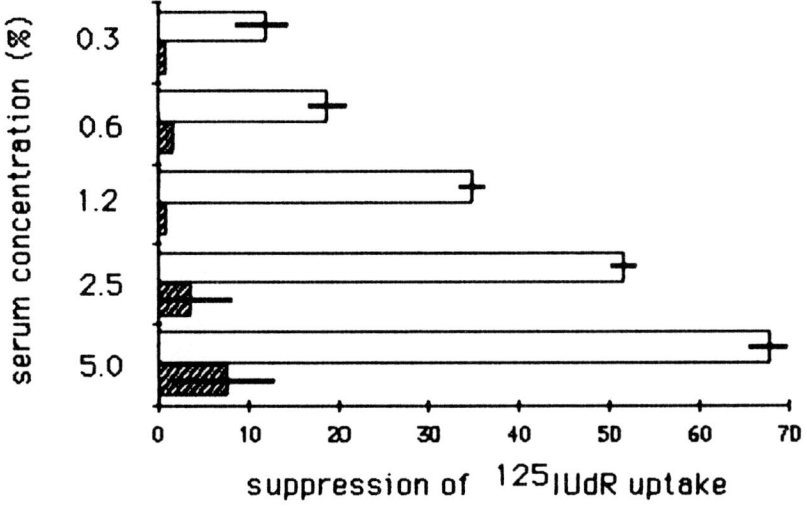

Figure 4. Suppressive effect of nondialysed sera from 6 week old NWL (☐, n=10) and OS (▨, n=30) chickens on the IL 2 mediated proliferation of lymphoblasts. The suppressive activity is expressed as percentual inhibition of ^{125}IUdR uptake by T lymphoblasts in presence of saturating concentrations of IL 2.

In conclusion, our data clearly show that the observed T cell hyperreactivity of OS chickens is due to aberrant immunoregulation, rather than to shifts in the precursor frequency of responder cells. This has also been suggested by recent limiting dilution analysis (data not shown).

The primary alteration leading to the enhanced T cell responsiveness of OS animals is the defect in a non specific suppressive activity in the CM of mitogen activated lymphocytes. We therefore postulate that the suppressive effect of crude CM, that is commonly found with Con A activated lymphocytes of several species, is important in the IL 2 production in normal conditions. Defects in this suppressor mechanism lead to immune dysregulation that is possibly involved in the development of spontaneous autoimmune reactions.

A strikingly similar defect in non specific suppressive activity was detected in the sera of OS animals. Although we do not yet know whether the suppression mediated by NWL serum represents the same mechanism as found in culture supernatant of lymphocytes, the close association between enhanced T cell function and the defect in this serum suppressor(s) suggests an important role for the quantitative outcome of T cell responses. In a recent ontogenetic study (Krömer et al.,1985b) we found that aged (3-6 yrs) NWL chickens lack the serum suppressor. Thus, OS chickens seem to be "prematurely aged" in this respect.

Experiments are presently underway to explore the cellular origin and chemical nature of the suppressor factor(s) responsible for the phenomena described.

ACKNOWLEDGMENT

These studies were supported by the Austrian Research Council (projects P4679 and S41/05).

REFERENCES

Kite JH, Tyler J, Pasquale J (1979). The immune response of obese strain chickens. In Milgrom F, Albini B (eds.): "Immunopathology. 6th International Convocation on Immunology" Basel: S. Karger, p 96.

Krömer G, Sundick RS, Schauenstein K, Hála K, Wick G (1985a). Analysis of lymphocytes infiltrating the thyroid gland of Obese Strain chickens. J Immunol in press.

Krömer G, Schauenstein K, Neu N, Stricker K, Wick G (1985b). In vitro T cell hyperreactivity in Obese Strain (OS) chickens is due to a defect in nonspecific suppressor mechanism(s). J Immunol in press.

Schauenstein K, Krömer G, Sundick RS, Wick G (1985). Enhanced response to Con A and production of TCGF by lymphocytes of Obese Strain (OS) chickens with spontaneous autoimmune thyroiditis. J Immunol 134:872.

Wick G, Boyd R, Hála K, Thunold S, Kofler H (1982). Pathogenesis of spontaneous autoimmune thyroiditis in Obese Strain (OS) chickens. Clin Exp Immunol 18:295.

BIOCHEMICAL MECHANISM(S) OF INTERLEUKIN 2 REGULATION OF LYMPHOCYTE GROWTH

William L. Farrar, Stuart W. Evans, Francis W. Ruscetti, Ezio Bonvini, Howard A. Young and Maria C. Birchenall-Sparks

Laboratory of Molecular Immunoregulation, BRMP, DCT, National Cancer Institute, NIH, Frederick Cancer Research Facility, Frederick, MD 21701 (W.L.F., S.W.E., F.W.R., H.A.Y., M.B.S) and Bureau of Biologics, National Institutes of Health, Bethesda, MD 20892 (E.B)

INTRODUCTION

Considerable advances in our understanding of the clonal expansion of antigen-sensitized T lymphocytes has been realized in recent years primarily from investigations which hybridized protein chemistry and cellular immunobiology. Since the original observation of Morgan et al. (1976) that conditioned medium from lectin-stimulated lymphocytes supported the continuous growth of their homologous lineage lymphocytes, rapid progress was made in the biochemical characterization and molecular cloning of T cell growth factor (Interleukin 2, IL-2).

The biological activity of IL-2 is believed to be initiated by a high affinity receptor-ligand interaction which leads to the stimulation of S phase progression and under certain circumstances, the release of additional immunomodulating lymphokines such as gamma interferon (IFNγ). Although important structural information has been derived from the nucleotide sequences of the cDNA clones of both IL-2 (Taniguchi et al., 1983) and its putative receptor, Tac (Leonard et al., 1984), relatively little information has been derived from these studies which suggest the biochemical mechanism(s) by which IL-2 regulates lymphocyte growth or gene expression. Here, we briefly describe some of the biochemical events stimulated by IL-2 which correlate with the induction of proliferation as well as transcriptional regulation of secretory proteins (IFNγ), IL-2 receptor (Tac), and early c-proto-oncogenes.

Recent studies have shown that both IL-2 and the multilineage colony stimulating factor, Interleukin 3 (IL-3), stimulate the activation of a unique protein phosphotransferase system, protein kinase C (PK-C) (Farrar and Anderson, 1985; Farrar et al., 1985a). Relevant to this observation are the studies of Castanaga et al. (1982) which suggested that PK-C is the enzymatic receptor for a potent class of tumor promoters, phorbol esters. The results of the PK-C activation studies with the proliferative interleukins suggested that tumor promoters, interleukins and certain oncogenes may share some common biochemical pathways which lead to cellular proliferation.

IL-2 Stimulation of PI Turnover

The physiological activation of PK-C is believed to occur as a result of the turnover and hydrolysis of phosphatidylinositol (PI). PI represents a relatively minor component of the total cellular phospholipid complement, but its relative rate of catabolism and turnover has been shown to increase in response to a variety of extracellular stimuli (Berridge, 1984). As a consequence of phosphoinositide hydrolysis is the formation of two metabolites (diacylglycerol and inositol trisphosphate), both of which may function as second messengers of the receptor mediated transmembrane signal apparatus. Inositol trisphosphate seems to act by mobilizing intracellular calcium, whereas diacylglycerol stimulates PK-C activation. Figure 1 demonstrates the accumulation of phosphatidylinositol (PI, panel A), phosphatidylinositol 4-phosphate (PIP, panel B), and phosphatidylinositol 4,5-bisphosphate CT6 murine lymphocytes (PIP_2, panel C). All three phosphoinositides are increased in a time dependent manner following the addition of IL-2 to ^{3}H-myo-inositol pulsed cells thereby indicating an increase in the rate of PI turnover. PIP_2 may be further metabolized both in the presence or absence of lithium to IP, IP_2 and IP_3 (data not shown). In the large majority of hormone and neurotransmitter biologies which have shown PI turnover and hydrolysis, a concomitant release of intracellular calcium or cationic influx has also been observed (Berridge, 1984). In the case of lymphokines, both IL-2 and IL-3 have been shown to stimulate increases in cytosolic

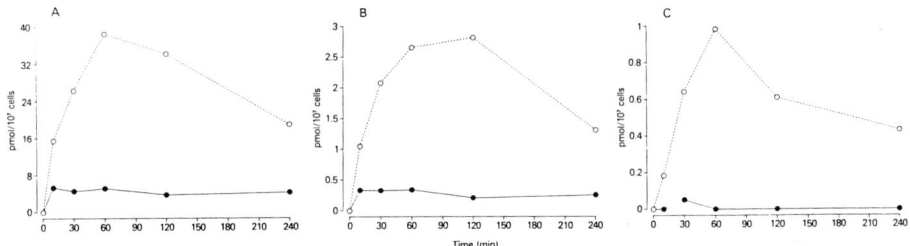

Figure 1. <u>IL-2 Stimulation of PI Turnover</u>. Panel A, PI; Panel B, PIP; Panel C, PIP_2; (o - o) plus IL-2, (● - ●) unstimulated. Chloroform-methanol extracted lipids were analyzed with single-dimension silica thin-layer chromatography.

$[Ca^{++}_i]$ as measured by QUIN-2 fluorescence (Rossio et al., 1985). The results of these studies suggested that IL-2 stimulates, as a result of receptor-coupled PI hydrolysis, a bifurcating signal pathway which results in the activation of PK-C and calcium mobilization.

Phosphoprotein substrates of PK-C

Protein phosphorylation has been long recognized as an exquisite mechanism of regulating protein and enzymatic functions (Cohen, 1982). Previously, our laboratory has identified that Tac, the putative IL-2 receptor, could serve as a direct substrate for PK-C (Farrar and Taguchi, 1985). Although the post-translational modification of receptors by protein kinases has resulted in altered ligand-binding affinity "states" in some systems (EGF, insulin, etc.), the phosphorylation of Tac by PK-C did not change the apparent high affinity binding characteristics for ^{3}H-leu-lys-IL-2 (Ruscetti and Farrar, unpublished observations).

Recent studies have identified a subcellular substrate of PK-C which is phosphorylated by either IL-2 or diacylglycerol stimulation of CT6 lymphocytes. Both IL-2 and a direct activator of PK-C, 1-olyeol-2-acetylglycerol (OAG), stimulated the phosphorylation of a 68 kd protein found in the cytoplasm and in loose association with plasma membrane. Two-dimensional analysis (Figure 2) shows the increased phosphorylation of the basic protein following stimulation of intact cells. The 68 kd substrate is phosphorylated with transient kinetics which approximates the temporal activation of PK-C (Farrar and Anderson, 1985). The 68 kd phosphoprotein is phosphorylated at threonine residues both in intact cells and in vitro and is also found in the cytoplasm of IL-3 or OAG treated myeloid cells dependent on IL-3 for growth (data not shown). Since both IL-2 and IL-3 appear to stimulate similar biochemical transmembrane signals (i.e., Ca^{2+} flux and PK-C activation) the identity of cellular substrates which are targets of the "second messenger" suggests a possible uniformity in the mechanism(s) regulating the growth of lymphoid and myeloid lineage cells.

IL-2 Regulation of Transcription

In addition to the effects on T lymphocyte proliferation, IL-2 has also been shown to facilitate the release of gamma interferon (IFNγ) from antigen-sensitized lymphocytes (Farrar et al., 1980). We examined whether IL-2, activators of PK-C, or calcium ionophores stimulated the

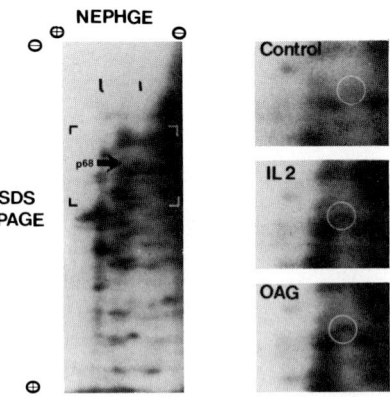

Figure 2. <u>IL-2 and Diacylglycerol Stimulate Phosphorylation of Identical Substrates.</u> Two-dimensional gel of intact CT6 cells phosphorylation patterns induced by IL-2 or the synthetic diacylglycerol, OAG. Phosphorylation of 68 kd substrate.

release of an intracellular prohormone IFNγ activity or
alternatively induce the transcription or accumulation of
IFNγ-mRNA (Figure 3). In order to address this question
a cell line, designated BUD-27, was derived from the IL-2-
dependent CT6 line. The BUD-27 are unique from CT6 in that
they exhibit the same number and affinity of IL-2 receptors
but no longer require IL-2 for proliferation (Farrar et al.,
1985b). BUD-27 cells, on the other hand, respond to IL-2
by the secretion of IFNγ. Dot-blot hybridization with
cDNA-IFNγ (Gray and Goeddel, 1983) of total RNA extractions
from stimulated BUD-27 cells revealed that transcription of
IFNγ-mRNA is increased by a variety of stimuli. Unstimulated BUD-27 (lane 1) cells exhibited no detectable IFNγ-
mRNA or antiviral activity (<4 units). Cells stimulated
with recombinant human IL-2 (lane 2), phorbol ester (lane 3),
and diacylglycerol (lane 4) had demonstrable IFNγ-mRNA
accumulation and corresponding antiviral activity. The
calcium ionophore, A23187, stimulated the highest relative
mRNA levels and bioactivities in a dose range of 1-10 μM
(lane 5-7). Therefore, IL-2, and direct activators of
either PK-C or calcium mobilization, stimulated IFNγ-mRNA
synthesis and consequent biological secretion.

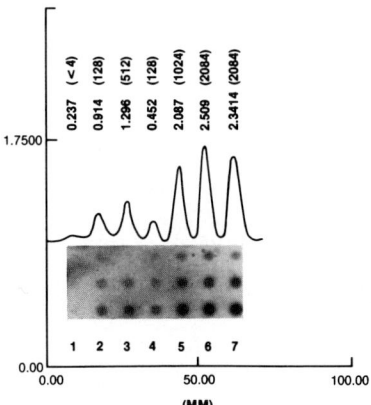

Figure 3. <u>IL-2 Stimulates IFNγ-mRNA Synthesis</u>. Various
stimulants were used to induce IFNγ-mRNA synthesis and
expression in BUD-27 cells. Lane 1, media; lane 2, IL-2;
lane 3, PMA; lane 4, OAG; lane 5, 1 μM A23187; lane 6, 10
μM A23187; lane 7, 1 μM + 50 μg OAG. Units of IFNγ
antiviral activity in parentheses.

Early c-proto-oncogenes have been suggested to be involved in the cell cycle response to certain growth peptides such as EGF and PDGF. We examined the nuclear runoff transcripts of three c-proto-oncogenes in CT6 cells in response to either IL-2 or phorbol ester (Figure 4). Both IL-2 and phorbol ester stimulated, in a temporal fashion, the same sequence of c-fos, c-myc and c-myb mRNA synthesis. The observation that a direct activator of PK-C, phorbol myristate acetate, stimulated a similar sequential pattern of oncogene mRNA synthesis suggested that the nuclear transcription of these early c-proto-oncogenes induced by IL-2 is mediated, in part, by the PK-C activation process.

Conclusions

IL-2 mediates its transmembrane signal apparatus by the stimulation of PI turnover which generates bifurcating biochemical signals which result in the mobilization of calcium and the activation of protein kinase C. The direct activation of PK-C by phorbol esters or diacylglycerol stimulates transcription of IFNγ-mRNA as well as the temporal expression of c-fos, c-myc, and c-myb proto-oncogenes. Whereas, IL-2 also regulates the expression of

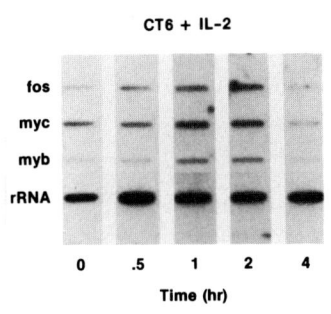
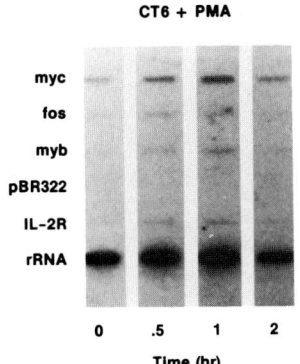

Figure 4. IL-2 and Phorbol Ester Stimulation of Early C-Proto-Oncogenes. IL-2 and PMA were used to stimulate CT6 c-proto-oncogene expression. Gene expression was analyzed by cDNA probe hybridization to nuclear-runoff transcripts.

the same gene transcripts, calcium may also play an important role in the proliferative response to the physiological stimuli.

REFERENCES

Morgan DA, Ruscetti FW, Gallo R (1976). Selective in vitro growth of T lymphocytes from normal human bone marrows. Science 193:1007-1010.

Taniguchi T, Matsui H, Jujita T, Takaoka C, Kashima N, Yoshimoto R, Manuro J (1983). Structure and expression of a cloned cDNA for human interleukin 2. Nature 302: 305-391.

Leonard WJ, Depper JM, Crabtree GR, Rudikoff S, Pumphrey J, Robb RJ, Kronke M, Svetlik PB, Peffer NJ, Waldmann, Greene WC (1984). Molecular cloning and expression of cDNA for the human interleukin 2 receptor: evidence for alternate mRNA splicing and the use of two polyandeylation sites. Nature 311:626-635.

Cohen N (1982). The role of protein phosphorylation in normal and hormonal control of cellular activity. Nature (London) 296:613-624.

Farrar WL, Anderson WB (1985). Interleukin 2-stimulates association of protein kinase C with plasma membrane. Nature 315:233-235.

Farrar WL, Thomas TP, Anderson WB (1985). Altered cytosol/membrane enzyme redistribution on interleukin 3 activation of protein kinase C. Nature 315:235-237.

Castagna M, Takai Y, Kaubuchi K, Sano K, Kikkawa U, Nishizuka Y (1982). Direct activation of calcium activated, phospholipid dependent, protein kinase by tumor-promoting phorbol esters. J Biol Chem 257:7987-7995.

Berridge MJ (1984). Inositol trisphosphate and diacylglycerol as second messengers. Biochem J 220:345-360.

Greenberg ME, Ziff EB (1984). Stimulation of 3T3 cells induces transcription of the c-fos proto-oncogene. Nature 311:433-438.

Farrar WL, Ruscetti FW, Young HA (1985b). 5-azacytidine treatment of a murine cytotoxic T cell line alters gamma interferon gene induction by IL-2. J Immunol 135:1551-1554.

Farrar WL, Johnson HM, Farrar JJ (1980). Regulation of the production of immune interferon and cytotoxic T lymphocytes by Interleukin 2. J Immunol 126:1120-1128.

Farrar WL, Taguchi M (1985). Interleukin 2 stimulation of
  protein kinase C membrane association: evidence for IL-2
  receptor phosphorylation. Lymph Res 4:87-93.
Rossio JL, Farrar WL, Ruscetti FW (1985). Calcium
  mobilization by specific recombinant ligands in IL-2 and
  IL-3 dependent cells in Role of Leukocytes in Host Defense,
  Eds. J. Oppenheim, D. Jacobs, Alan R. Liss, Inc., NY, NY
  (this volume).
Gray PW, Goeddel DV (1983). Cloning and expression of
  murine immune interferon cDNA. Proc Natl Acad Sci 80:
  5842-5846.

REGULATION OF C-MYC EXPRESSION AND T LYMPHOCYTE PROLIFERATION BY INTERLEUKIN 2 AND INHIBITORS

John C. Reed, Michael B. Prystowsky, Brian V. Jegasothy, Richard G. Hoover, and Peter C. Nowell

Departments of Pathology and Dermatology (B.V.J.), University of Pennsylvania, Philadelphia PA 19104

INTRODUCTION

The regulation of T lymphocyte proliferation is achieved through a balance between stimulatory and suppressive signals generated by soluble factors and by cell-cell recognition events. Central to the stimulation of T cell growth are the production of interleukin 2 (IL2) and the expression of receptors for this growth factor, both of which occur in G_1 phase of the cell cycle following exposure of T cells to antigen or to lectin mitogen (Greene & Robb, 1985). Besides IL2, recent studies suggested a role for the proto-oncogene c-myc in the regulation of the proliferation of non-neoplastic T cells (Kelly et al., 1983). How the events of IL2 binding to its receptor and of c-myc gene expression interact in the control of lymphocyte growth is unknown. We thus investigated the effects of purified recombinant IL2 (rIL2) on the accumulation of c-myc mRNA in activated T lymphocytes. We also employed various inhibitory agents, including an immunosuppressive lymphokine, IDS ("Inhibitor of DNA synthesis"), to study the regulation of c-myc expression, IL2 receptor expression, IL2 production, and other events involved in T cell activation and proliferation.

RESULTS

Earlier, we extended the initial observations of Kelly et al. (1983) regarding the expression of the cellular proto-oncogene c-myc in normal T cells. We found that rIL2 augments and anti-Tac antibody (anti-IL2 receptor) diminishes the levels of c-myc mRNA in activated T cells (Reed et al., 1985a). This suggested that accumulation of c-myc mRNA may be induced in T cells both at the $G_0 \to G_1$ phase transition when antigen or lectin mitogen binds to resting (G_0 phase) T cells, and during G_1 phase of the cell cycle when IL2 interacts with its cellular receptor on activated (G_1 phase) T cells.

To test this hypothesis further, we first performed a careful study of the time course of accumulation of c-myc mRNA in peripheral blood mononuclear cells (PBMC) cultures stimulated with phytohemagglutinin (PHA). In 3 of five experiments (Fig. 1A) we observed a biphasic response, consistent with the notion that accumulation of c-myc mRNA is induced at two points in the cell cycle. As a second approach, we investigated the effects of rIL2 on c-myc expression in a cloned murine T cell, L2 (Prystowsky et al., 1985). Even when quiescent, L2 cells have elevated RNA content relative to unstimulatyed splenocytes, express IL2 receptors, and proliferate in response to IL2. Thus, quiescent L2 cells are best regarded as early G_1 phase cells. When resting L2 cells were stimulated with rIL2, we observed a very rapid accumulation of c-myc mRNA that reached maximal levels within 1-2 hours (Fig. 1B). The combined data from experiments using PBMC and L2 cells demonstrate conclusively that IL2 can stimulate expression of c-myc in activated (G_1 phase) T cells.

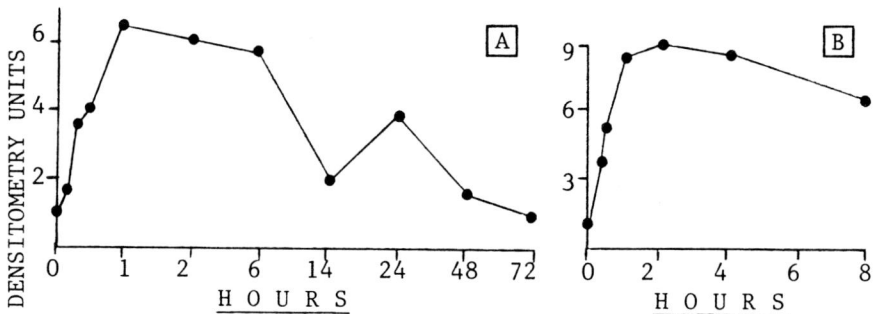

Figure 1. Total RNA was isolated from either (A) PBMC cultured with PHA-P (1 ug/ml) or (B) L2 cells cultured with rIL2 (100 U/ml) for various times; relative levels of c-myc mRNA were determined by RNA blot analysis with scanning densitometry.

Lectin mitogens stimulate T lymphocytes through their receptors for specific antigen (presumably), whereas IL2 stimulates through IL2 receptors. Though the molecular events involved in signal transduction upon binding of specific ligand to antigen receptors or to IL2 receptors remain poorly understood, at least some events, such as elevation of cytosolic Ca^{2+} (Weiss et al., 1984; Farrar, personal communication) and activation of protein kinase C (Farrar & Anderson, 1985), are common to both antigen receptor and IL2 receptor pathways. We have also observed that stimulation of PBMC through the antigen receptor with PHA or through the IL2 receptor with rIL2 induces expression of some of the same genes. For example, levels of IL2 receptor mRNA are upregulated both by PHA stimulation of resting (G_0 phase) PBMC and by IL2 stimulation of activated (G_1 phase) PBMC (Reed et al., 1985b).

To investigate whether lectin mitogens and IL2 induce accumulation of c-myc mRNA via common or independent pathways, we employed the protein synthesis inhibitor cycloheximide (CHX) and the immunosuppressive agent cyclosporin A (CsA). When quiescent L2 cells were stimulated in the presence of CHX either with concanavalin A (ConA) or with IL2, no decrease in the levels of c-myc mRNA was observed (Figs. 2A, 2B). Thus both ConA and IL2 induce c-myc mRNA accumulation without requirement for protein synthesis. When CsA was added to L2 cell cultures, however, IL2 but not ConA stimulated accumultaion of c-myc mRNA. These findings indicate that c-myc expression is regulated in T cells by at least two pathways, one IL2-independent and CsA-sensitive, the other IL2-dependent and CsA-resistant.

Besides IL2 receptors, the expression of transferrin receptors in late G_1 phase of the cell cycle represents a critical event for activated T cells to undergo the G_1-->S phase transition (Neckers & Cossman, 1984). To investigate the effects of transferrin receptor-mediated signals on c-myc expression, we used a monoclonal antibody, 42/6, to block binding of serum transferrin to its receptors on activated T cells. Adding 42/6 antibody to PHA-stimulated PBMC cultures did not produce a diminution of the levels of c-myc mRNA, but rather elevated them (Fig. 2C). Experiments with the DNA synthesis inhibitor hydroxyurea (HU) produced similar results (Fig. 2D). These data, combined with the time course studies (Fig. 1A), provide indirect evidence that 42/6 and HU, by blocking the G_1-->S phase

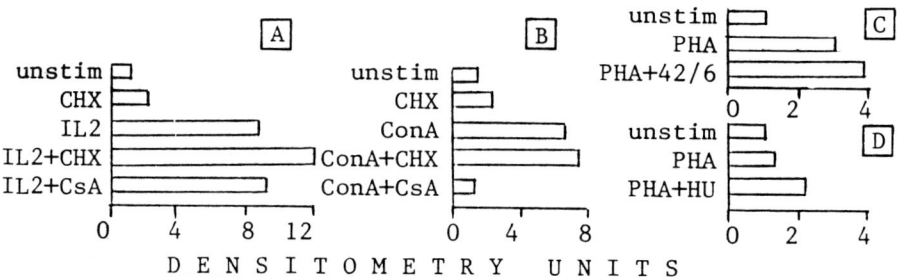

Figure 2. Levels of c-myc mRNA, relative to unstimulated cells, were measured by scanning densitometry after RNA blot analysis: (A) L2 cells cultured for 1 hr with CHX (15 ug/ml), rIL2 (1000 U/ml), CsA (1 ug/ml); (B) L2 cells, 8 hr with ConA (10 ug/ml); (C) PBMC, 24 hr with PHA-P (1 ug/ml), 42/6 (0.2 ug/ml); (D) PBMC, 48 hr with HU (1 mM).

transition, prevent activated T cells from reaching a point in S phase where an unknown signal is generated that downregulates c-myc expression. These data also suggest why some investigators failed to find a difference in c-myc mRNA levels in exponentially growing cells compared to density-arrested cells (Thompson et al., 1985). If density-arrested cells are blocked in late G_1 phase of the cell cycle, then the levels of c-myc mRNA could be equivalent in density-arrested and in exponentially growing cells.

Indirect support for a late G_1 phase block in activated T cells comes from studies we performed with IDS, an immunosuppressive lymphokine. IDS is produced by PBMC cultured at high density and stimulated with ConA. IDS has been purified to molecular homogeneity and distinguished from several other inhibitory lymphokines (Jegasothy & Battles, 1981). Given the failure of IDS to inhibit production of IL2 and expression of receptors for IL2 and for transferrin, IDS appears to block proliferation of activated T cells in late G_1 phase of the cell cycle. A summary of results for IDS and other inhibitors of T cell proliferation appears in Table 1.

Table 1. Summary of results for inhibitors of PHA-induced proliferation of PBMC.

Inhib.	IL2R*	IL2§	TFR*	DNA#	c-myc mRNA	c-fos mRNA	IL2R mRNA	TFR mRNA
OKT11A	+	+	+	+	+	+	+	ND
CsA	+	+	+	+	+	+	+	ND
DEX	+	+	+	+	+	+	+	ND
anti-Tac	-	-	+	+	+	ND	+	ND
CHX	ND	ND	ND	+	-	-	-	+
42/6	-	-	-	+	-	-	-	-
HU	-	-	-	+	-	-	-	-
IDS	-	-	-	+	ND	ND	ND	ND

(+ = inhibition; - = failure to inhibit; ND = not done)
*IL2 and transferrin receptor expression determined by indirect immunofluorescence; §IL2 production determined by bioassay; #DNA synthesis determined by ^{3}H-thymidine incorporation. DEX is 10^{-4} M dexamethasone; OKT11A is anti-p50 antibody (0.5 ug/ml).

DISCUSSION

We have presented evidence that accumulation of c-myc mRNA is regulated by two pathways in T lymphocytes. Although signal transduction mediated through antigen and IL2 receptors clearly shares common elements, there are also some differences. For example, in other experiments (not shown here), we have observed that lectin mitogens and rIL2 induce expression of an overlapping but non-identical set of genes in T lymphocytes. Stimulation of resting (G_0) T cells via their antigen receptors with PHA or with OKT3 antibody induces expression of c-myc, c-fos, IL2 receptors, and IL2. In contrast, stimulation of activated (G_1 phase) T cells via the IL2 receptor with rIL2 results in increased expression of c-myc, IL2 receptors, and transferrin receptors, but not in IL2 and only slightly in c-fos (unpublished observations).

Precisely how IL2 mediates cellular proliferation is unknown, but the evidence available to date suggests that interaction of this growth factor with its receptor on activated T cells results in a cascade of events, mediated at least in part by protein kinase C, that ultimately leads to alterations in gene expression. The data presented here, coupled with the fact that c-myc expression has been implicated in the regulation of the growth of normal and neoplastic cells, raise the possibility that some of the stimulatory effects of IL2 on T cell proliferation are mediated through c-myc. Accordingly, constitutive expression of the c-myc oncogene in T cell leukemias may represent a mechanism for achieving factor-independent growth.

REFERENCES

Farrar WL, Anderson WB (1985) Interleukin 2 stimulation of protein kinase C plasma membrane association. Nature 235: 233-235.

Greene WC, Robb RJ (1985) Receptors for T cell growth factor: Structure, function, and expression in normal and neoplastic cells. Contemp Topics Mol Immunol 10: 1-34.

Jegasothy BV, Battles DR (1981) Immunosuppressive lymphocyte factors. III. Complete purification and partial characterization of human Inhibitor of DNA Synthesis. Mol Immunol 18: 395-401.

Kelly K, Cochran BH, Stiles CD, Leder P (1983) Cell-specific regulation of the c-myc gene by lymphocyte mitogens and platelet-derived growth factor. Cell 35: 603-610.

Neckers LM, Cossman J (1984) Transferrin receptor induction in mitogen-stimulated human T lymphocytes is required for DNA synthesis and cell division and is regulated by Interleukin 2(TCGF). IN: Thymic Hormones and Lymphokines (ed. Goldstein), Plenum Press, NY, 383-398.

Prystowsky MB, Otten G, Pierce SK, Shay J, Olsham J, Fitch FW (1985) Lymphokine production by cloned T lymphocytes. IN: Lymphokines 12: 13-38 (ed. Pick), Plenum Press, NY.

Reed JC, Nowell PC, Hoover RG (1985a) Regulation of c-myc mRNA levels in normal human lymphocytes by modulators of cell proliferation. Proc Natl Acad Sci 82: 4221-4224.

Reed JC, Greene WC, Hoover RG, Nowell PC (1985b) OKT11A antibody inhibits and recombinant interleukin 2 (IL2) augments IL2 receptor expression at a pretranslational level. J Immunol, in press.

Thompson CB, Challoner PB, Neiman PE, Gioroudine M (1985) Levels of c-myc mRNA are invariant through the cell cycle. Nature 314: 363-366.

Weiss A, Imboden J, Shoback D, Stobo J (1984) Role of T3 surface molecules in human T cell activation: T3-dependent activation results in an increase in cytoplasmic free calcium. Proc Natl Acad Sci 81: 4169-4173.

PATTERNS OF PROTEIN SYNTHESIS FOLLOWING IL2 STIMULATION OF CLONED T HELPER LYMPHOCYTES

Daniel E. Sabath and Michael B. Prystowsky

Department of Pathology and Laboratory Medicine,
University of Pennsylvania School of Medicine,
Philadelphia, PA 19104

INTRODUCTION

Interleukin 2 (IL2) is released from lectin or antigen stimulated T lymphocytes, and causes T cells bearing IL2 receptors to proliferate. Recent work from several laboratories has shown that IL2 stimulation results in increased potassium conductance (Lee et al., 1985), increased c-myc transcription (Kelly et al., 1983; Reed et al., 1985), activation of the lipoxygenase pathway (Farrar and Humes, 1985), association of protein kinase C with the plasma membrane (Farrar and Anderson, 1985), induction of transferrin receptors (Neckers and Cossman, 1983), induction of IL2 receptors (Depper et al., 1985), and secretion of gamma interferon (Reem and Yeh, 1984). In this study we show that IL2 causes an overall increase in protein synthesis as well as sequential changes in the patterns of protein synthesis as the cells progress through the cell division cycle.

METHODS

The derivation and maintenance of the murine L2 cell line has been described previously (Glasebrook et al., 1981). L2 cells separated over Ficoll-Hypaque were cultured at 10^6 cells in 1 ml with 100 units/ml rIL2 (Cetus Corp., Emeryville, CA).

For cell cycle analysis, rIL2-stimulated cells were lysed in 0.1% sodium citrate (w/v) at pH 7.0 containing 50 ug/ml propidium iodide. DNA content was quantitated using a FACS IV. To determine the percentage of cells in G1, S, and G2+M, histograms of linear fluorescence intensity vs. cell number were deconvoluted into ten Gaussian curves.

To examine rates of protein synthesis, 10^6 rIL2-stimulated L2 cells were pulse labeled for one hour in methionine-free medium containing 50 uCi/ml [35-S]-methionine ([35-S]-met, specific activity >800 Ci/mmol). The cells were then washed in cold PBS, lysed with 100 ul of extraction buffer (0.01 M Tris pH 7.4, 0.15 M NaCl, 0.5% NP-40), and incubated on ice for 20 min. Cell lysates were separated by SDS polyacrylamide gel electrophoresis (SDS-PAGE) and exposed to X-ray film for 1-7 days at -70°C. The autoradiographs were scanned with a Hoefer Model GS300 densitometer connected to a Waters M840 data reduction system. A 5 ul aliquot was TCA precipitated and assayed for radioactivity to determine total protein synthesis.

RESULTS

Seven daya after previous stimulation with antigen, about 90% of unstimulated L2 cells had G0/G1 DNA content (Table I). DNA content of L2 cells stimulated with rIL2 for 5 hr was not changed. At 19 hr 38% of the cells were just beginning to enter S phase. By 27 hr, 67% of the cells were distributed throughout early, middle, and late S phase, and 7% were in G2+M. At 46 hr, the cells were distributed throughout all phases of the cell cycle, and at 68 hr, the distribution of cells was returning to that of a resting population. In experiments using the mitotic inhibitor colchicine, greater than 85% of rIL2-stimulated L2 cells entered the cell division cycle. These data suggest that the first round of division is relatively

Table I. DNA content of rIL2 stimulated L2 cells

Time (hours)	G1 (%)	S (%)	G2+M (%)
0	90	9	1
5	94	5	1
20	61	38	2
27	27	67	7
46	20	54	26
68	66	25	10

synchronous. Therefore, changes in protein synthesis can be defined for G1 activation and G1 to S phase transition.

In a parallel set of experiments, L2 cells were pulse labeled with [35-S]-met to determine the synthetic rate of various proteins during G1 activation and the G1-S phase transition. Total protein synthesis was maximal at 20-24 hr, just as the cells were beginning DNA synthesis (Table I). The maximal rate of incorporation was increased about four-fold over baseline (Table 2). Separation of proteins by one-dimensional (1D) SDS-PAGE suggested that there were three patterns of protein synthesis (Fig. 1). Type I

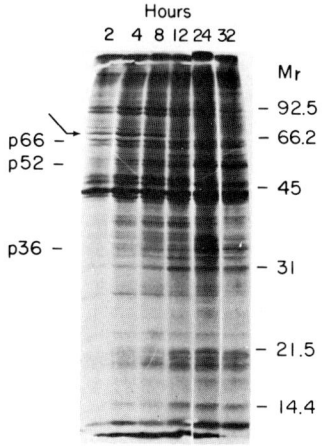

Figure 1. SDS-PAGE analysis of [35-S]-met pulse labeled proteins after rIL2 stimulation of L2 cells. p66, p52, and p36 are bands representing single proteins.

proteins, represented by p66, were synthesized at near maximal rates early after stimulation, and their rates of synthesis were maintained through the 32 hr time course. Type II proteins, represented by p52 and p36, were characterized by increasing rates of synthesis early after rIL2 stimulation that continued to increase between 12 and 24 hr after stimulation. A third pattern, Type III, in which the rate of synthesis was high early after stimulation and low by 12 hr was observed occasionally (Fig. 1, arrow). Two dimensional (2D) gel analysis confirmed the existence of three patterns of protein synthesis, including the existence of seven Type III proteins that were not visualized using 1D gels (data not shown). In addition, changes observed in about ten of the bands seen on 1D gels were shown to be attributable to changes in single proteins on 2D gels.

Three bands that represented single proteins on 1D gels were analyzed further using densitometry to quantify the rIL2-induced changes in their rates of synthesis. In a third experiment, the rates of synthesis of these three representative proteins, as well as total TCA precipitable cpm, were quantitated (Table 2). Synthesis of the type I protein p66 reached greater than 60% of its maximal rate by 4 to 8 hr after rIL2 stimulation and, like overall

Table 2 Rates of synthesis of rIL2-induced proteins

Time (hours)	Total	p66	p52	p36
0	[1][a]	[1][b]	[1][b]	[1][b]
4	1.7	3.4	2.8	5.4
8	2.0	2.7	6.4	5.9
12	1.9	3.4	7.0	12.2
16	2.6	3.9	8.1	16.1
20	3.1	4.4	12.1	18.4
24	3.8	4.4	13.6	18.5
32	2.9	3.2	9.7	10.3

[a]relative TCA precipitable cpm with t=0 defined as 1.
[b]relative density with t=0 defined as 1.

protein synthesis, reached a maximal synthetic rate of 4- to 5-fold over baseline at 20 to 24 hr. The rates of synthesis of the Type II proteins p52 and p36 increased continuously for the first 20 to 24 hr after stimulation, reaching maximal rates of 14- to 18-fold over those in unstimulated cells. In this particular experiment, no Type III proteins were detectable by 1D gel analysis.

Attempts were made to identify the Type II proteins by immunoprecipitation. They were not precipitated or removed from the total cellular extract by antisera to p53, to the 39 kD lysosomal major excreted protein (MEP), or to the IL2 receptor. Additionally, it was noted that the Type II proteins p52 and p36 had half lives of greater than 7 hr. No further characterization has been accomplished at this time.

DISCUSSION

Sequential gene activation following IL2 stimulation has been demonstrated in lymphocytes by a number of laboratories. Following IL2 stimulation, one of the earliest events is transcription of the oncogene c-myc (Reed et al., 1985). Later the genes for the IL2 receptor (Depper et al., 1985) and transferrin receptor are activated (Neckers and Cossman, 1983). Similarly, in PDGF-stimulated fibroblasts, c-fos is transcribed within minutes, followed by transcription of c-myc (Muller et al., 1984). In addition to there being an ordered sequence of gene activation, there is evidence that early protein products muct be synthesized before later genes are activated. For example, IL2- or PDGF-induced transcription of c-myc mRNA (Reed et al., 1985; Muller et al., 1984) does not require prior protein synthesis, while prior protein synthesis is required before PDGF-induced MEP mRNA can be transcribed (Frick et al., 1985). It is possible that some of the early oncogenes like c-myc cause directly or indirectly the activation of later genes like MEP or Type II proteins.

From this study it is apparent that there are specific sequences of protein synthesis during IL2 stimulated proliferation of L2 cells. Type I proteins reach near maximal rates of synthesis early after stimulation, and continue to be synthesized through the G1-S transition. Type III proteins are expressed early after rIL2 stimulation, and are synthesized at minimal rates when Type I and Type II proteins are being synthesized maximally. Type II proteins are synthesized at higher relative rates than Type I proteins and reach their maximal rates of synthesis later after stimulation. These proteins may be important in making the G1-S transition or preparing the cell for division. Since Type I and Type III proteins are expressed early after stimulation, they may regulate the later expression of Type II proteins. The availability of homogeneous cell populations (L2 cells) and pure stimuli (recombinant IL2) will allow the further dissection of the events occurring between the first membrane signal and eventual cell division.

REFERENCES

Depper JM, Leonard WJ, Drogula C, Krönke M, Waldmann TA, Greene WC (1985) Interleukin 2 (IL-2) augments transcription of the IL-2 receptor gene. Proc Natl Acad Sci USA 82:4230-4234.

Farrar WL, Anderson WB (1985) Interleukin 2 stimulates association of protein kinase C with plasma membrane. Nature 315:233-235.

Farrar WL, Humes JL (1985) The role of arachidonic acid metabolism in the activities of interleukin 1 and 2. J Immunol 135:1153-1159.

Frick KK, Doherty PJ, Gottesman MM, Scher CD (1985) Regulation of the transcript for a lysosomal protein: evidence for a PDGF-modulated gene program. Mol Cell Biol, in press.

Glasebrook AL, Sarmiento M, Loken MR, Dialynas DP, Quintans J, Eisenberg L, Lutz CT, Wilde D, Fitch FW (1981) Murine T lymphocyte clones with distinct immunological functions. Immunol Rev 54:225-266.

Kelly K, Cochran BH, Stiles CD, Leder P (1983) Cell-specific regulation of the c-myc gene by lymphocyte mitogens and platelet-derived growth factor. Cell 35:603-610.

Lee SC, Sabath DE, Deutsch C, Prystowsky MB (1985) Increased voltage-gated potassium conductance during interleukin 2 stimulated proliferation of a mouse helper T-lymphocyte clone. Submitted for publication.

Muller R, Bravo R, Burckhardt J, Curran T (1984) Induction of c-fos gene and protein by growth factors precedes activation of c-myc. Nature 312:716-720.

Neckers L, Cossman J (1983) Transferrin receptor induction in mitogen-stimulated human T lymphocytes is required for DNA synthesis and cell division and is regulated by interleukin 2. Proc Natl Acad Sci USA 80:3494-3498.

Reed JC, Sabath DE, Hoover RG, Prystowsly MB (1985) Recombinant interleukin 2 regulates levels of c-myc mRNA in a cloned murine T lymphocyte. Mol Cell Biol, in press.

Reem GH, Yeh N-H (1984) Interleukin 2 regulates expression of its receptor and synthesis of gamma interferon by human T lymphocytes. Science 225:429-430.

Identification and Characterization of a Released Form of
the Interleukin-2 Receptor.

Laurence A. Rubin M.D., FRCPC, Carole C. Kurman, B.S.,
M. Elizabeth Fritz, B.S., Robert Yarchoan, M.D., and
David L. Nelson, M.D.
From the Immunophysiology Section, Metabolism Branch (LAR,
CCK, MEF, DLN) and the Clinical Oncology Program (RY),
National Cancer Institute, National Institutes of Health,
Bethesda, MD 20205

INTRODUCTION

   The availability of hybridoma-derived monoclonal antibodies has greatly facilitated the recognition and characterization of cell surface molecules expressed by certain neoplastic cells and some normal cells at various stages of activation and/or maturation (Bull WHO, 1984). These antibodies have also clarified some the complex events involved in both normal and aberrant cell growth and differentiation.

   Interleukin-2 (IL-2), is a lymphokine synthesized and secreted by activated T cells which plays a pivotal role in the regulation of the immune response. (Smith, 1980). This molecule causes the growth of T cells by binding to specific high affinity receptors (IL-2R) newly expressed on the surface of activated lymphocytes. (Leonard et al. 1983). Cellular activation is a prerequisite for the expression of both the IL-2R and its ligand (Greene and Robb, 1985). Several monoclonal antibodies which recognize the human IL-2R have been produced, and using one such monoclonal anti-IL-2R antibody, anti-Tac, (Uchiyama et al, 1981) IL-2R have been consistently identified on the surface of lymphoid cells in certain leukemias (Waldmann et al, 1984).

We have developed an enzyme linked immunosorbent assay (ELISA) to specifically quantitate IL-2R. In addition to the expected finding of cell associated IL-2R, we have identified a soluble form of this molecule released into the culture supernatants of activated normal lymphocytes and constitutively released by certain lymphoid tumor cell lines in vitro. In this report, we describe these observations, as well as the finding of soluble IL-2R in vivo in the sera of healthy controls at low but measurable levels, and at markedly elevated levels in the sera of patients with certain lymphoreticular malignancies.

METHODS

ELISA for Soluble IL-2R
Alternate columns of wells of microtiter plates were coated with 150 ul of a 1 ug/ml solution of anti-Tac in pH 9.6 carbonate buffer or buffer alone. Following washing, 100 ul of sample was added to coated and control wells, incubated for two hours and the washing repeated. 100 ul of fluorescein isothiocyanate (FITC) conjugated 7G7B6 (Rubin et al, 1985a) was then added to all wells, incubated for two hours, and the washing repeated. All wells then received 100 ul of alkaline phosphatase-conjugated rabbit anti-FITC, and following a one hour incubation the plates were washed and 100 ul of the substrate p-nitrophenyl phosphate (Sigma 1mg/ml) in diethanolamine buffer pH. 9.8 was added to the wells. The conversion of substrate to product was measured spectrophotometrically at 405 nM. The absorbance in the control wells was subtracted from the experimental wells and this absorbance was compared to the absorbances determined for a standard curve generated by adding varying amounts of IL-2R to wells as previously described (Yarchoan et al, 1981) The IL-2R standard was the cell-free supernatant of an in vitro passaged T-cell line (IL-2 CTC) which was assigned a level of 1000 IL-2R/ml.

Cell Cultures/Cell Lines
Cultures of activated human PBMC were prepared as previously described (Rubin et al, 1985A). Cells and supernatant were separated by centrifugation, and the cells extracted in PBS containing 1% Triton X-100. Cell lines were maintained and prepared as previously described (Rubin et al., 1985b).

Molecular weight estimation
Biosynthetically labeled soluble and cell-associated IL-2R from HUT 102 cell cultures were prepared in cysteine/

methionine-free McCoy's 5A medium (GIBCO) with 2% dialyzed
FCS to which 125 µ Ci/ml of both [^{35}S]cysteine and
[^{35}S]methionine were added. After an overnight incubation,
cells and supernatant were separated by centrifugation, and
detergent extracts of the cells prepared. Immunoprecipitation was performed by incubation with 1 ug of anti-Tac or a
control mouse G_{2a} antiserum for 2 hr at 4° C, followed by
a 1-hr incubation with 10% Staphylococcus aureus and analysis on a 12.5% NaDodSO$_4$ polyacrylamide gel.

Sephadex G-200 gel filtration was performed using serum
from a patient with elevated circulating IL-2R levels.
Following molecular sieving, the individual fractions (2.5
ml) were lyophilized, resuspended in 100 ul of distilled
water, and assayed by ELISA to determine IL-2R content.

Patient Population

For these initial studies, frozen sera from patients with a
variety of malignant diseases obtained from the reference
serum bank of the Metabolism Branch, National Cancer Institute, National Institutes of Health were examined retro-
spectively. The sera were from patients seen at the NIH as
well as samples sent for immunologic assessment by outside
physicians. Similarly stored normal volunteer serum were
also tested.

RESULTS
    Initial studies on in vitro PHA activated normal PBMC
revealed rapid (<24 hr) production of both supernatant and
cellular IL-2R as measured by ELISA. The assay was sensitive, with both supernatant and cellular IL-2R detectable
above background levels at cell culture concentrations as
low as 3×10^4 cells/ml. Furthermore, the soluble nature
of the released IL-2R was confirmed by passage through
0.22 micron filters and ultracentrifuged at 100,000 X G
for 1 hr without loss of reactivity. The assay was specific
for soluble IL-2R, in that wells coated with control antisera, and reacted with anti-IL-2R antibodies after sample
addition scored negative by ELISA. In addition, activation
of PBMC with a variety of specific as well as nonspecific
stimuli resulted in the generation of supernatant as well
as cellular IL-2R (Rubin et. al. 1985b).

We also assessed whether supernatant IL-2R was the result of cell death, lysis and release of cell associated IL-2R. For these studies, normal PBMC were activated with PHA for 24 hrs, then subjected to three cycles of freeze/thawing, or sham treated, and returned to the same IL-2 and IL-2R containing media for additional periods of in vitro culture. The level of supernatant IL-2R was determined by ELISA and represents the Units of IL-2R per 10^6 cultured PBMC.

TABLE I

Soluble IL-2R is not released from killed IL-2R positive cells in vitro

Treatment	Supernatant IL-2R Levels on Day		
	1	2	3
None	187	674	1265
Freeze/thaw	187	195	158

As can be seen in Table I, no additional accumulation of supernatant IL-2R was noted as a result of cell death.

As part of our initial in vitro studies characterizing released soluble IL-2R, we tested the supernatants of a number of different human lymphocytic cell lines. (Table II). The culture supernatants of T cells infected with the lymphotrophic retrovirus, HTLV-I, contained markedly elevated levels of soluble IL-2R. In contrast, supernatants from an HTLV negative and non IL-2 dependent T cell line, JURKAT, contained <31.25 U/ml of soluble IL-2R. While most pre-B and B-cell culture supernatants which we examined exhibited no detectable levels of released IL-2R, one Epstein-Barr Virus transformed B-lymphoblastoid cell line released measurable amounts of this soluble receptor.

TABLE II

Analysis of various cell lines for the presence of cellular and supernatant IL-2R

Cell Line	Cell Type	Cellular IL-2R (U/ml)	Supernatant IL-2R (U/ml)
IL-2 CTC	T cell (HTLV-)	1,250	1,000
JURKAT	T cell (HTLV-)	31.3	<31.3
MJ	T cell (HTLV+)	9,430	4,638
HUT 102B2	T cell (HTLV+)	5,413	10,715
NALM-1	pre-B	<31.3	<31.3
SU-DHL9	B	55	<31.3
EBV-2	B	55	<31.3
EBV-3	B	205	65.0

Molecular Weight Estimation. Figure 1:

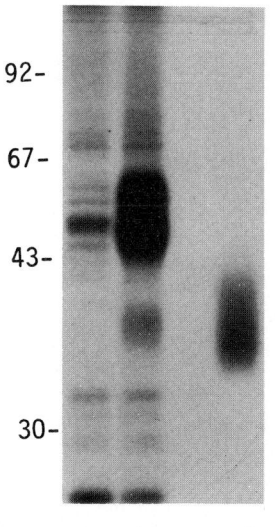

SDS-PAGE Analysis of cellular and supernatant biosynthetically labelled IL-2R from HUT 102 cell cultures. Lanes a) and c) control antibody; lanes b) and d) anti-Tac immunoprecipitation. Mr markers are listed in the left hand column. Supernatant IL-2R (lane d) is a moleculle of Mr=35-40,000, approximately 15,000 daltons smaller than the cell associated receptor from these HUT 102 cell cultures (lane b).

Figure 2   Sephadex G-200 gel filtration of serum IL-2R. A uniform peak value of IL-2R is noted at an approximate molecular weight less than gammaglobulin but greater than human albumin.

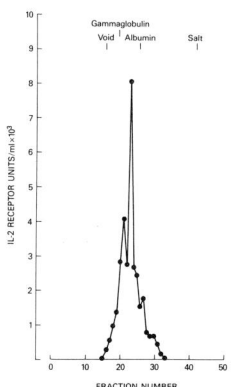

To investigate the in vivo counterpart of this in vitro observation, the serum levels of soluble IL-2R in patients with a variety of malignant diseases, as well as a group of normals, were determined.

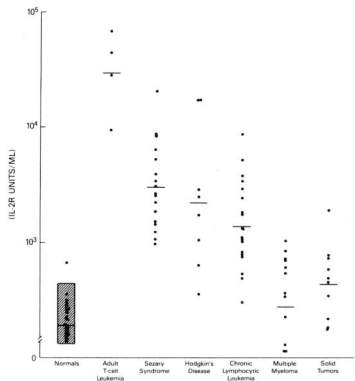

Figure 3.   The geometric mean for each group listed is denoted by a bar.   The hatched area represents 2 standard deviations above and below the mean value for the normal controls.   Results are recorded as IL-2R units/ml as described in methods.

DISCUSSION

Utilizing two monoclonal antibodies which recognize distinct epitopes on the IL-2R, an ELISA was constructed to quantitatively measure soluble IL-2R (IL-2R). In addition to the expected finding of IL-2R in the detergent extracts of lectin or antigen activated peripheral blood mononuclear cells, the cell free supernatants of such cultures were found to contain a released form of the IL-2R. HTLV-I positive T cell lines studied were found to constitutively release large quantities of IL-2R into their culture supernatants. HTLV-I negative and IL-2 independent T, as well as most B and pre B cell lines examined, were negative for released and cell associated IL-2R. Immunoaffinity purification and SDS polyacrylamide gel electropheresis of soluble IL-2R from HUT 102B2 culture supernatant revealed a molecule of apparent $M_r=35-40,000$, approximately 15,000 daltons smaller than the surface receptor on these cells.

With the ELISA described here, we have also detected a soluble form of the IL-2R molecule in the sera of healthy controls and in considerably elevated amounts in the sera of patients with some malignant disorders. The presence of low levels of circulating IL-2R in the control group is not entirely unexpected, since the immune system undergoes constant challenge by foreign antigens, presumably resulting in a low level of continual lymphocyte activation with the resultant release of soluble IL-2R. Similarly, the elevated levels of serum IL-2R in patients with non-lymphoid solid organ cancers, whose neoplasms would not be expected to synthesize IL-2R, suggests that the generation of this molecule in these cases is more likely a reflection of host response to the tumor.

The most markedly elevated levels of serum IL-2R were found in patients with HTLV-1 positive Adult T-cell Leukemia. Infection of T-cells *in vitro* with this retrovirus results in abnormally high levels of both cell associated and released IL-2R (Greene and Robb, 1985; Rubin et. al. 1985b). Thus the serum IL-2R in these patients is most probably produced by the malignant cells themselves.

Further investigations will be required to correlate the serum and cellular IL-2R levels in patients with lymphoreticular neoplasia and to look for changes in these levels in patients undergoing various therapies. This preliminary report suggests that serum IL-2R measurement might prove to be a valuable and relatively simple seroepidemiologic tool, as well as a means of following cancer patients in whom abnormal levels of soluble serum IL-2R have been identified. Additional studies will be necessary to elucidate what role this soluble molecule might play in the pathophysiology of these and related disorders.

Acknowledgements: Dr. Rubin is a recipient of a fellowship from the Arthritis Society of Canda.

REFERENCES

First International Workshop on Human Leukocyte Differentation Antigens(1980). Bull WHO 5:809-11.

Greene WC, Robb RJ (1985). Receptors for T-cell growth factor: Structure, function and expression on normal and neoplastic cells. Contemp Top Mol Immunol. 10:1-34.

Leonard WJ, Depper JD, Robb RJ, Waldmann TA, Greene WC (1983). Characterization of the human receptor for the T cell growth factor. Proc Nat'l Acad Sci USA. 80: 6957-61.

Rubin LA, Kurman CC, Biddison WE, Goldman ND, Nelson DL (1985a). A monoclonal antibody, 7G7/B6, that binds to an epitope on the human IL-2 receptor distinct from that recognized by IL-2 or anti-Tac. Hybridoma. 4:91-102.

Rubin LA, Kurman CC, Fritz ME et al. (1985 b). Soluble Interleukin-2 receptors are released by activated lymphocytes *in vitro*. J. Immunol. (in press)

Smith KA (1980). T-cell growth factor. Immunol Rev. 51:337-57.

Uchiyama T, Broder S, Waldmann TA (1981). A monoclonal antibody reactive with activated and functionally mature human T cells. J Immunol. 126:1393-97.

Waldmann TA, Greene WC, Sarin PS, et al (1984). Functional and phenotypic comparison of HTLV positive adult T cell leukemia with HTLV negative Sezary leukemia and their distinction using anti-Tac. J Clin Inv. 73:1711-18.

Yarchoan R, Murphy BR, Strober W, Clements ML, Nelson DL (1981). *In vitro* production of anti-influenza virus antibody after intranasal innoculation with cold-adapted influenza virus. J. Immunol. 127:1958-63.

EVIDENCE OF INTERLEUKIN 2-INDEPENDENT PROLIFERATION OF NON-TRANSFORMED T CELLS

Jay P. Siegel, D. Bruce Burlington and Theresa L. Gerrard

Division of Virology, Office of Biologics Research and Review, Center for Drugs and Biologics, Food and Drug Administration, Bethesda, Maryland 20205

When resting T lymphocytes are activated, they produce and secrete interleukin 2 (IL 2), express IL 2 receptors, and proliferate. The presence of IL 2 (exogenous or endogenous) and the expression of IL 2 receptors have been demonstrated in essentially all systems in which T cells proliferate; and the use of tissue culture media containing IL 2 has allowed the growth of a wide variety of cloned, nontransformed T cell lines. For these reasons, it has frequently been hypothesized that the action of IL 2 on IL 2 receptors may be required for all T cell proliferation. Alteratively there may exist a signal (or signals) sufficient to induce proliferation of T cells independently of IL 2. The demonstration of IL 2-independent proliferation is made difficult by the fact that signals which induce proliferation of T cells also induce IL 2 production, IL 2 receptor expression, and IL 2-dependent proliferation. A number of investigators have employed antibodies either to IL 2 or to the IL 2 receptor in order to determine whether the IL 2-IL 2 receptor interaction is necessary for T cell proliferation (Gillis et al., 1981; Depper et al. 1983; Koretzky et al., 1983; Malek et al., 1984, Bettens et al., 1984). This methodology is limited because antibodies to the IL 2 receptor do not block the receptor completely and irreversibly, but rather compete with IL 2 itself for binding sites, and thus do not fully block IL 2 actions under many conditions. Similarly, antibodies to IL 2 do not fully block the ability of IL 2 to bind to its receptor and to activate T cells. Thus the results of such experiments are difficult to interpret.

In the present report, we describe studies in which human T cells were activated with mitogens or allogeneic cells while using a monoclonal antibody to the IL 2 receptor, anti-TAC, to interfere with the binding of IL 2 with its receptor and the drug, cyclosporine A, to block production of IL 2 (Elliott et al., 1984). Invariably we found that a significant portion of the lectin- or alloantigen-induced proliferation of fresh T cells was resistant to these agents, even under conditions in which anti-TAC blocked a high proportion of IL 2-induced proliferation in control cultures and conditions in which no IL 2 production was detectable. These findings are consistent with the hypothesis that the proliferative response of T cells is in part independent of IL 2.

METHODS

Peripheral blood mononuclear cells (PBMC) were depleted of plastic adherent cells and nylon wool adherent cells to yield a T-enriched cell population. T-enriched cells were further depleted of cells buoyant on 50% Percoll and of cells adherent to plates coated with IgG-Fc to yield small T cells containing less than 0.1% esterase positive cells. In some experiments, cells from a T cell line specific for allogeneic cells of HLA-DR2 haplotype were used as responders. This line was established and grown in the presence of irradiated allogeneic cells without exogenous IL 2 but was also capable of proliferating in response to IL 2. B cells from an Epstein-Barr virus-transformed HLA-DR2 positive line were gamma irradiated (5000 R) and used as stimulators in some experiments.

Freshly isolated lymphocytes were placed in 96 well flat-bottomed microtiter plates at 2×10^5 cells/well for use as responders. The allo-specific T cell line was used at 2×10^4 cells/well. The stimuli used were purified phytohemagglutinin (PHA), concanavalin A (Con A), or the B cell line used at 2×10^5 cells/well. In some experiments recombinant human IL 2 (Cetus Corp., Emeryville, CA) was used. Responses were modified by exposing cells to anti-TAC at 10 µg/ml and/or cyclosporine A for 30 minutes prior to and thoughout the period of stimulation. Thymidine incorporation was measured during a 6 hour pulse with ^{3}H-methyl thymidine.

IL 2 activity was determined using a microassay of thymidine incorporation by a murine IL 2-dependent lymphocyte line, CTLL 2, (Gillis et al., 1978) modified as previously described (Siegel et al., 1985). The primary reference standard for IL 2 was provided by the Biological Response Modifiers Program of the National Cancer Institute. Samples containing cyclosporine A were ultrafiltered using Centricon 10 microconcentrators (Amicon Corp., Danvers, MA) and rediluted with phosphate-buffer saline repeatedly prior to assay. Preliminary experiments indicated that this procedure was effective in removing cyclosporine A and in concentrating IL 2.

SUMMARY OF RESULTS

In the first series of experiments, PBMC were stimulated with PHA at 0.5 or 5.0 µg/ml. Anti-TAC at 10 µg/ml and/or cyclosporine A at 2 µg/ml were added to the cells prior to stimulation. Anti-TAC had little effect on PHA-induced proliferation; cyclosporine A inhibited 50-70% of the proliferative response; and the combination inhibited 60-70% of proliferation.

To assess and control for the efficacy of anti-TAC in blocking IL 2-dependent responses, we wished to create a population of T cells which had not yet entered the cell proliferation cycle but which had the ability to proliferate in response to IL 2. We accomplished this by culturing highly purified small T cells for 24 hours in medium supplemented with Con A at 2.0 µg/ml. Next these cells were washed and stimulated with either IL 2 (10 U/ml) or high-dose Con A (20 µg/ml). In the absence of anti-TAC, IL 2 and Con A stimulated an equivalent amount of thymidine incorporation. However, while anti-TAC blocked approximately 80% of the IL 2-induced proliferation, the same concentration blocked less than 20% of the Con A-induced proliferation.

In the following experiments, the effectiveness of cyclosporine A in blocking IL 2 production was assessed. Allogeneic B cells were used as the stimulus and T-enriched cells were used as responders. IL 2 levels in the supernatant fluids were measured after removal of cyclosporine A and concentration of IL 2 as described under methods. At 0.2 µg/ml, cyclosporine A resulted in a decrease in peak IL 2 content of the supernatant fluids from 31 U/ml to

0.25 U/ml; 2.0 µg/ml of cyclosporine A resulted in there being no detectable IL 2 (<0.1 U/ml) in the supernatant fluids. Nevertheless approximately 40% of the proliferative response persisted despite the presence of cyclosporine A at either concentration.

Cyclosporine-resistant, IL 2-independent proliferation may be more relevant in the initiation of a T cell response than later in the response. To test this hypothesis, the degree of cyclosporine-resistant proliferation was compared for freshly isolated T-enriched cells vs. a T cell line specific for HLA-DR2 alloantigen. The stimulus for both types of responders was allogeneic, HLA-DR2 positive B cells. Whereas the proliferative response of the T cell line was completely abrogated by cyclosporine A at 2.0 µg/ml, the response of the freshly isolated cells was inhibited by only approximately 70%.

DISCUSSION

In this study we examined the proliferation of activated, nontransformed T cells to determine whether an IL 2-independent component exists. Using anti-TAC, a monoclonal antibody to the IL 2 receptor, to block the interaction of IL 2 with its receptor, we found that the lectin-induced proliferation of T lymphocytes was relatively resistant to anti-TAC compared with the IL 2-induced proliferation of identically prepared cells. Using cyclosporine A to block IL 2 production, we found that 30 to 40% of the alloantigen-induced proliferation of freshly activated T cells persisted in the absence of detectable IL 2 production. By contrast, the alloantigen-induced proliferation of an allospecific T cell line was entirely blocked by cyclosporine A. These findings suggest that both IL 2-dependent and IL 2-independent proliferation of T cells occur and that perhaps the IL 2-independent mechanisms are more important during the initiation of a T cell response than in the ongoing proliferation of activated T cells.

To prove the existence of an IL 2-independent component of the proliferation of activated T cells is technically complicated by the fact that these T cell populations also undergo IL 2-dependent proliferation. Anti-TAC was effective in blocking the IL 2-induced proliferation of pre-activated T cells. However, the relative resistance to anti-TAC of the lectin-induced proliferation by the same cells may have resulted from increased expression of IL 2 receptors, greater IL 2 concentration at the cell surface (although IL 2 was not detected in the supernatant fluids), and/or greater responsiveness of the cells to IL 2 rather than from IL 2-independent proliferation. Also, we cannot excude the possibility that the cyclosporine-resistant proliferation resulted from small amounts of IL 2 secreted at the cell surface and bound to IL 2 receptors without achieving detectable levels in the supernatant fluids. Nevertheless we believe our findings strongly suggest the presence of IL 2-independent proliferation and warrant further investigation into this phenomenon.

A number of investigators have addressed the possibility of IL 2-independent T cell proliferation. Lugo et al. (1985) demonstrated that a significant portion of spontaneously proliferating murine thymocytes lack IL 2 receptors; however, they speculated that the antigen-induced proliferation of mature T cells is entirely IL 2-dependent. Malek et al. (1984) reported that PHA and IL 1-induced proliferation of murine thymocytes was only poorly inhibited by antibody to the IL 2 receptor early during culture (days 2 and 3) despite low IL 2 receptor density and no significant IL 2 in the supernatant fluids thus suggesting some IL 2-independent proliferation. Koretzky et al. (1983) reported that human T cell proliferation induced by the calcium ionophore, A23187, was not inhibited by anti-TAC thus suggesting a mechanism by which an IL 2-independent proliferative signal might act. Several investigators have observed the partial blocking of the mitogen-induced proliferation of mature T cells by antibody to IL 2 on the IL 2 receptor and have speculated with varying emphasis on the roles of IL 2-independent proliferation versus incomplete blocking of IL 2-dependent proliferation (Gillis et al., 1981; Depper et al., 1983; Koretzky et al., 1983; Malek et al., 1984; Bettens et al., 1984). Our data lend additional weight to the arguments for IL 2-independent proliferation.

IL 2-independent proliferation of T cells may occur in a population of cells distinct from those which proliferate in response to IL 2 or it may exist as an alternative mechanism of proliferation in the same cells. It may occur only for a limited period after cell activation or there may exist conditions which promote long-term IL 2-independent proliferation of nontransformed T cells. However, whichever of these proposed types of IL 2-independent proliferation of T cells may occur, its identification and study is likely to be important in understanding and ultimately manipulating the regulation of human immune responses.

REFERENCES

Bettens F, Kristensen F, Walker C, Schwulera U, Bonnard GD, DeWeck AL (1984). Lymphokine regulation of activated (G_1) lymphocytes. II. Glucocorticoid and anti-TAC-induced inhibition of human T lymphocyte proliferation. J Immunol 132:261-265.

Depper JM, Leonard WJ, Robb RJ, Waldmann TA, Greene WC (1983). Blockade of the interleukin-2 receptor by anti-TAC antibody: inhibition of human lymphocyte activation. J Immunol 131:690-696.

Elliott JF, Lin Y, Mizel SB, Bleackley RC, Harnish DG, Paetkau V (1984). Induction of interleukin 2 messenger RNA inhibited by cyclosporine A. Science 226:1439-1441.

Gillis S, Ferm MM, Ou W, Smith KA (1978). T cell growth factor: parameters of production and a quantitative microassay for activity. J Immunol 120:2027-2032.

Gillis S, Gillis AE, Henney CS (1981). Monoclonal antibody directed against interleukin 2. I. Inhibition of T lymphocyte mitogenesis and the in vitro differentiation of alloreactive cytolytic T cells. J Exp Med 154:983-988.

Koretzky GA, Daniele RP, Greene WC, Nowell PC (1983). Evidence for an interleukin-independent pathway for human lymphocyte activation. Proc Natl Acad Sci USA 80:3444-3447.

Lugo JP, Krishnan SN, Sailor RD, Koen P, Malek T, Rothenberg E (1985). Proliferation of thymic stem cells with and without receptors for interleukin 2: implications for intrathymic antigen recognition. J Exp Med 161:1048-1062.

Malek TR, Ortega R. G, Jakway JP, Chan C, Shevach EM (1984). The murine IL 2 receptor. II. Monoclonal anti-IL 2 receptor antibodies as specific inhibitors of T cell function in vitro. J Immunol 133:1976-1982.

Siegel JP, Djeu JY, Stocks NI, Masur H, Gelmann EP, Quinnan GV (1985). Sera from patients with the acquired immunodeficiency syndrome inhibit production of interleukin-2 by normal lymphocytes. J Clin Invest 75:1957-1964.

INTERLEUKIN 2 IS A GROWTH FACTOR FOR B LYMPHOCYTES

John W. Lowenthal, Rudolf H. Zubler, Noboru Hashimoto, Markus Nabholz and H. Robson MacDonald

Ludwig Institute for Cancer Research, Lausanne Branch (J.W.L., H.R.M.) and Swiss Institute for Experimental Cancer Research (R.H.Z., N.H., M.N.), 1066 Epalinges, Switzerland.
Present address for R.H.Z. and N.H. is Division of Hematology, Department of Medicine, Hôpital Cantonal Universitaire, CH-1211 Geneva, Switzerland.

INTRODUCTION

The polypeptide hormone Interleukin 2 (IL2) plays a critical regulatory role in the induction and maintenance of the immune response. It has been shown that the growth promoting activity of IL2 is mediated through specific receptors which are expressed on the surface of activated T lymphocytes (Robb et al., 1981). Resting lymphocytes do not express receptors for, and hence do not respond to IL2, but upon stimulation with antigen or mitogen, large numbers of receptors are expressed within 24 h (Smith, 1984 ; Lowenthal et al., 1985a). Interaction of IL2 with its receptor induces the progression of resting cells into the cell cycle, resulting in several rounds of cell division. We have recently shown that IL2 can support the growth of appropriately activated murine B cells, as well as their differentiation into antibody secreting cells (Zubler et al., 1984), thereby dispelling the original notion that IL2 can act only on T cells. We show here that B cells stimulated with Lippopolysaccharide (LPS) and anti-immunoglobulin antibodies (anti-Ig) express both high and low affinity IL2 receptors, and this expression is quantitatively similar to that which we (Lowenthal et al., 1985b) and others (Robb et al., 1984) have previously reported for a variety of T cell types.

RESULTS

We have previously shown that purified murine B cells stimulated with LPS and anti-Ig respond to pure IL2 by undergoing proliferation and differentiation into antibody secreting cells (Zubler et al., 1984). B cells stimulated in this manner become homogeneously positive for IL2-receptor expression within 3 days, as measured by staining with a monoclonal anti-murine IL2 receptor antibody, PC61 (Fig. 1A). Resting B cells or cells stimulated with LPS alone or anti-Ig alone are negative for IL2 receptor expression and are consequently unable to respond to IL2.

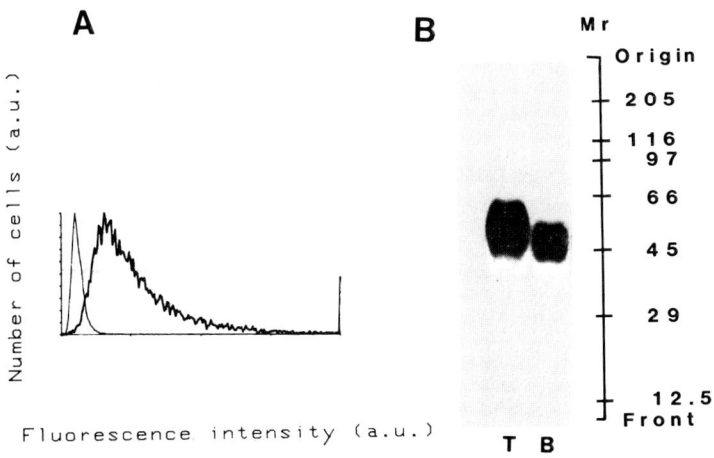

Figure 1. A. Most activated B cells express IL2 receptors. B cells were stimulated with LPS and anti-Ig and grown for 3 days in the presence of IL2. Cells were stained with directly biotinylated-PC61 and analyzed on the FACS (Lowenthal et al. 1985b).

B. PC61 immunoprecipitates IL2 receptors of similar molecular weight from activated B and T cells. PC61 immunoprecipitates were obtained from surface-labelled lysates of LPS and anti-Ig activated B cells and Con A activated T cells and were analyzed by SDS-PAGE under reducing conditions.

IL2-dependent proliferation of B-blasts can be completely inhibited in the presence of PC61. We have shown elsewhere that the amount of PC61 required to inhibit B cell proliferation was the same as that needed to block proliferation of the IL2-dependent T cell clone CTLL (Lowenthal et al., 1985b). Furthermore, PC61 immunoprecipitates IL2 receptors of similar molecular weight from activated B and T cells (Fig. 1B).

Using computer Scatchard plot analysis of equilibrium IL2 binding data we show that B cells, like T cells, can be induced to express two classes of IL2 receptor (Fig. 2). A minority of the receptors (approximately 2000 per cell) are of a high affinity class (dissociation constant, K_d of 20 pM) and the remaining 90% of receptors have around a 100-fold lower affinity for IL2.

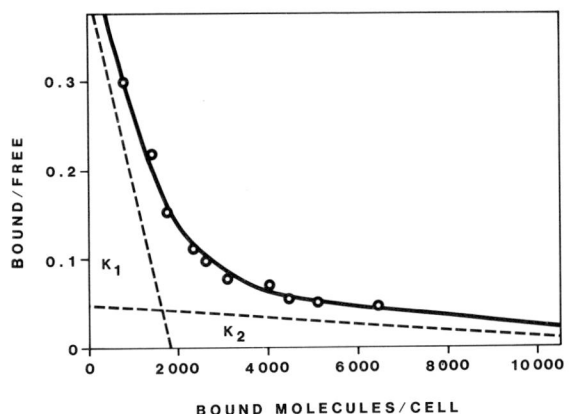

Figure 2. B cells activated with LPS and anti-Ig express both high and low affinity IL2 receptors. B cells were incubated at 4°C in the presence of various amounts of radiolabelled IL2 for 60 min. Cells were then spun through an oil gradient and the bound and free cpm was determined by scintillation counting. Computer-generated binding componants of the high (K1) and low (K2) affinity IL2 receptors after correction for non specific binding is shown. Similar results have been obtained with Con A activated T cells (Lowenthal et al., 1985b).

We have previously shown that he binding of IL2 to both classes of receptor is completely inhibited in the presence of PC61 (Lowenthal et al., 1985b). The finding that high and low affinity IL2 receptors have at least one determinant (PC61) in common suggests that both classes of receptor have a similar molecular structure. In terms of receptor number and affinity, the expression of IL2 receptors by B and T cells are strikingly similar (see Table 1). This dissociation of high from low affinity receptors has been reported for a variety of other types of polypeptide hormones and growth factors, and may reflect a highly conserved mode of hormone-receptor interaction. Activated B cells, like activated T cells, show a transient expression of high and low affinity IL2-R. Table 1 shows that maximum receptor expression occured on day 3, and declined 3-5 fold by day 7. Cell proliferation ceases in both of these populations by day 10-12 despite the addition of IL2.

TABLE 1. Expression of high and low affinity IL2 receptors on activated B and T lymphocytes.

	Cell type	IL2 receptors/cell		$Kd\ (pM)^a$	
		high affinity	low affinity	high affinity	low affinity
day 3	B-Blasts	1900	17,000	25	1280
day 7	B-Blasts	375	5800	27	2150
day 3	T-Blasts	3300	36,500	21	1440
day 7	T-Blasts	1050	13,500	21	1830

[a] dissociation constant.

Equilibrium binding of radiolabelled IL2 to activated-B cells (LPS plus anti-Ig) and -T cells (Con A) was carried out as described (Lowenthal et al. 1985b). The number of high and low affinity IL2 receptors and dissociation constants were calculated by computer Scatchard plot analysis. Cells were harvested on day 3 and day 7 and the number of IL2-receptors was measured. Mean values from 2-4 experiments are shown.

The biological function of the low affinity IL2 receptor is not known. It is apparent that they are not involved in the growth-promoting activity of IL2 because IL2-dependent B and T cells proliferate in vitro in the presence of low concentrations of IL2, sufficient to cause occupancy of only the high affinity receptors.

CONCLUSION

By several independent criteria, the IL2 receptors expressed by LPS-anti-Ig activated B cells and activated T cells are similar. Quantitative IL2 binding revealed that B blasts, like a variety of independently-derived types of activated T cells, express two classes of IL2 binding sites; one has a high affinity for IL2 and the other a 50-100-fold lower affinity. Binding to both classes can be inhibited by the same monoclonal anti-IL2 receptor antibody. The ratio of the number of low to high affinity sites per cell for B blasts is within the range found for activated T cells. In addition, studies using PC61 antibody show that 1) 95% of activated B and T cells express IL2 receptors, 2) IL2 dependent proliferation of both cell types is inhibited at similar concentrations of PC61 antibody and 3) similar molecular weight bands are immunoprecipitated from activated T and B cells with PC61. The finding that activated B cells respond to IL2 by undergoing proliferation and differentiation and that the expression of IL2 receptors is essentially the same as that found on activated T cells suggests that IL2 may have an even more extensive role in the regulation of the immune response than originally thought. On the basis of these results, we propose that IL2 may be a universal growth factor for cells of both the T and B lymphocyte lineage.

REFERENCES

Lowenthal JW, Tougne C, MacDonald HR, Smith KA, Nabholz M (1985a). Antigenic stimulation regulates the expression of IL2 receptors in a cytolytic T cell clone. J Immunol 134:931-939.

Lowenthal JW, Zubler RH, Nabholz M, MacDonald HR (1985b). Similarities between interleukin 2 receptor number and affinity on activated B and T lymphocytes. Nature 315: 669-672.

Robb RJ, Munck A, Smith KA (1981). T cell growth factor receptors. Quantitation, specificity and biological relevance. J Exp Med 154:1455-1464.

Robb RJ, Greene WC, Rusk CM (1984). Low and high affinity cellular receptors for interleukin 2. Implications for the level of Tac antigen. J Exp Med 160:1126-1146.

Smith KA (1984). T cell growth factor. A. Rev. Immunol. 2:319-333.

Zubler RH, Lowenthal JW, Erard F, Hashimoto N, Devos R, MacDonald HR (1984). Activated B cells express receptors for, and proliferate in response to pure interleukin 2. J Exp Med 160:1170-1183.

R.H.Z. and M.N. were supported by funds of the Swiss National Science Foundation.

INTERLEUKIN 1 (IL 1) AS A POSSIBLE AUTOCRINE SIGNAL: EXISTENCE OF SPECIFIC IL 1 RECEPTORS ON HUMAN EPSTEIN BARR VIRUS TRANSFORMED B LYMPHOCYTES

Kouji Matsushima

Laboratory of Molecular Immunoregulation,
Biological Response Modifiers Program, DCT,
NCI, Frederick, MD 21701

INTRODUCTION

We have previously reported that various kinds of human B lymphocytes produce low levels of IL 1-like thymocyte comitogenic and fibroblast proliferation activities (Matsushima et al., 1985 a, b, c). Moreover, there are several reports concerning the augmenting effects of IL 1 on the proliferation and differentiation of B lymphocytes (Howard, 1983, Lipsky et al., 1983). It is particularly relevant to establish IL 1 as an autocrine signal in human B lymphocyte proliferation, especially since the constitutive production of IL 1 by Epstein-Barr virus (EBV)-transformed B (EBV-B) lymphocytes may contribute to the immortalization of EBV-B lymphocytes. Therefore, we examined EBV-B cell lines the existence of specific IL 1 receptors and the effects of IL 1 on the proliferation of EBV-B lines.

RESULTS

Properties of IL 1 Produced by EBV-B Cell Lines:

Every human EBV-B lines so far tested has constitutively produced varying levels of IL 1 activities as described (Matsushima et al., 1985a). The m.w. of the IL 1 derived from one of the EBV-B lines (FMO) was 25 kd and the pI was 5.5, which differs from the properties of human monocyte derived IL 1 (Matsushima et al., 1985b). To ascertain whether there is immunological cross-reactivity between human monocyte-derived IL 1 and EBV-B derived IL 1, the effects of anti-IL 1 antibody (Kelley et al., 1984) were studied. This antibody was prepared by immunizing a rabbit with both partially purified human monocyte derived pI 5 and pI 7 IL 1. The effects of this antibody were tested on murine thymocytes cultured with pure pI 5, or pure pI 7, human IL 1 derived from a myelomonocytic (THP-1) cell line (Matsushima, manuscript in preparation), partially purified FMO-derived IL 1 or partially purified VDS-O-derived IL 1. As shown in Table 1, the thymocyte comitogenic activity of both THP-1-derived IL 1s and VDSO-derived IL 1 was completely neutralized by anti-IL 1, but FMO-derived IL 1 was only partially neutralized, suggesting that VDS-O-derived IL 1 is immunologically similar to monocyte-derived IL 1, whereas FMO-derived IL 1 is antigenically distinct.

TABLE 1. Immunological Cross Reactivity Among Different IL 1s*

Source of IL 1		Normal IgG (Δ cpm)	Anti-IL 1 (Δ cpm)	% Inhibition
THP-1	pI 7.0, 17 kd	31,000	100	99
THP-1	pI 4.9, 17 kd	12,000	150	100
VDS-O	pI 5, 20 kd	38,000	400	99
FMO	pI 5.5, 25 kd	27,000	6,100	77

*C3H/HeJ murine thymocytes at 1.5×10^6 cells/well were cultured with about 3 U/ml IL 1 in the presence of 5 ug/well normal rabbit IgG or anti-IL 1 for 3 days. For the final 16 hr, thymocyte cultures were pulsed with 0.5 uCi ^{3}H-TdR.

Exsistence of Specific IL 1 Receptors on EBV-B Lines:

Pure human monocyte derived IL 1 (17 kd, pI 7) (Matsushima et al., 1985d) was labelled with ^{125}I by the Bolton Hunter method without an apparent loss of biological activity (~4×10^7 U/mg on thymocyte comitogenic assay). Eight human EBV-B lines examined bound ^{125}I-IL 1 to various degrees. One of the eight lines, a pre-B type line (VDS-O) (Tosato, 1985), which bound the highest amount of ^{125}I-IL 1, was studied further. The binding of ^{125}I-IL to this line was specifically inhibited by both unlabelled pure human monocyte-derived pI 7, 17 kd IL 1 and partially purified monocyte-derived pI 5, 17 kd IL 1 with the same efficency, but recombinant α-IFN failed to inhibit the binding of ^{125}I-IL 1. Maximal binding of ^{125}I-IL 1 occurred within 20 min at 4°C. Scatchard plot analyses revealed that the receptor number ranged from 100-200/cell with a Kd (dissociation constant) of 2.4-5.0 x 10^{-10}M.

Effect of unlabelled pI 7.0-IL 1, pI 5.0-IL 1 and α-IFN, on the binding of ^{125}I-IL 1 (pI 7.0) to EBV-B cells.

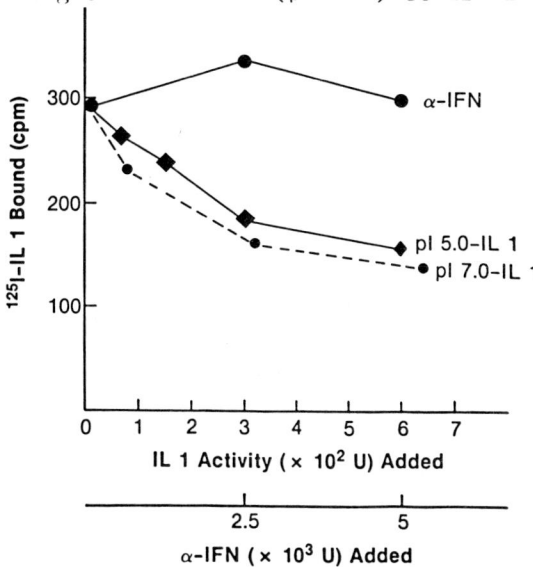

Figure 1. Binding of ^{125}I-IL 1 (2 ng = 20,000 cpm) in the presence of various doses of recombinant human α-IFN, partially purified pI 5.0 human IL 1 or purified pI 7.0 human IL 1 to 2 x 10^7 VDS-O cells in 1 ml at 4°C for 30 min.

Effects of IL 1 on the Proliferation of VDS-O-Cells:

As shown in Figure 2, both purified monocyte-derived (pI 7, 17 kd) IL 1 and partially purified VDS-O cell-derived IL 1 increased the ^{3}H-TdR uptake by VDS-O cells in a dose dependent fashion. About 0.5 U/ml of IL 1 resulted in 50% of the maximal proliferative response of VDS-O cells to IL 1. We could not detect any effect of IL 1 on immunoglobulin production by VDS-O cells.

Effects of IL 1 on the Proliferation of VDS-0 Cells.

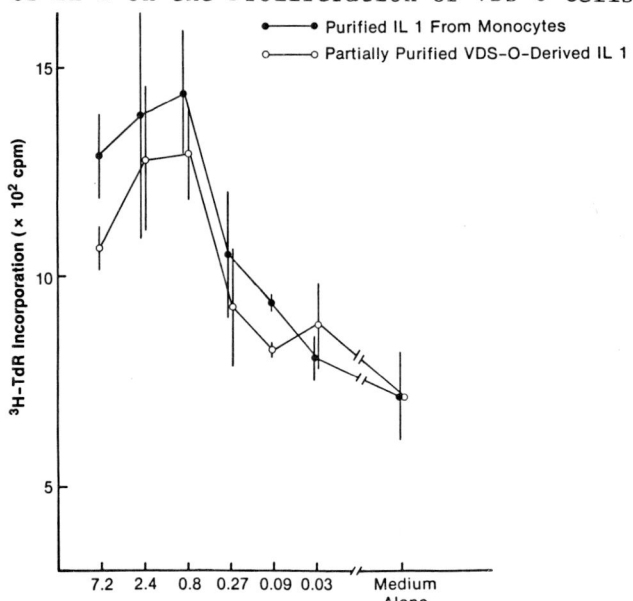

Figure 2.   2.5 X 10^3 cells/0.2 ml RPMI 1640, 0.5% Ultroser (synthetic serum, LKB) were cultured for 5 days. For the final 24 hr 0.5 μCi ^{3}H-TdR was added.

DISCUSSIONS AND CONCLUSIONS

We recently succeeded in purifying both pI 7, 17 kd and pI 5, 17 kd IL 1 to homogeneity from human myelomonocytic THP-1 cells (Matsushima et al., manuscript in preparation), confirming the existence of at least two forms of human IL 1 (March et al., 1985). Furthermore, as described in this paper, EBV-B cell line FMO-derived IL 1 is immunologically distinct from either monocyte-derived pI 5 or 7 IL 1. Therefore it is crucial to use completely purified FMO and VDS-0 derived-IL 1 to establish whether or not these EBV-B cell derived IL 1 compete for the same receptors on B lymphocytes. Although the receptor number on B cell lines is low, similar observation has been reported (Dower et al., 1985). We cannot exclude the possibility that the IL 1 receptor on B cells are already occupied by the autologously produced IL 1. However, perhaps only a few functional receptors are needed to trigger cell responses, since IL 1 at 10^{-12}M stimulated 50% of the response of B cells.

In conclusion, the production of IL 1 like activities by EBV-B lines (Matsushima 1985a), the exsistence of specific IL 1 receptors and the proliferative response of an EBV-B cell line to IL 1, suggest that IL 1 maybe an autocrine signal contributing to the immortalization of EBV-B lymphocytes. This hypothesis requires further evaluation by testing the effects of inhibitors of IL 1 on the growth of EBV-B cells.

ACKNOWLEDGEMENTS

I gratefully acknowledge Ms. M. M. Kelley (Du Pont Co.,) for providing anti-human IL 1 serum; Dr. G. Tosato for providing EBV-B lines; Drs. T. Kasahara, C. Faltynek and J. J. Oppenheim for reviewing this manuscript; and Ms. Louise Shaw for preparing this manuscript.

REFERENCES

Matsushima K, Kuang Y-D, Tosato G, Hopkins SJ, Oppenheim, JJ (1985a). B cell-derived interleukin 1 (IL 1)-like factor. (1) Relationship of production of IL 1-like factor to accessory function of Epstein Barr virus-transformed B-lymphoblast lines. Cell Immunol, 94:406-417.

Matsushima K, Tosato G, Benjamin D, Oppenheim JJ (1985b). B cell-derived interleukin 1 (IL 1)-like factor. (2) Sources, effects, and biochemical properties. Cell Immunol, 94:418-426.

Matsushima K, Procopio A, Abe H, Ortaldo JR, Oppenheim JJ (1985c). Production of interleukin 1 activity by normal human peripheral blood B lymphocytes. J Immunol 135: 1132-1136.

Howard M, Mizel SB, Lachman L, Ansel J, Johnson B, Paul WE (1983). Role of interleukin 1 in anti-immunoglobulin induced B cell proliferation. J Exp Med 157:1529-1563.

Lipsky PE, Thompson PA, Rosenwasser LJ, Dinarello C (1983). The role of interleukin 1 in human B cell activation: Inhibition of B cell proliferation and the generation of immunoglobulin secretory cells by antibody against human leukocyte pryogen. J Immunol 130:2708-2716.

Kelly MM, Rosenmiller ME, Dauleno AJ, Newton RC (1984). Development of an antibody specific for human interleukin 1. Lymphokine Res 3:251 (Abst).

Matsushima K, Durum SK, Kimball ES, Oppenheim JJ (1985d). Purification of human interleukin 1 from human monocyte culture supernatants and identity of thymocyte comitogenic factor, fibroblast proliferation factor, acute phase protein inducing factor, and endogenous pyrogen. Cell Immunol 92:290-301.

Tasato G, Marei G, Heidman CA, Wane F, Pike SE, Siminovitch K. (1985). Epstein-Barr virus immortalization of normal B cell precursors with ineffectively rearranged Ig genes. Fed. Proc. Abst. 3325.

March CJ, Mosley B, Larsen A, Cerretti P, Braedt G, Price V, Gillis S, Henney CS, Kronheim SR, Grabstein K, Conlon PJ, Honn TP, Cosman D (1985). Cloning sequence and expression of two distinct human interleukin-1 complementary DNAs. Nature 315:641-647.

Section III. Growth Regulation in Normal and Abnormal Leukocytes

SODIUM ION INFLUX: AN ESSENTIAL EARLY SIGNAL IN LYMPHOCYTE PROLIFERATION

A. Severini, K.V.S. Prasad, W.L. Greer and J.G. Kaplan

Department of Biochemistry, University of Alberta, Edmonton, Canada

INTRODUCTION

An early and indispensable event in the proliferative activation of lymphocytes is a rapid increase in the rate of uphill monovalent cation transport (Kaplan, 1978) through the Na^+K^+-ATPase. Two hypotheses have been advanced to account for the phenomenon. According to the first, mitogen effects an increase in cation pump sites by a mechanism not involving protein synthesis (Quastel and Kaplan, 1975). According to the second, mitogenic stimulation provokes an increase in concentration of intracellular Na^+, $[Na^+]_i$, which causes increase in their number (Segel et al., 1979); indeed, it is known that the Na^+K^+-ATPase has a third power dependence on $[Na^+]_i$ (Glynn and Karlish, 1975).

We now show that both of these hypotheses are correct. In pig lymphocytes, the rapid increase in cation pumping following treatment with mitogen is shown to be due to a rise in $[Na^+]_i$ that occurs within a few minutes of activation - in fact, as soon as it can be measured. Some hours later an increase in number of pump sites occurs, even in presence of inhibitors of protein synthesis. Finally, we show that the increase in $[Na^+]_i$ is a sufficient signal to the nucleus to cause the repair of some 3000 DNA strand breaks, known to be an early and essential event in iymphocyte proliferation (Johnstone and Williams, 1982; Greer and Kaplan, 1984). It is likely that this signal to the nucleus is mediated through a rise in cell NAD^+ level.

MATERIALS AND METHODS

Pig lymphocytes were isolated from peripheral blood and cultured essentially as described by Kay et al. (1975). K^+ uptake was measured by incubating the cells for 1 and 5 min at 37°C, in the presence of 5 µCi/ml ^{86}RbCl and 5 mM of K^+; the uptake was terminated by spinning 100 µl aliquots through a silicon oil mixture; the pellet was counted in a β-counter. Na^+ uptake was measured using 5 µCi/ml of ^{22}NaCl as tracer in the presence of 120 mM Na^+; the procedure was similar to that used for K^+ influx, but 80 µl of isotonic sucrose-buffer were placed at the bottom of the microfuge tube in order to dilute the extracellular space. $[Na^+]_i$ was measured by emission flame photometry, in samples processed as described for Na^+ uptake. Intracellular water volume (Kletzein et al., 1975) was 0.037 µl/10^6 cells. Kinetics of ^{3}H-ouabain binding was measured by incubating the cells for 6 hours at 37°C, in the presence of a range of ouabain concentrations from 0.056 µM to 1.6 µM; non-specific binding of ouabain was determined at 4°C. Total number of ^{3}H-ouabain-binding sites was determined by incubating the cells for 20 min at 37°C, in the presence of 2.4 µM ouabain; incubation was carried out in K^+-free buffer. Na^+K^+-ATPase activity was measured as described (Charnock et al., 1977) in cells permeabilized by hypotonic shock.

Mouse splenocytes were isolated and cultured and DNA strand breaks and NAD^+ determined as described by Greer and Kaplan (1984), Nisselbaum and Green (1969) and Kroger and Grahn (1983).

RESULTS AND DISCUSSION

Active K^+ influx increased by 237 ± 89% (average ± SD of 4 experiments) after stimulation of pig lymphocytes with optimal mitogenic concentration of Con A (50 µg/ml).
Fig. 1 shows a typical experiment in which K^+ influx increased within 10 min of mitogen addition without significant early change in number of ouabain binding sites, as measured by rapid saturation binding of 2.4 µM ^{3}H-ouabain. However, an increase in ouabain binding took place after 2 hours of activation. The average increase after 5 h of incubation with Con A was 75 ± 45% (average ± SD of 8 experiments). Comparison between the time course of increase in K^+ uptake and ouabain binding sites indicated that the two

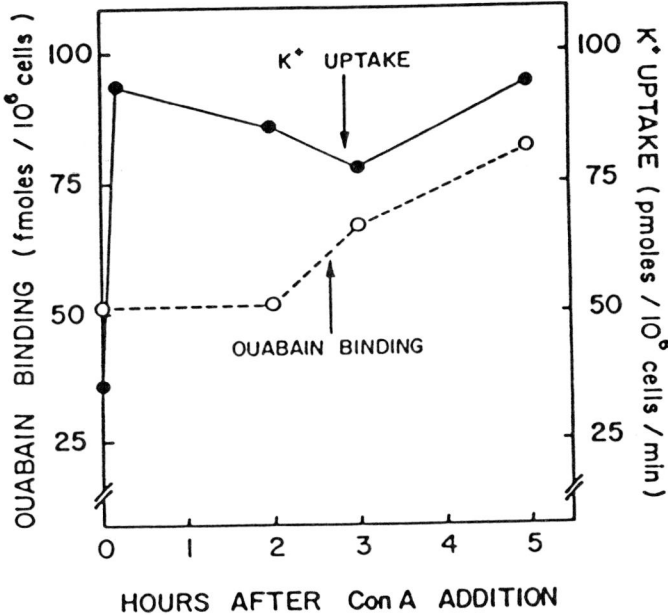

Figure 1. Time course of effects of Con A.

events are independent and that two distinct mechanisms are involved. In the early stages, the increase of K^+ influx was accompanied by a simultaneous increase in Na^+ influx and $[Na^+]_i$ as shown in Table 1. The activation of Na^+ influx was due mostly to the Na^+/H^+ antiport as shown by the effect of 1 mM amiloride during the 5 min of measurement. Moreover, treatment with 500 μM amiloride during the incubation with Con A also prevented the increase in $[Na^+]_i$. Incubation in low Na^+ medium totally prevented the Con A induced increase in $[Na^+]$.

In order to establish whether the increase in $[Na^+]_i$ was responsible for the activation of Na^+K^+-ATPase-mediated K^+ influx after Con A stimulation, we measured the effect of inhibition of the rise in $[Na^+]_i$ on K^+ influx by treatment with amiloride or incubation in low-Na^+ medium; both prevented the increase in K^+ influx. On the other hand, increase in $[Na^+]_i$, obtained by incubation in the presence of the Na^+ ionophore monensin (30 μM), activated the Na^+K^+-ATPase-mediated K^+ influx. Table 1 shows that the early

TABLE 1. Na^+ uptake, $[Na^+]c$ and K^+ influx in resting and activated pig lymphocytes

Culture conditions	A	B	[Na]c mM	C
-Con A	59.1±10.2	21.1	17.6±3.8	26.1± 5.0
+Con A	84.8± 6.5	46.7	37.8±5.2	56.9±15.2
+Con A + 100 µM amiloride	58.1±10.1	2.3	15.6±1.5	31.2±15.8
+Con A in low Na^+ medium	-	-	19.5±3.1	16.9± 3.3
-Con A + 20 µM monensin	-	-	123.6±5.7	153.2± 1.6

A: Total Na^+ uptake (pmoles/10^6 cells/min).
B: Amiloride inhibitable Na^+ uptake (pmoles/10^6 cells/min).
C: Ouabain inhibitable K^+ uptake (pmoles/10^6 cells/min).

Cells were incubated for 20 minutes in the condition indicated. Amiloride-inhibitable Na^+ uptake and ouabain-inhibitable K^+ uptake represent the difference between the uptakes measured in the presence and in the absence of 1 mM amiloride or 2 mM of ouabain, respectively.

activation of Na^+K^+-ATPase-mediated K^+ influx is caused by the increase in $[Na^+]_i$, which, in turn, is caused by the activation of an amiloride-sensitive Na^+ influx. On the other hand, the late increase in number of ouabain-binding sites was not affected by inhibition of $[Na^+]_i$ increase in 5 h stimulated cells; monensin-induced rise in $[Na^+]_i$ for 5 h in resting cells did not cause a change in number of these sites (Severini et al.).

Kinetics of ouabain binding in resting and 5 h activated pig lymphocytes, showed an increase in V_{max}, without change in affinity for ouabain (Severini et al., in preparation), as already reported for human lymphocytes (Quastel and Kaplan, 1975; Averdunk and Lauf, 1975). This and other data rule out the possibility that the increase in ouabain binding was due to change in affinity for ouabain of Na^+K^+-ATPase or to an increase in non-specific uptake of ouabain.

Na^+K^+-ATPase activity in permeabilized cells, measured in the presence of optimal concentrations of Mg^{++}, Na^+, K^+ and ATP, was increased after 5 h of incubation of the intact cells with Con A (Table 2). We also measured optimal K^+ influx in the presence of 20 µM monensin which increased $[Na^+]_i$ in both resting and activated cells. As shown in Table 2, the increase in ouabain-binding sites appears to be proportional to both the increase in Na^+K^+-ATPase activity in permeabilized cells and the increase of K^+ influx, measured under condition of optimal $[Na^+]_i$. Taken together,

TABLE 2. Ouabain-binding sites, Na^+,K^+-ATPase activity in permeabilized cells and optimal K^+ uptake in resting and activated pig lymphocytes

	A	B	C
-Con A	65.7 (39.8×10^3)	19.6	156.5
+Con A	93.7 (56.8×10^3)	27.7	200.9
% increase	46.6%	41.3%	45.5%

A: Ouabain binding (fmoles/10^6 cells).
B: Na^+,K^+-ATPase activity (nmoles Pi/10^6 cells/h).
C: Ouabain inhibitable K^+ uptake (pmoles/10^6 cells/min).

Cells were incubated in the presence and in the absence of Con A for 5 hours. K^+ influx was measured after incubation for 10 min in the presence of 20 μM monensin, in order to increase [Na]c up to 120 mM, in both resting and activated cells.

The number of ouabain-binding sites per cell is indicated in brackets.

these results indicate that the increase in ouabain-binding observed after 5 h of activation in the presence of Con A reflects an increase in the number of active Na^+K^+-ATPase molecules. We have strong, indirect evidence that indicates that the rise in pump sites is essential to subsequent events of the proliferative cycle (Severini et al., in preparation). It is interesting that, like the rapid increase in Na^+K^+-ATPase (Kaplan, 1978), the mitogen-induced increase in pump sites occurred in the presence of anisomycin and other inhibitors of protein synthesis (Severini et al., in preparation); indeed inhibition of protein synthesis was itself sufficient to induce an increase in cation pump sites, even in absence of mitogen. We speculate that proliferation causes arrest in the synthesis of an unstable protein that either blocks the external ouabain site of the Na^+K^+-ATPase or that prevents the incorporation of the latter into the plasma membrane.

Another early essential requirement in the cascade of events leading to mitogenic activation of lymphocytes is repair of DNA strand breaks. Johnstone and Williams (1982) showed in human peripheral blood and we found using mouse spleen (Greer and Kaplan, 1984) and pig peripheral blood (Greer and Kaplan, 1985) that resting lymphocytes contained a large number of DNA strand breaks which must be repaired through a system that requires ADP ribosylation before blast transformation and DNA synthesis can occur. The cellular level of NAD^+, the substrate for ADP ribose polymerase, was limiting in resting lymphocytes for ADP ribosylation and thus for repair of the endogenous strand breaks (Greer and Kaplan, 1984). There was a 2-fold increase in NAD^+ level within 45 min of Con A stimulation and repair was induced with nicotinamide in the growth medium in the absence of Con A. Table 3 indicates that the increase in NAD^+ level, and the consequent increase in strand break repair after mitogenic stimulation of mouse lymphocytes were triggered by elevated levels of Na^+. Soon after Con A stimulation there was a 2-fold increase in the cellular concentration of Na^+. This correlates with a transient 2-fold increase in NAD^+ level, and a decrease in the number of DNA strand breaks. The same observations were made if Na^+ levels were increased by incubation with monensin or with ouabain. However, if the cells were incubated with Con A in low Na^+ medium, the increase in cellular NAD^+ did not occur; neither did strand break repair. The increase in NAD^+ and repair could not be induced by monensin in low Na^+ medium.

TABLE 3. Effect of Na^+ on cellular levels of NAD^+ and repair of DNA strand breaks

Treatment	$[Na^+]c$ (mM) at 2 h	NAD^+ (μM)	#DNA strand breaks repaired/genome at 2 h
Resting	19.1±1.6	.040±0.1	-
Con A	31.4±2.9	.096±0.2	3136±262
Monensin	104.8±8.4	.072±0.1	4291±1940
Ouabain	43.4±5.7	.076±0.2	4269±1256
Low Na^+	5.0	.032	-
Low Na^+ + Con A	5.0	.031	645±596
Low Na^+ + Monensin	24.0	.045	1400±736

The rise in NAD^+ levels was transient (at 40-60 min with Con A; 120 min with monensin; 30 min with ouabain). Low Na^+ medium contained 9 mM Na^+, compared to 120 mM in control.

We conclude that increase in both Na^+ influx and $[Na^+]_i$ is an essential early signal in proliferation. This signal is sufficient to cause activation of pre-existing Na^+K^+-ATPase sites and repair of DNA strand breaks; both events are necessary if the subsequent events of proliferation are to occur. However, the increase in influx is not involved in or necessary for the rise in cation pump sites that occurs at 3-5 h of mitogenic activation.

REFERENCES

Averdunk R, Lauf PK (1975). Effects of mitogens on sodium-potassium transport, ^{3}H-ouabain binding, and adenosine triphosphatase activity in lymphocytes. Exp Cell Res 93: 331-342.
Charnock JS, Simonson LP, Almeida AF (1977). Variation in sensitivity of the cardiac glycoside receptor characteristics of Na,K-ATPase to lipolysis and temperature. Biochim Biophys Acta 465:77-92.
Glynn IM, Karlish SSD (1975). The sodium pump. Ann Rev Physiol 37:13-55.
Greer WL, Kaplan JG (1984). Regulation of repair of naturally occurring DNA strand breaks in lymphocytes. Biochem Biophys Res Commun 122:366-372.
Greer WL, Kaplan JG (1985). Regulation of lymphocyte proliferation by a continuous production and repair of DNA strand breaks. In: ADP ribosylation of proteins. F.R. Althaus, H. Hiltz and S. Shall, eds., Springer Verlag, Berlin, pp 417-423.
Johnstone AP, Williams GT (1982). Role of DNA breaks and ADP ribosylation activity in eukaryotic differentiation demonstrated in human lymphocytes. Nature (London) 30: 368-370.
Kaplan JG (1978). Membrane cation transport and the control of proliferation of mammalian cells. Ann Rev Physiol 40: 19-41.
Kay JE, Ahern T, Lindsay VJ, Sampson J (1975). The control of protein synthesis during the stimulation of lymphocytes by phytohemagglutinin. III. Poly(r) translation and the rate of polypeptide chain elongation. Biochim Biophys Acta 378:241-250.
Kletzein RF, Pariza W, Becker JE, Potter VR (1975). A method using 3-0-methyl-D-glucose and phloretin for the determination of intracellular water space of cells in monolayer culture. Anal. Biochem 68:537-544.
Kroger H, Grahn H (1983). Influence of dexamethasone phosphate upon the DNA- and the NAD-metabolism of concanavalin A stimulated T-lymphocyte. Int J Biochem 15:211-215.
Nisselbaum JS, Green S (1969). A simple ultramicro method for determination of pyridine nucleotides in tissues. Anal. Biochem 68:537-544.

Quastel MR, Kaplan JG (1975). Ouabain binding to intact lymphocytes. Exp Cell Res 94:351-362.

Segel JB, Simon W, Lichtman MA (1979). Regulation of sodium and potassium transport in phytohemagglutinin-stimulated human blood lymphocytes. J Clin Invest 64: 834-841.

Severini A, Prasad KVS, Kaplan JB (in preparation).

CALCIUM MOBILIZATION BY SPECIFIC RECOMBINANT LIGANDS IN
IL 2 AND IL 3 DEPENDENT CELL LINES[1]

Jeffrey L. Rossio, William L. Farrar and Frank
W. Ruscetti

Program Resources, Inc. (J.L.R.) and Laboratory
of Molecular Immunoregulation, Division of
Cancer Treatment, National Cancer Institute
(W.L.F., F.W.R.), NCI-Frederick Cancer Research
Facility, Frederick, Maryland 21701

INTRODUCTION

Among the best characterized of the lymphokines secreted by T lymphocytes are the interleukins. These polypeptide molecules regulate the growth and differentiation of both lymphocytes and hematopoietic cells. The full peptide structures of two of these lymphokines, interleukin 2 (IL 2) and interleukin 3 (IL 3) have been determined (Taniguchi, et al., 1983; Devos, et al., 1983). IL 2 has specificity primarily for mature T lymphocytes (Ruscetti and Gallo, 1981). IL 3, on the other hand, has been characterized as a multi-colony stimulating factor which can induce the proliferation and differentiation of multipotential bone marrow stem cells (Prystowsky, et al., 1984). These two lymphokines exhibit no structural homologies, nor do they share target cell specificities However, it has been shown that both of these molecules function by interacting with specific high affinity cell surface receptors on their target cells. This interaction

[1]This project has been funded at least in part with Federal funds from the Department of Health and Human Services under contract number N01-CO-23910 with Program Resources, Inc. The contents of this publication do not necessarily reflect the view or policies of the Department of Health and Human Services, nor does mention of trade names, commercial products, or organization imply endorsement by the U.S. Government.

can result in the proliferation of the the target cell (Gillis, et al., 1978).

Relatively little is known at this time concerning the physiological mechanisms which mediate cellular responses in target cells after ligand-receptor binding. However, our laboratory has recently shown that both IL 2 and IL 3 share the property of inducing the redistribution of intracellular protein kinase C, a novel phosphotrasferase, in specific receptor-bearing cells (Farrar and Anderson, 1985). Protein kinase C is a Ca^{++}-phospholipid dependent enzyme which has been shown to be activated (fixed to membrane) by the phorbol esters or the phosphatidyl-inositol metabolite diacylglycerol (Watson and Lapetina, 1985). Thus, at least one intracellular event following ligand binding to receptor is common in Il 2 and IL 3-mediated cellular stimulation.

This paper presents evidence that another event, increase in intracellular levels of free calcium, also is seen in both IL 2 and IL 3 stimulated cells.

METHODS

Two cell lines were employed in this study. Line CT-6 is an IL 2 dependent line (Gillis, et al., 1978), which was grown under standard conditions in the presence of 5 units/ml commercial IL 2 (Cellular Products, Inc., Buffalo, N.Y.). Line FDC-P1 is IL 3-dependent (Dexter, et al., 1978), and was grown using 5 percent of supernatant from the WEHI-3 cell line as an IL 3 source.

Intracellular free calcium levels were measured using the fluorescent molecule Quin-2 as described by Beaven, et al. (1984). Cells were labelled with Quin-2-AME (esterified form) for 1 hour, and were washed and evaluated by spectrofluorimetry for free Quin. Calcium concentration was estimated as described by Hesketh, et al. (1983) and Tsien (1980), using an estimated dissociation constant of 115 nM. Maximal and minimal fluorescence were read after treatment of cells with Triton X-100 detergent and $MnCl_2$, respectively.

Recombinant ligands were added to rested cells as described in the Results Section. Recombinant IL 2 was obtained from Biogen Research (Cambridge, MA). Recombinant IL 3 was obtained from Dnax Corp. (Palo Alto, CA).

IL 2 receptor numbers were measured using affinity-purified unlabeled and ($[^3H]$-leu,lys)-labeled IL 2 from the Jurkat cell line (Smith, et al., 1983). The number of binding sites per cell was estimated by Scatchard analysis after subtraction of nonsaturable binding in the presence of 150-fold excess ligand. Receptors were measured on CT-6 cells, and on human T cells cultured in the presence of IL 2.

RESULTS

Both the murine cell line CT-6, which is totally dependent upon IL 2 for growth, and FDC-P1, which is similarly dependent upon IL 3, exhibited high levels of intracellular calcium during culture (Table 1). Normal, resting T lymphocytes, for comparison, exhibit intracellular calcium levels of about 100-120 nM. In order to demonstrate elevations of intracellular calcium in the CT-6 and FDC-P1 cell lines, it was necessary to bring the cells to a quiescent state. This was done by removal of the lymphokine growth factor from the cells for a period of time sufficient to utilize any lymphokine present. Calcium levels were observed to drop to resting levels, without any loss of cell viability, within 48 hours of lymphokine deprivation. At this point, addition of recombinant ligand caused a marked increase in intracellular free calcium levels, as shown in Table 1. Significantly, only the homologous ligand induced increased levels of calcium. That is, IL 2 was able to induce increased free calcium levels only in CT-6 cells, and not in FDC-P1. Conversely, FDC-P1 cells responded only to IL 3, and not to IL 2.

Most of the free intracellular calcium increase could be blocked by the addition of the calcium chelator EGTA, indicating that the calcium present in the external medium is important to the development of high intracellular calcium levels.

TABLE 1. Effects of Recombinant Lymphokines on Interleukin-Dependent Cell Lines

Growth Conditions	Intracellular $[Ca^{++}]$[a]	
	CT-6	FDC-P1
Growing Cells	227.0	159.1
Rested Cells	114.3	116.0
+IL 2 (100 U)	315.9	118.0
+IL 3 (100 U)	110.1	202.4
+factor + EGTA[b]	144.0	107.9

[a] Intracellular calcium in nM, determined 3 minutes after ligand addition.
[b] EGTA was added to 2 mM to cells along with homologous lymphokine.

The response to ligand in these two cell lines was of the threshold type; about 1 unit of lymphokine was enought to induce calcium increases, and further lymphokine addition did not result in any additional rise in the calcium levels (Table 2).

Table 2. Threshold Nature of Ligand-Induced Calcium Increases on CT-6 and FDC-P1 Cells

Units of Homologous Lymphokine Added	Intracellular $[Ca^{++}]$ Levels (nM)	
	CT-6	FDC-P1
None	114.3	116.0
1 Unit	116.5	191.1
5 Units	110.0	210.5
10 Units	306.1	208.8
50 Units	308.1	185.1
100 Units	315.9	202.4

A unique characteristic of the CT-6 cell line is that the high-affinity IL 2 receptors on its cell surface do not appear to disappear or modulate in the presence of the ligand. This is in marked contrast to the situation with normal T cells, in which IL 2 appears to down-regulate membrane receptors of cells within a few days (Figure 1). This phenomenon has not been investigated as yet in the FDC-P1 cell line.

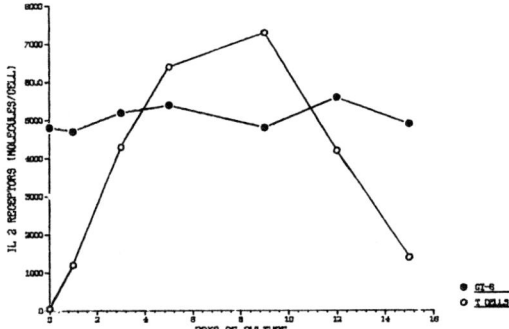

Figure 1. Il 2 Receptors on CT-6 Cells and Normal Human T Cells During Culture in IL 2.

DISCUSSION

The exact role of intracellular calcium in the growth of lymphokine receptor-bearing cells is not yet clear. Others have shown that stimulation of T cell lines or human T cells with antibody to the T cell antigen receptor (anti-T3) or other T cell receptors (T11) can result in increased intracytoplasmic calcium levels (Imboden, et al., 1985; Weiss, et al., 1984). Their results indicate, as do ours, that calcium may play a role in early steps of lymphocyte activation. Blockage of the lymphokine stimulation with EGTA suggests that intracellular calcium stores are not sufficient to produce the observed cell activation.

An important point in this study is that the cell lines studied, CT-6 and FDC-P1, are totally lymphokine dependent for growth, but lymphokine is the only growth signal required. These cells apparently are suspended in a state analagous to that of a mitogen or antigen-treated normal T cell. They exhibit high levels of intracellular calcium, in agreement with the studies quoted earlier. The only way to observe calcium effects in these cells is to rest them free of lymphokine until this high level of calcium is reduced. Only at this time can the lymphokine-induced calcium stimulation be seen. This may make these cells valuable models for studying growth factor-receptor interactions.

Finally, it is interesting to note that two divergent cell types, responding to completely unique and non-cross-reacting lymphokine growth factors, seem to share intracellular biochemical mechanisms of activation. This is true for both the protein kinase C system, as we have shown previously, and for the apparent role of intracellular calcium.

REFERENCES

Beaven MA, Rogers J, Moore JP, Hesketh TR, Smith GA, Metcalf JC (1984). J Biol Chem 259:7129.
Devos R, Plaetinck G, Cheroutre H, Simons G, Degrave W, Tavernier J, Remaut E, Fiers W (1983). Nuc Acids Res 11:4307.
Dexter TM, Garland D, Scott D, Scolnick E, Metcalf J (1980). J Exp Med 152:1036.
Farrar WL, Anderson WB (1985). Nature 315:233.
Gillis S, Ferm M, Ou W, Smith KA (1978). J Immunol 120:2027.
Hesketh TR, Smith GA, Moore JP, Taylor MV, Metcalf JC (1983). J Biol Chem 258:4876.
Imboden JB, Weiss A, Stobo JD (1985). J Immunol 134:663.
Prystowsky MB, Otten G, Naujokas MF, Vardiman J, Ihle JN, Goldwasser E, Fitch FW (1984). Am J Path 117:171.
Ruscetti FW, Gallo RC (1981). Blood 57:379.
Smith KA, Favata MF, Oroszlan S (1983). J Immunol 131:1808.
Taniguchi T, Matsui H, Fujita T, Takaoka C, Kashima N, Yoschimoto R, Januro J (1983). Nature 302:305.
Tsien RY (1980). Biochem 19:2396.
Watson SP, Lapetina EG (1985). Proc Nat Acad Sci 82:2623.
Weiss AJ, Imboden J, Shoback D, Stubo J (1984). Proc Nat Acad Sci 81:4169.

REQUIREMENTS FOR THE INITIAL ACTIVATION AND CELL CYCLE PROGRESSION OF NAIVE T CELLS.

Laurie Davis and Peter E. Lipsky

The Harold C. Simmons Arthritis Research Center and The Department of Internal Medicine, University of Texas Health Science Center at Dallas, and The Immunology Graduate Program, Southwestern Graduate School, Dallas, Texas 75235

INTRODUCTION

The activation of resting T lymphocytes by antigen or mitogen requires accessory cell (AC) signals. Mitogen-driven T cell activation provides a model for study in which a majority of T cells are induced to enter the cell cycle. Mitogens bind a number of T cell surface structures including those associated with the antigen receptor, while AC deliver an additional set of signals required to initiate a proliferative response. The nature of the AC signals required for mitogen-induced activation of resting T cells remains incompletely understood. A number of studies, however, have demonstrated that many cell types can function as AC in mitogen responses (Lipsky and Kettman, 1982). Moreover, several reports have shown that the macrophage (Mϕ) product interleukin 1 (IL 1) or chemical agents such as 4β-phorbol 12-myristate 13-acetate (PMA) can provide some of the AC signals. In addition, it has become apparent that T cells may differ in their AC requirements for activation, depending on their phenotype or position in the cell cycle.

The goal of the current studies was to delineate the activation requirements of resting G_0 T cells. In order to accomplish this, a T cell population was prepared from the lymph nodes of one-month old, unprimed guinea pigs. The animals used in these studies were free from infections making it possible to obtain a uniform population of resting T cells that were small, lacked surface activation antigens and were in the G_0 stage of the cell cycle when assayed by staining with acridine orange (AO). The cell culture conditions were also altered to make AC signals limiting. Thus, low density cultures were employed when the role of intact AC was examined.

RESULTS

Initial experiments established that intact AC were necessary for mitogen-induced DNA synthesis (Table 1). Thus, when cells were cultured at low density, the addition of intact AC was necessary to initiate responses. PMA or IL 1 alone was not effective. By contrast, when cells were cultured at high density, either PMA or Mϕ supernatant potentiated mitogen responses, and together they appeared to have a synergistic effect. However, intact AC were more effective than either of these soluble mediators in promoting T cell responses. Thus, while both IL 1 and PMA appeared to have enhancing activities, the mitogen responses of resting T cells required intact AC.

AO staining (Darzynkiewicz et al., 1976) was employed to delineate the signals involved in T cell activation. As can be seen in Table 2, mitogen or PMA alone activated few cells in low cell density cultures, whereas PMA in combination with mitogen was able to stimulate a small percentage of the cells to enter the early G_1 phase of the cell cycle. In high den-

Table 1. Mϕ but not IL 1 or PMA Support Mitogen-Induced T Cell DNA Synthesis in Low Density Cultures.

Addition:	Low Density		High Density	
	PHA	PHA+PMA	PHA	PHA+PMA
	(^{3}H-thymidine incorporation cpm x 10^{-3})			
Nil	0.1 ± 0.0	0.1 ± 0.0	0.7 ± 0.0	13.3 ± 1.5
Cont Supt	0.1 ± 0.0	0.1 ± 0.0	1.4 ± 0.0	15.9 ± 1.9
Mϕ Supt	0.1 ± 0.0	0.2 ± 0.0	12.0 ± 1.2	57.5 ± 6.6
Mϕ	5.9 ± 0.1	5.5 ± 0.1	73.9 ± 3.8	97.5 ± 5.2

T cells were cultured at high (5×10^4/well) or low density (5×10^3/well) alone or with control or IL 1 containing Mϕ supernatant, or peritoneal exudate Mϕ (5×10^4/well). The cells were harvested after 48 hours. ^{3}H-thymidine incorporation of T cells alone or with PMA ± Mϕ supernatant was less than 400 cpm.

Table 2. The Effect of PMA on T Cell Activation.

Addition:	Cell Cycle Analysis (% Activation)	
	Low Density	High Density
Nil	0.5 ± 0.4	0.9 ± 0.1
PHA	2.5 ± 1.0	20.2 ± 9.2
PMA	2.9 ± 1.4	3.0 ± 1.5
PHA+PMA	7.6 ± 1.7	90.5 ± 7.8

T cells cultured for 24 hours at high (1×10^5/well) or low cell density (1×10^4/well) were analyzed for cellular RNA and DNA content by AO staining. The % activation indicates cells in the G_1, S, and G_2+M phases of the cell cycle. The data are the mean ± SEM of three experiments.

sity cultures, PMA plus mitogen stimulated most of the T cells to enter the cell cycle.

The role of AC in the induction of activation antigen expression was also examined. A monoclonal antibody, 5C3, which recognizes a determinant associated with the IL 2 receptor on guinea pig T cells was employed (Malek et al, 1983). This antigen is expressed by activated but not resting T cells. In high density cultures, only a small number of cells expressed the 5C3 antigen when cultured alone or with mitogen (Table 3). A much greater number were induced to express the 5C3 antigen when cultured with PMA alone or with the combination of PMA and mitogen. Of importance,

Table 3. The Induction of 5C3 Expression by PMA.

Addition:	High Density	Low Density	
	T Cells Alone	Alone	+Mφ
	(Percent 5C3 positive cells)		
Nil	4	10	19
PHA	11	17	36
PMA	30	54	65
PHA+PMA	47	43	66

T cells were cultured at high (1×10^5/well) or low density (5×10^3/well) for 24 to 48 hours.

Table 4. Kinetics of the Effect of PMA on Proliferation.

PMA Added: (Hours)	Con A-induced ^{3}H-thymidine incorporation	
	36 Hours	72 Hours
	(cpm x 10^{-3})	
No PMA	12.4 ± 0.8	88.2 ± 5.7
Initiation	50.7 ± 1.3	211.2 ± 15.3
12	14.6 ± 1.2	72.5 ± 5.5
24	14.0 ± 0.8	65.1 ± 4.4

T cells (1×10^5/well) were cultured with AC (1×10^4/well) and Con A (5 ug/ml) for 36 or 72 hours.

PMA alone or in combination with mitogen, was also able to induce the expression of the 5C3 antigen on T cells in low density cultures. Although intact AC could increase the number of T cells expressing the 5C3 antigen, IL 1 did not. IL 1 could, however, increase the amount of 5C3 antigen expressed by the activated cells (data not shown).

The next experiments compared the effect of PMA and IL 1 in high density cultures containing small numbers of AC. To determine when PMA and IL 1 were active, cultures were stimulated with mitogen and PMA or IL 1 was added at varying times thereafter. PMA was able to augment mitogen stimulated T cell responses only when it was present at the initiation of culture; by 12 hours it was no longer able to induce increased DNA synthesis (Table 4). By contrast, IL 1 was comparably effective at increasing DNA synthesis when added

Table 5. Kinetics of the Effect of IL 1 on T Cell Responses During the Initial Cell Cycle.

Addition:	Time of Addition:	PHA induced T Cell DNA Synthesis	
		Control	PMA
		(cpm x 10^{-3})	
Nil		0.3 ± 0.0	8.3 ± 0.9
Mφ Supt	Initiation	2.5 ± 0.0	24.9 ± 2.7
	12 Hours	1.4 ± 0.1	18.7 ± 0.4

T cells (1×10^5/well) were cultured for 30 hours.

Table 6. IL 1 Promotes T cell DNA Synthesis.

Addition:	Stimulus	AO Analysis		^{3}H-Thymidine Incorporation
		%G_1	%S+G_2+M	
				(cpm x 10^{-3})
Nil	Nil	0.3	0.1	0.0 ± 0.0
	PHA	3.2	0.5	0.3 ± 0.0
	PMA	0.3	0.1	0.1 ± 0.0
	PHA+PMA	23.8	7.7	1.4 ± 0.2
Mφ Supt	Nil	0.2	0	0.1 ± 0.0
	PHA	3.6	0.6	4.6 ± 0.2
	PMA	0.8	0.3	0.6 ± 0.1
	PHA+PMA	31.1	8.9	6.0 ± 0.8

T cells (1×10^5/well) were cultured alone or with IL 1 containing Mφ supernatant. AO analysis was carried out at 20 hrs and ^{3}H-thymidine incorporation was measured after 48 hrs.

at the initiation of culture or 12 hours later (Table 5). Thus, PMA promotes responsiveness by delivering an early signal whereas IL 1 appears to be involved in enhancing subsequent events. An additional set of experiments confirmed this conclusion. In high density cultures of T cells containing small numbers of AC, PMA was able to induce a significant number of mitogen-stimulated cells to enter the G_1 phase of the cell cycle and also promoted DNA synthesis (Table 6). IL 1 alone, however, had only a minimal effect on initial T cell activation, but significantly augmented DNA synthesis in the presence or absence of PMA.

DISCUSSION

The role of AC during mitogen-triggered activation of a resting population of T lymphocytes was investigated. While intact AC were necessary for the responses and promoted them maximally, PMA and IL 1 could convey distinct enhancing influences but only in the presence of small numbers of intact AC. PMA but not IL 1 could induce an early stage of activation in mitogen-stimulated low density T cell cultures as measured by increased RNA synthesis and the expression of the activation antigen 5C3. Of note, PMA could promote the expression of activation antigens in the absence of mitogen or AC. PMA could also promote later stages of mitogen-stimulated T cell activation in the presence of intact AC and could synergize with the effects of IL 1. In this model, the major and unique effect of IL 1 was to augment T cell DNA synthesis late during the first cell cycle. These results are compatible with a model of the activation of resting T cells in which at least three separate AC signals play a role. Intact AC appear to convey all of these signals. An early acting PMA-like signal is required to activate the cells to enter the cell cycle. A second signal which may be delivered through cell contact is required to drive the cells into the later G_1 phase of the cell cycle. This signal could only be delivered by intact AC and not by PMA or other soluble factors. A third late acting signal augments DNA synthesis and appears to be mediated by the Mϕ product, IL 1.

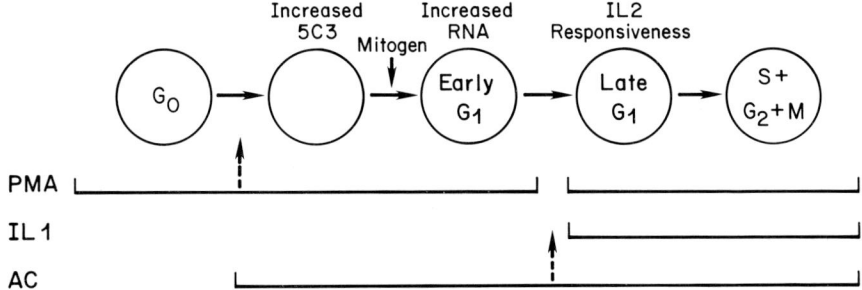

Figure 1. AC influences in mitogen induced T cell proliferation. The dotted arrows indicate unique effects of the accessory signal.

REFERENCES

Lipsky PE, Kettman JR (1982). Accessory cells unrelated to mononuclear phagocytes and not of bone marrow origin. Immunol. Today   3:36-42.

Darzynkiewicz Z, Traganos F, Sharpless T, Melamed MR (1976). Lymphocyte stimulation: A rapid multiparameter analysis. Proc. Natl. Acad. Sci. 73:2881-2884.

Malek TR, Robb RJ, Shevach EM (1983). Identification of a membrane antigen that is distinct from the interleukin 2 receptor and that may be required for interleukin 2-driven proliferative responses. J. Immunol. 130:747-755.

STRUCTURE AND SOME FUNCTIONAL ASPECTS OF hnRNP COMPLEXES IN LECTIN-STIMULATED LYMPHOCYTES

Birgit Henrich, Helmut Werr, Hans-Erich Wilk and Klaus P. Schäfer

Ruhr-Universität Bochum, Lehrstuhl für Biochemie, D-4630 Bochum 1, FRG

INTRODUCTION

During transcription and post-transcriptional processing heterogeneous nuclear RNA is associated with nuclear proteins in the form of ribonucleoprotein complexes (hnRNP). HnRNP complexes of 30-40S containing a set of mostly basic core proteins (M_r 30-42,000) in association with fragments of hnRNA form essential substructures of these complexes (1, 2). It has been assumed that they mainly have structural functions rendering the long hnRNA transcripts more manageable and protecting them from unspecific degradation. If core protein function is really confined to such a passive role then we would not expect to detect any change in the number, amount and post-translational modifications of the core proteins e.g. during the cell cycle or after response to a proliferative signal.

In this communication we show that 40S hnRNP complexes from bovine lymphocytes contain the same conserved set of proteins as found in other mammalian cells. The amount of hnRNP core proteins in the nuclei is coupled to the rate of hnRNA synthesis. One major core protein (A1 (3, 4)) is strongly reduced in 40S hnRNP from resting cells but appears gradually after lectin stimulation. All of the major core proteins show multiple charge isomers caused partly by phosphorylation. A similar pattern is seen in other non-proliferating cells (e.g. rat liver (5)). The number of charge isomers is reduced, however, in mitogenically stimulated lymphocytes. The results support the hypothesis that the modification of the hnRNP core proteins acts as an element of control for hnRNP assembly and hence hnRNA degradation and/or processing according to the metabolic need of the cell.

METHODS

All experimental methods have been described in detail elsewhere (11, 12).

RESULTS

The Amount of 40S hnRNP Complexes Increases after Lectin Stimulation Together with snRNA Synthesis

HnRNA synthesis, after a lag phase of about 6 h (6) shows a steady increase after lectin stimulation for up to 40 h (Fig. 1 A). A parallel increase of 40S RNP material is observed when identical numbers of nuclei are extracted from resting and stimulated cells (7). Since, on the other hand, the free core proteins are not present in large amounts in the soluble nucleoplasmic protein pool we have to assume that along with increasing rates of hnRNA synthesis the stimulated lymphocyte has to synthesize increasing amounts of the core proteins de novo to meet this demand.

SnRNAs as components of snRNP complexes are found in association with hnRNP complexes (8). An active role of the snRNPs in hnRNA splicing has been suggested (8, 9, 10). It was therefore of interest to determine the response of snRNA synthesis to lectin stimulation. Lymphocytes were pulse labeled for 2 h with [^{3}H]uridine at various times after lectin addition. Equal amounts of total cellular RNA were analyzed. SnRNA synthesis is part of a concerted reaction during which the synthesis of all kinds of RNA is stimulated after the initial lag phase (Fig. 1 B). The reduced level of snRNAs in resting lymphocytes is achieved not by a reduced half life of the snRNA but rather by a reduced rate of production. In accordance with this a pulse/chase experiment demonstrates that snRNAs are equally stable in resting and lectin-stimulated cells (Fig. 1 C).

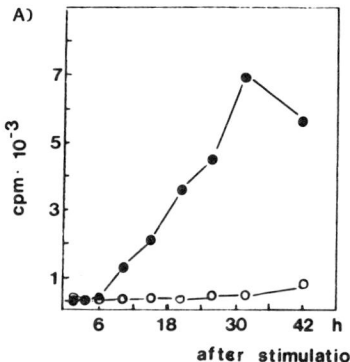 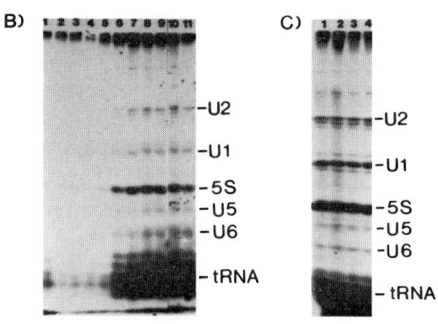

Figure 1: Small nuclear RNA synthesis in lymphocytes after lectin stimulation

A) Rate of transcription in bovine lymphocytes after concanavalin A addition (O------O). 5 · 10⁶ cells were labeled with 5 µCi [³H]uridine for 30 min. (O------O) control with resting lymphocytes.
B) Synthesis of snRNAs after lectin addition. 2.5 · 10⁸ cells were labeled as in A for 2 h at different times after lectin addition (1 (0 h), 2 (2 h), 3 (4 h), 4 (5 h), 5 (6 h) 6 (10 h), 7 (15 h), 8 (20 h), 9 (25 h), 10 (30 h), 11 (45 h). Total cellular RNA was isolated and fractionated by 10% PAGE.
C) Stability of snRNAs in lectin-stimulated lymphocytes. Lymphocytes were labeled for 16 h with 1 µCi/ml [³H]uridine. The cells were then <chased> for 0, 18, 28 and 42 h (lane 1 to 4). Total cellular RNA was analyzed by 10% PAGE. In resting cells an identical behavior of the snRNAs was found.

Methylation of Core Proteins Shows No Changes after Lectin Stimulation

The presence of the methylated amino acid N^G,N^G-dimethylarginine in the nuclear hnRNP complexes has been shown (1, 2, 12). Two thirds of the total dimethylarginine in nuclear protein is found in the hnRNP proteins. Methylation has been implemented as a modulator of RNA-protein interaction (13). Methylation was achieved by incubation of lymphocytes with [^{3}H-methyl]methionine for 16 h. Total hnRNP proteins were hydrolyzed and their amino acid composition determined. Identical specific radioactivity (dpm/nmol CH_3) was found in methionine and dimethylarginine indicating that methylation of arginine closely follows core protein synthesis. No change in this value was seen after lectin stimulation although absolute incorporation of methyl groups (sum of methionine and dimethylarginine) went up about 2 to 4-fold (Fig. 2).

In agreement with HeLa cells (12) we found that protein A1 is the major acceptor of methyl groups in the A group proteins in lymphocytes. This was determined by directly hydrolyzing the proteins contained in respective spots from two-dimensional gels. In A1 46% of total methyl group radioactivity (derived from methionine) is incorporated into methylated arginine but only 16% is found in this amino acid in A2.

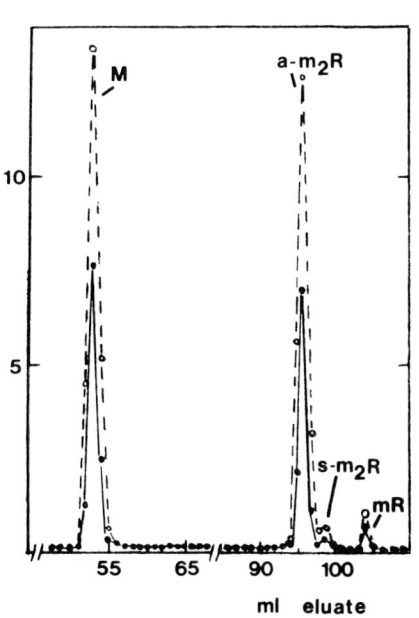

Figure 2: Methylated arginines in 40S hnRNP proteins

40S hnRNP proteins from [^{3}H-methyl] methionine - labeled resting (──────) and 50 h stimulated (- - - - -) lymphocytes, respectively, were hydrolyzed in 6 N HCl for 24 h and hydrolysates analyzed. M = position of methionine; am_2R = position of asymmetric dimethylarginine; sm_2R = position of symmetric dimethylarginine; mR = position of monomethylarginine.

The Core Proteins Are Modified
Phosphorylation Cannot Explain All Charge Isomers

On two-dimensional gels the core proteins of mammalian hnRNP particles exhibit multiple charge isomers (5, 11). In vitro carbamoylation has demonstrated that the charge isomers originate from integer shifts of single charges (12). Earlier experiments had indicated that phosphorylation was a possible candidate (2). Recently, we have shown that (with the exception of B1c, C1 and C2) the core proteins of HeLa cells are phosphorylated in vivo. We therefore performed in vivo and in vitro experiments to examine the extent of phosphorylation and possible changes after lectin stimulation in lymphocytes. In vitro labeling was done exploiting the presence of an endogenous protein kinase in 40S hnRNP preparations (12).

We never found qualitative differences in the phosphorylation pattern between resting and stimulated lymphocytes, neither in vivo nor in vitro. In addition, under both conditions the same proteins were labeled with the only exception of the basic core protein C1 which was only phosphorylated in vivo. In particular, the acidic core protein C3 (together with C3x) was heavily phosphorylated (Fig. 3).

Both of the major core proteins A1 and A2 show phosphorylated charge isomers. On two-dimensional gels, A1 is found in two conformeric forms A1 and A1x (12). As found in HeLa cells, labeling of A1 is restricted to conformer A1x (Fig. 3). In contrast to HeLa cells, however, where we find phosphorylation of A1 as well as A1x under in vitro conditions, A1 is never labeled in lymphocytes in vitro. The significance of this finding is not clear at the moment. The labeling pattern of the core protein A2 indicates that phosphorylation may not be the only charge isomerizing modification of the core proteins. In agreement with HeLa protein A2, only the second satellite spot carries a radioactive phosphate group (Fig. 3). The assumption of a second kind of modification is in agreement with the fact that the acidic protein C2, which has several satellite spots, is not phosphorylated. Since there is no increase in M_r from the mother proteins through all satellites, a rather small chemical group must be added during modification. Acetylation is a probable candidate.

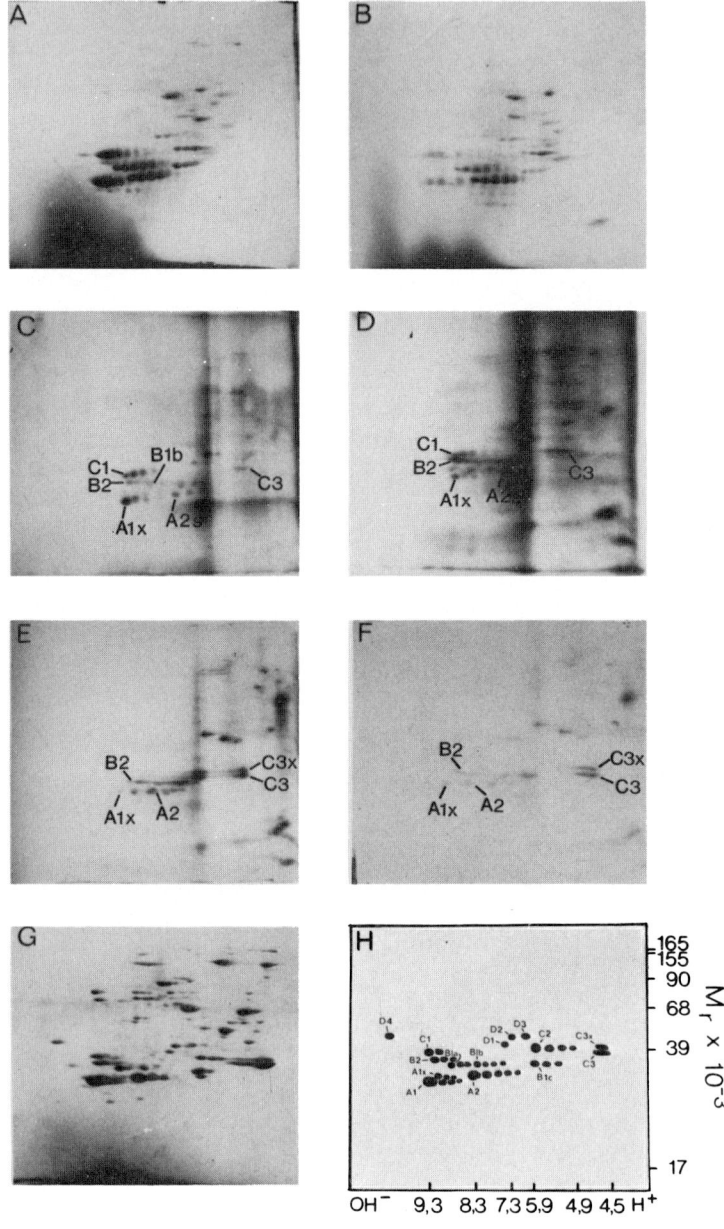

Figure 3: Two-dimensional gel electrophoretic analysis of various hnRNP fractions

A, B) NEPHGE analysis of 40S hnRNP proteins from resting (B) and stimulated (A) lymphocytes.
C, D) Resting (D) and stimulated (C) lymphocytes were labeled with [^{32}P]orthophosphate in vivo. 40S hnRNP fractions were analyzed by NEPHGE.
E, F) NEPHGE analysis of in vitro phosphorylated 40S hnRNP proteins from resting (F) and stimulated (E) lymphocytes. Labeling was performed with 10 μCi [γ-^{32}P]ATP for 30 min at 37℃.
G) NEPHGE analysis of a 40S hnRNP fraction from HeLa cells.
H) Nomenclature of core proteins.

DISCUSSION

In lymphocytes, lectin addition leads to a drastic increase of hnRNA synthesis (and other RNA species as well) after an initial lag phase of 4 to 6 h (14)(Fig. 1 A). Concomitantly, we observe an increase in the amount of 40S hnRNP complexes. In addition, lectin stimulation leads to several other changes: (i) an induction of core protein A1 synthesis and incorporation into hnRNP complexes making it a major constituent in growing lymphocytes (Fig. 3 A/B), (ii) a decrease of the charge isomerizing modifications of most of the core proteins (manuscript in preparation), and (iii) an increase in snRNA synthesis (Fig. 1 B). In conclusion, A1 does not seem to be necessary for 40S hnRNP core complex formation. Its function must therefore transcend that of a mere packaging protein for hnRNA. Other evidence suggests that A1 may have helix-destabilizing properties.

2d PAGE analysis shows that most of the core proteins can serve as substrates for protein kinases, either in vivo or in vitro (Fig. 3). This is in agreement with the behavior of core proteins from HeLa cells (12). Serine and threonine are the acceptor amino acids for the phosphate groups in these kinase reactions. 2d analysis also shows that phosphorylation alone cannot explain the complete pattern of charge isomers, especially with respect to proteins A2 and C2 (Fig. 3 C/D). A good candidate for a necessary second modification is acetylation. In other proteins, e.g. the histones, it has been shown to be involved in the modulation of protein properties together with phosphorylation (15). Indeed, preliminary experiments indicate that incubation of lymphocytes with sodium butyrate (an inhibitor of histone deacetylase) increases the amount of charge isomers of the core proteins slightly (data not shown). Our data suggest that the degree of charge isomerization of the core proteins is inversely related to the rate of cell proliferation (Fig. 3 A/B/G).

In vitro reconstitution of core complexes has demonstrated that the higher charge isomers are selectively excluded from 40S RNP complexes (manuscript in preparation). Obviously, charge isomerization reduces the ability of the respective core proteins to assemble into RNP complexes in vitro. However, since the higher charge isomers are present in RNP complexes isolated from nuclei, it seems that, in vivo, the modifications are used to destabilize pre-existing RNP complexes. Thus, in lymphocytes, after lectin stimulation, a rapid response of the processing apparatus would be possible by a simple change in the activity of the modifying/demodifying enzyme(s).

ACKNOWLEDGEMENT

This study has been supported by the Fonds der Chemischen Industrie and a grant from the Deutsche Forschungsgemeinshaft to K.P.S. and a Graduate Fellowship of the Consejo Nacional de Investigaciones Cientificas y Tecnologicas (CONICIT), Caracas, Venezuela, to I. G. de K.

REFERENCES

(1) Beyer, A L, Christensen, M E, Walker, B W, LeStourgeon, W M (1977).
Identification and characterization of the packaging proteins of core 40S HnRNP particles. Cell 11:127-138.
(2) Karn, J, Vidali, G, Boffa, L C, Allfrey, V G (1977). J Biol Chem 252:7307-7322.
(3) Schäfer, K P, Gabaldon de Koch, I, Wilk, H-E, Kecskemethy, N (1983).
'Post-transcriptional RNA processing and the activation of lymphocytes. In Parker, J W, O'Brien, R L (eds): 'Intercellular communication in leucocyte function', New York: Wiley & Sons, pp 395-403.

(4) LeStourgeon, W M, Beyer, A L, Christensen, M E, Walker, B W, Poupore, S M, Daniels, L P (1978).
The packaging proteins of core hnRNP particles and the maintenance of proliferative cell states. Cold Spring Harbor Symp Quant Biol 42:885-898.
(5) Peters, KE, Comings, DE (1980).
Two-dimensional gel elctrophoresis of rat liver nuclear washes, nuclear matrix, and hnRNA proteins. J Cell Biol 86:135-155.
(6) Hauser, H, Knippers, R, Schäfer, KP, Sons, W, Unsöld, H-J (1976).
Effect of colchicine on RNA synthesis in concanavalin A stimulated bovine lymphocytes. Exp Cell Res 102:79-84.
(7) Gabaldon de Koch, I, Wilk, H-E, Schäfer, K P (1981).
Con A-stimulated bovine lymphocytes: a model to study protein and RNA components of nuclear ribonucleoprotein particles. In Resch, K, Kirchner, H (eds): 'Mechanisms of lymphocyte activation', Amsterdam: Elsevier/North Holland, pp 222-225.
(8) Lerner, M R, Boyle, J A, Mount, S M, Wolin, S L, Steitz, J A (1980).
Are snRNPs involved in splicing? Nature (Lond) 283:220-224.
(9) Rogers, J, Wall, R (1980).
A mechanism for RNA splicing. Proc Natl Acad Sci USA 72:1877-1879.
(10) Oshima, Y, Itoh, M, Okada, N, Miyaha, T (1981).
Novel models for RNA splicing that involve a small nuclear RNA. Proc Natl Acad Sci USA 78:4471-4474.
(11) Wilk, H-E, Angeli, G, Schäfer, K P (1983).
In vitro reconstitution of 35S RNP complexes. Biochemistry 22:4592-4600.
(12) Wilk, H-E, Werr, H, Friedrich, D, Kiltz, H H, Schäfer, K P (1985).
The core proteins of 35S hnRNP complexes. Eur J Biochem 146:71-81.
(13) Carter Jr, C W, Kraut, J (1974).
Proc Natl Acad Sci USA 71:283-287.
(14) Kecskemethy, N, Schäfer, K P (1982).
Lectin-induced changes among polyadenylated and non-polyadenylated mRNA in lymphocytes. Eur J Biochem 126:573-582.
(15) McGhee, J D, Felsenfeld, G (1980).
Nucleosome structure. Annu Rev Biochem 49:1115-1156.

CHROMOSOME AND GENETIC CHANGES IN LEUKEMIA

Peter C. Nowell, Beverly S. Emanuel, and Carlo M. Croce

Department of Pathology and Laboratory Medicine, University of Pennsylvania (P.C.N.), Department of Pediatrics, Children's Hospital of Philadelphia (B.S.E.), and the Wistar Institute of Anatomy and Biology (C.M.C.), Philadelphia, Pennsylvania 19104.

INTRODUCTION

Studies of leukemia and lymphoma have provided most of the cytogenetic information on human tumors. These investigations have had practical applications in diagnosis and prognosis, and have also contributed significantly to our understanding of fundamental tumor biology. In the last several years, cytogenetic techniques have been combined with molecular genetic approaches to extend such investigations to the level of individual genes involved in human carcinogenesis and mechanisms underlying their altered function. This brief review will focus primarily on this aspect of the cytogenetics of hematopoietic tumors, with emphasis on our own recent studies.

The specific findings in leukemia and lymphoma, however, should be viewed in the context of certain generalizations that can be made about karyotypic abnormalities in neoplasia. It is now clear, from studies in many laboratories (e.g., Yunis, 1983; Rowley, 1984), that most tumors have chromosome abnormalities, and that these are not usually present in other cells of the body. Also, in a given tumor, all the neoplastic cells typically have the same cytogenetic change, or related changes. This has provided strong evidence that most neoplasms arise from a single altered cell in which a critical somatic genetic change has occurred. That change apparently confers on the progenitor cell a selective growth advantage, allowing its progeny to expand as a neoplastic "clone."

It is also generally true that chromosome abnormalities are extensive in advanced tumors, and that, although karyotypic alterations frequently differ between individual tumors, there are nonrandom patterns. The first of these two statements has been the basis of considerable speculation and investigation on the role of sequential somatic changes in the biological and clinical progression of tumors over time and on the heterogeneity within tumor cell populations. Neoplastic cells frequently show increased genetic instability, and are thus more likely than normal cells to generate genetic variants. It has been suggested that occasionally such a variant cell may have more aggressive biological characteristics, and so its progeny may grow out as the predominant malignant population, providing the basis for clinical tumor progression (Nowell, 1983). Studies of chronic myelogenous leukemia (CML) have provided some of the best evidence in support of this view. In this disease, the cells in the early indolent stage typically show only the Philadelphia chromosome, but the terminal accelerated phase of CML apparently results from overgrowth of this initial population by one or more subclones having additional karyotypic changes. A similar sequence of events has been documented in other leukemias. Hematopoietic neoplasms, as well as other types of malignancy, have also been utilized to demonstrate cytogenetically the co-existence of multiple variant subpopulations within advanced tumors, thus providing at least one explanation for the heterogeneity common in late malignancies.

It is the recognition of nonrandom karyotypic patterns in many hematopoietic neoplasms, however, that has led to much of the very recent interest in tumor cytogenetics. With improved staining methods, it has been recognized that specific alterations in chromosomes are associated, with various degrees of consistency, with specific disorders (Yunis, 1983; Rowley, 1984). It has been hypothesized that these nonrandom karyotypic changes indicate sites in the genome where genes important in carcinogenesis may be located. In some instances the consistent abnormality has been the gain or loss of a whole chromosome, or parts of a chromosome, suggesting a critical role for gene dosage in oncogenesis. Other nonrandom abnormalities, recognizable cytogenetically, have recently been identified as gene amplification units, and these may appear as elongated homogeneously staining regions (HSR's), small extra-chromosomal paired chromatin bodies (double minutes, DM's), and abnormally banded regions (ABR's) (Biedler et al., 1983). The most extensively investigated alterations in leukemia and lymphoma, however, have been specific reciprocal chromosome translocations, without apparent gain or loss of genetic material. It was hypothesized that their importance in carcinogenesis might result from position effects, with the translocation bringing an inactive (proto-) oncogene into juxtaposition with activating sequences elsewhere in the genome (Klein, 1981). This hypothesis has now been examined in detail in several leukemias and lymphomas, and these studies will be summarized before proceeding to a brief discussion of other types of nonrandom karyotypic alterations.

CHROMOSOME TRANSLOCATIONS IN LEUKEMIA AND LYMPHOMA

Lymphocytic tumors

The most extensive evidence concerning activation of a human proto-oncogene by chromosome translocation has come from studies of Burkitt's lymphoma. In most cases of this tumor there is a reciprocal translocation between chromosomes 8 and 14. In a minority there are variant translocations involving chromosomes 8 and 22 or chromosomes 2 and 8. In all instances the breakpoint on chromosome 8 is the same, in the terminal portion of the long arm (band q24). The genes for the human immunoglobulin heavy and light chains have been mapped to chromosome regions involved in these translocations: the heavy chain locus to band 14q32, the lambda light chain genes to band 22q11, and the kappa light chain genes to band 2p11. At the same time, the human homologue of the retroviral v-myc oncogene was mapped to the terminal portion of 8q, suggesting that this gene, as well as the immunoglobulin genes, might be significant in the pathogenesis of Burkitt's lymphoma (Croce & Nowell, 1985).

This possibility has now been investigated in several laboratories (Croce & Nowell, 1985; Leder et al., 1983; Rabbitts et al., 1984). It has been demonstrated that in each of these translocations a transcriptionally active and rearranged immunoglobulin gene is brought into juxtaposition with the c-myc gene, resulting in deregulation of the oncogene. In the case of the common t(8;14) translocation, the immunoglobulin heavy chain locus is split, and the c-myc oncogene, with or without structural alteration, is brought into association with it. In the variant translocations, the kappa or lambda immunoglobulin gene is translocated to the 3' end of the c-myc oncogene, which remains on chromosome 8, usually without structural alteration.

These various rearrangements are still being investigated, but it appears that in each instance the c-myc proto-oncogene comes under the influence of enhancers in or adjacent to the immunoglobulin loci, resulting in deregulation of expression of the oncogene. The c-myc gene product is a nucleoprotein, apparently having a normal function in growth regulation of lymphocytes and other cells. Studies of the translocated c-myc gene, on the 14q+ chromosome of Burkitt tumor cells, indicate that it can still be regulated in an appropriate cellular background (e.g., a fibroblast), but when under the influence of an enhancing element in a B cell at the proper stage of differentiation, it does not respond to normal regulatory mechanisms (Croce & Nowell, 1985). These findings concerning the c-myc gene in Burkitt's lymphoma have provided strong evidence for tumorigenic effects of a structurally unaltered, but deregulated, oncogene. However, the exact role of the myc gene product in the pathogenesis of the lymphoma remains uncertain, as well as the contribution of other factors such as chronic infection with malaria and with the Epstein-Barr virus.

Translocations in other B cell tumors

A significant proportion of other human lymphomas and chronic B cell leukemias have characteristic translocations that also involve the terminal portion of 14q (band q32) (Yunis, 1983; Rowley, 1984). Although the "donor" site is different from that of the Burkitt tumor, being on either the long arm of chromosome 11 (q13) or the long arm of chromosome 18 (q21), it seemed likely that these rearrangements might also involve the immunoglobulin heavy chain locus.

No candidate oncogene has been mapped to the relevant regions of 11q and 18q, but we have recently used neoplastic cells from patients with B cell tumors having either the t(11;14)(q13;q32) translocation or the t(14;18)(q32;q21) translocation to molecularly clone the breakpoints involved (Tsujimoto et al., 1985a,b). DNA probes flanking the breakpoints on chromosomes 11 and 18 were then used to detect rearrangements of the homologous sequences in B cell lymphomas and leukemias carrying the translocation under study. The breakpoints were found to be clustered within short segments either on chromosome 11 or on chromosome 18, and the breakpoint on chromosome 14 was consistently within the immunoglobulin heavy chain locus. These findings suggested that previously unknown oncogenes, located on chromosomes 11 and 18, might be involved in these rearrangements in a manner analogous to the c-myc gene in the t(8;14) translocation.

These two putative new oncogenes, tentatively named bcl-1 and bcl-2, are currently being characterized. The findings to date indicate that in both cases the translocation is into the J-region of the immunoglobulin locus on chromosome 14. Furthermore, in the breakpoint regions of the translocated sequences of chromosomes 11 and 18, we have identified several short signal sequences typically used in V-D-J joining during normal rearrangement within the heavy chain locus. This observation has suggested that following chromosome breakage there may be an increased probability of the specific t(11;14) or t(14;18) translocation occurring, with the recombinase system normally involved in immunoglobulin gene rearrangement erroneously utilizing the chromosome 11 or chromosome 18 signal sequence (Tsujimoto et al., 1985a,b). We have also used the bcl-2 gene probe to identify a 6 kb RNA transcript, and determined that levels of this transcript are tenfold higher in leukemic cells with the t(14;18) translocation than in neoplastic B cells without it, suggesting deregulation of the bcl-2 gene.

These studies of chromosomal translocations involving the immunoglobulin heavy chain locus as an activating site in various B cell tumors are continuing. There are also several nonrandom translocations that have been described in association with acute lymphocyte leukemia (ALL) that are just beginning to be investigated at the molecular level. In some cases of ALL, there is a t(9;22) translocation with breakpoints in the same regions as the typical t(9;22)(q34;q11) rearrangement that produces the

Philadelphia (Ph) chromosome in chronic myelogenous leukemia (CML) (Yunis, 1983; Rowley, 1984). Preliminary data suggest that the chromosome 22 breakpoint in Ph-positive ALL is not the same as in CML, but the details of this rearrangement need clarification (Cannizzaro et al., 1985). Similarly, it has been suggested that a characteristic t(1;19)(q21;p13) translocation associated with pre-B cell acute leukemia might involve the insulin receptor gene that has recently been mapped to 19p13 (Yang-Feng et al., 1985). Since this gene has homologies with both the c-src and the c-erbB oncogenes, the possibility of altered insulin receptor function having an oncogenic effect warrants exploration. Another gene that might also be a candidate for involvement, the ski oncogene, has recently been mapped to the region of the breakpoint on the long arm of chromosome 1 in this translocation (E. Stavnezer, personal communication).

There are also a group of cases of childhood ALL characterized by a t(4;11)(q21;q23) translocation involving the terminal portion of the long arm of chromosome 11, to which the c-ets oncogene has been mapped (deTaisne et al., 1984). Since several other neoplasms (e.g,., acute monocytic leukemia, Ewing's tumor) have also been shown to have translocations involving this site, the possibility of altered structure or function of the c-ets oncogene is now under study.

Translocations in T cell tumors

Karyotypic and molecular studies have been less extensive in T cell neoplasms than in B cell tumors. Several recent findings, however, have suggested that the approaches used for the study of oncogenes in B cell neoplasia may now be profitably extended to these tumors also. The genes coding for several chains of the T cell antigen receptor have been mapped, and translocations involving these chromosomal regions have been reported in various T cell tumors (Hecht et al, 1984; Ueshima et al., 1984; Sadmori et al., 1985). The gene for the alpha subunit of the T cell receptor has been mapped to chromosome 14 (band 14q11) (Croce et al., 1985), a site frequently involved in translocations and inversions in T cell tumors (Ueshima et al., 1984); the beta chain gene has been mapped to the terminal portion of 7q (7q32-35);

and other subunit genes may be located at 7p13 and 14q32 (Isobe et al., 1985; Morton et al., 1985).

All four of these chromosomal sites appear to be unusually fragile in human T cells, perhaps reflecting the effects of somatic recombination in the generation of the T cell receptor (Isobe et al., 1985; Morton et al., 1985), but their possible activating role in neoplasia, or the putative oncogenes that might be involved, have not been defined. This is particularly true of the 14q32 region, where the various chromosome rearrangements noted thus far in T cell tumors suggest that activating genes (immunoglobulin gene? T cell receptor gene?) as well as one or more proto-oncogenes may all be located within this short chromosomal segment (Ueshima et al., 1984; Croce et al., 1985; Nowell et al., 1985).

Another interesting finding has been the recognition in some acute T cell leukemias of a translocation from the short arm of chromosome 11 (band p13) to the proximal (q11) region of chromosome 14 (Williams et al., 1984). No known oncogene is implicated, but our analysis of this rearrangement indicates that it does split the alpha chain of the T cell receptor (Erikson et al., 1985). If studies of other nonrandom alterations in T cell neoplasia show similar involvement of T cell receptor genes, information concerning oncogenes important in the development of these tumors should soon follow.

TRANSLOCATIONS IN NONLYMPHOCYTIC LEUKEMIAS

The chromosomal translocation in nonlymphocytic leukemia that has been most extensively studied with respect to oncogene involvement is the characteristic t(9;22) (q34;q11) rearrangement that produces the Philadelphia (Ph) chromosome in most typical cases of chronic myelogenous leukemia (CML) (Yunis, 1983; Rowley, 1984). Mapping of the chromosomal breakpoints in this translocation has indicated that the c-abl proto-oncogene is regularly translocated from its normal site on chromosome 9 to a very restricted region of chromosome 22. The term "breakpoint cluster region," or BCR, has been applied to this critical segment (Groffen et al., 1984).

Several laboratories have reported on recent studies of the c-abl oncogene in CML, indicating production of a novel 8 kb mRNA, larger than the normal transcript. Cloning of the joining region on chromosome 22 has shown that the altered RNA is in fact a hybrid molecule containing both BCR and abl sequences (Shtivelman et al., 1985). Furthermore, this transcript appears to code for an abnormal protein of higher molecular weight and having tyrosine kinase activity, which has not been demonstrated with the normal product. It has been suggested that the altered BCR-abl product, if it proves to be a cell surface protein, might represent a hybrid growth factor receptor with altered regulatory effects (Shtivelman et al., 1985). Unlike the Burkitt tumor translocations, where the myc gene product appears unaltered, the recent findings in CML suggest that this may represent a tumorigenic chromosomal translocation with an oncogene product that is modified both in structure and function.

Other nonlymphocytic leukemias

Several types of acute nonlymphocytic leukemia are associated with specific chromosomal translocations. Although the possibility of involvement of known oncogenes has been suggested, and possible activation mechanisms, none has yet been completely documented. For instance, in nearly every case of acute promyelocytic leukemia (APL), there is a characteristic t(15;17)(q22;q21) translocation (Yunis, 1983; Rowley, 1984). The c-erbA oncogene has been mapped closely proximal to the breakpoint on chromosome 17, suggesting is "activation" through juxtaposition with a critical sequence on chromosome 15, but no candidate activating gene or mechanism has yet been demonstrated (Dayton et al., 1984).

There is also a characteristic t(8;21)(q22;q22) translocation in a subgroup acute myelogenous leukemia (AML). The c-mos oncogene is proximal to the breakpoint on chromosome 8, but there is no evidence of its involvement (Rowley, 1984). Attempts are under way to identify and characterize the involved DNA sequence on band 8q22, as well as a possible activating sequence on chromosome 21. We recently studied a case of acute nonlymphocytic leukemia with an unusual t(17;21)(q21;q22) translocation in which the breakpoints on chromosomes 17 and 21 appeared to be identical, respectively, with those of the t(15;17) of APL and the t(8;21) of AML (Dayton et al., 1984). In this case, as in APL, the erbA oncogene was closely proximal to the breakpoint on chromosome 17, and this suggested that perhaps the activating sequence in this rearrangement, as well as in AML, was derived from chromosome 21, but direct evidence is lacking.

In one form of acute myelomonocytic leukemia (AMMoL) there is a characteristic inversion of chromosome 16 or else a t(16;16) translocation, involving bands p13 and q22. Interruption of the metallothionein gene complex in band 16q22 has been demonstrated in these cases, with the possibility that these genes might activate a proto-oncogene from the 16p13 region (LeBeau et al., 1985). As with the the other acute nonlymphocytic leukemias, however, data on the altered function of involved genes have not yet been obtained.

OTHER CHROMOSOME ALTERATIONS IN LEUKEMIA AND LYMPHOMA

As mentioned previously, there are other types of karyotypic abnormalities, in addition to reciprocal translocations, that have been identified as occurring non-randomly in human leukemias and lymphomas. The most common are gain or loss of a whole chromosome or a segment of a chromosome. Less frequent have been HSRs, DMs, and ABRs that appear to represent gene amplification units.

In earlier studies of cell lines, it was demonstrated that these latter cytogenetic structures represented, in some cases, multiple copies of genes necessary for cell growth under specific culture culture conditions, and also that they might be relatively labile alternative forms of gene amplification (Biedler et al., 1983; Balaban-Malenbaum & Gilbert, 1977; Kaufman et al., 1979). Although these structures do not show the same consistent localization within the genome as the nonrandom translocations, deletions, and additions, they can involve human homologues of retroviral oncogenes. They have been most common in certain solid tumors, such as neuroblastoma (Schwab et al., 1983; Alitalo et al., 1983), but have occasionally been recognized in hematopoietic neoplasms. For example, in the HL-60 cell line, originally established from a patient with acute promyelocytic leukemia, there are from 20 to 40 copies of the c-myc gene (Dalla Favera et al., 1982). In some sublines of HL-60 cells, these amplified copies appear to be present in the form of an ABR on chromosome 8, the normal location of c-myc (Nowell et al., 1983), and in other sublines the amplification has been in the form of DMs or an HSR on another chromosome (Nowell et al., 1983; Wolman et al., 1985). We have also shown that multiple copies of the c-abl oncogene in the K562 cell line (from a case of CML) are associated in an ABR located on what appears to be a modified Philadelphia chromosome (Selden et al., 1983). It remains to be determined how important this type of oncogene modification may be in the development of hematopoietic tumors in vivo.

The same is true with respect to the altered gene dosage resulting from gain or loss of a chromosomal segment. Trisomy 8 is the commonest cytogenetic abnormality in human acute leukemia (Yunis, 1983; Rowley, 1984), and trisomy 12 is the most frequent alteration in the B cell form of chronic lymphocytic leukemia (Juliusson et al., 1985). Loss of all or part of chromosomes 5 and 7 is a very common finding in myeloid preleukemia and leukemia (Rowley, 1984). Presumably, the selective advantage gained by the cell carrying such alterations results from gain or loss of one or more "oncogenes," but to date the specific gene(s) have not been identified in any of these circumstances. It has been recently shown, however, that trisomy 7 in malignant melanoma cell lines correlates with expression on the cell surface of the epidermal growth factor receptor (Koprowski et al., 1985), a portion of which is coded for by the erbB oncogene and which has been mapped to 7p12. This observation suggests that similar phenotypic changes, with associated growth regulatory effects, may also be demonstrable in hematopoietic tumors that have gained or lost a single dose of a critical gene.

CONCLUSIONS

Cytogenetic studies on human leukemia and lymphoma during the past decade have provided important evidence on the critical role of somatic genetic change in the initiation and progression of these neoplasms. Recent combination with molecular genetic approaches has further demonstrated the value of karyotypic alterations as

indicators of the location of specific genes involved in
tumorigenesis. Most work has been done on chromosomal
translocations, and the findings in Burkitt's lymphoma and
CML have shown that this type of somatic genetic rearrangement represents one mechanism by which oncogene
function can be significantly altered. These data have
also demonstrated differences in different tumors. In
Burkitt's lymphoma, a usually unaltered c-myc oncogene
appears to be deregulated by its juxtaposition to a
rearranged and transcriptionally active immunoglobulin
gene. In CML, altered function of the c-abl oncogene
apparently results from a new gene product, derived from a
hybrid gene formed in the translocation event.

Limited data from other hemic neoplasms and from
tumors of other organs indicate that translocation
represents only one mechanism by which oncogene function
may be significantly altered. At the chromosome level,
gains and losses of single gene copies can be recognized,
as well as gene amplification units. Other studies have
shown that additional forms of somatic genetic alteration,
such as point mutation and promoter insertion, may be
critical in some carcinogenic pathways. For any specific
leukemia or lymphoma, it may be necessary to identify a
series of genetic alterations and host factors that interact in ultimately leading to clinical disease. Despite
these difficulties, its seems likely that molecular
genetic investigation of the nonrandom chromosome
abnormalities in human hematopoietic tumors will continue
to be one of the most profitable approaches to our
improved understanding of the pathogenesis of these
disorders.

REFERENCES

Alitalo K, Schwab M, Lin CC, Varmus HE, Bishop JM (1983)
    Homogeneously staining chromosomal regions contain
    amplified copies of an abundantly expressed cellular
    oncogene (c-myc) in malignant neuroendocrine cells from
    a human colon carcinoma. Proc Natl Acad Sci USA 80:
    1707-1711.
Balaban-Malenbaum G, Gilbert F (1977) Double minute chro-
    mosomes and the homogeneously staining regions in chro-
    mosomes of a human neuroblastoma cell line. Science
    198: 739-741.

Biedler JL, Malera PW, Spengler BA (1983) Chromosome abnormalities and gene amplification: comparison of antifolate-resistent and human neuroblastoma cell systems. In Rowley JD, Ultmann JE (eds): "Chromosomes and Cancer: From Molecules to Man," New York: Academic Press, pp 117-138.

Cannizzaro LA, Nowell PC, Belasco JB, Croce CM, Emanuel BS (1985) The breakpoint in 22q11 in a case of Ph-positive acute lymphocytic leukemia interrupts the immunoglobulin light chain gene cluster. Cancer Genet Cytogenet, in press.

Croce CM, Nowell PC (1985) Molecular basis of human B cell neoplasia. Blood 65: 1-7.

Croce CM, Isobe M, Palumbo A, Puck J, Ming J, Tweardy D, Erikson J, Davis M, Rovera G (1985) Gene for alpha chain of human T-cell receptor: localization on chromosome 14 region involved in T-cell neoplasms. Science 227: 1044-1047.

Dalla Favera R, Wong-Staal F, Gallo RC (1982) Onc-gene amplification in promyelocytic leukaemia cell line HL-60 and primary leukaemic cells of the same patient. Nature 299: 61-63.

Dayton AI, Selden JR, Laws G, Dorney DJ, Finan J, Tripputi P, Emanuel BS, Rovera G, Nowell PC, Croce CM (1984) A human c-erbA oncogene homologue is closely proximal to the chromosome 17 breakpoint in acute promyelocytic leukemia. Proc Natl Acad Sci USA 81: 4495.

deTaisne C, Gegonne A, Stehelin D, Bernheim A, Berger R (1984) Chromosomal localization of the human proto-oncogene c-ets. Nature 310: 581-583.

Erikson J, Williams DL, Finan J, Nowell PC, Croce CM (1985) The locus for the alpha chain of the T cell receptor is split by the t(11;14)(p13;q11) chromosome translocation in T cell leukemias. Science, in press.

Groffen J, Stephenson JR, Heistercamp N, DeKlein A, Barton CR, Grosveld G (1984) Philadelphia chromosomal breakpoints are clustered within a limited region, bcr, on chromosome 22. Cell 36: 93-99.

Hecht F, Morgan R, Hecht BK-M, Smith SD (1984) Common region on chromosome 14 in T-cell leukemia and lymphoma. Science 226: 1445-1446.

Isobe M, Emanuel BS, Erikson J, Nowell PC, Croce CM (1985) Location of gene for beta subunit of human T cell receptor at band 7q35, a region prone to rearrangements in T cells. Science 228: 580.

Juliusson G, Robert K-H, Ost A, Friberg K, Biberfeld P, Nilsson B, Zech L, Gahrton G (1985) Prognostic information from cytogenetic analysis in chronic B-lymphocytic leukemia and leukemic immunocytoma. Blood 65: 134.

Kaufman RJ, Brown PC, Schimke RT (1979) Amplified digydrofolate reductase genes in unstably methotrexate-resistant cells are associated with double minute chromosomes. Proc Natl Acad Sci USA 76: 5669-5673.

Klein G (1981) The role of gene dosage and genetic transpositions in carcinogenesis. Nature 294: 313-318.

Koprowski H, Herlyn M, Balaban G, Parmiter A, Ross A, Nowell P (1985) Expression of the receptor for epidermal growth factor correlates with increased dosage of chromosome 7 in malignant melanoma. Somatic Cell Molec Genet, in press.

LeBeau MM, Diaz MO, Karin M, Rowley JD (1985) Metallothionein gene cluster is split by chromosome 16 rearrangements in myelomonocytic leukaemia. Nature 313: 709-711.

Leder P, Battey J, Lenoir G, Moulding C, Murphy W, Potter H, Stewart T, Taub R (1983) Translocations among antibody genes in human cancer. Science 222: 765.

Morton CC, Duby AD, Eddy RL, Shows TB, Seidman JG (1985) Genes for beta chain of human T-cell antigen receptor map to regions of chromosomal rearrangement in T cells. Science 228: 582-585.

Nowell P (1983) Tumor progression and clonal evolution: the role of genetic instability. In German J (ed): "Chromosome Mutation and Neoplasia," New York: Alan R. Liss, pp 413-432.

Nowell P, Finan J, Dalla Favera R, Gallo R, ar-Rushdi A, Ramanczuk P, Selden J, Emanuel B, Rovera G, Croce C (1983) Association of amplified oncogene c-myc with an abnormally banded chromosome 8 in a human leukemia cell line. Nature 306: 494-497.

Nowell PC, Vonderheid EC, Besa EC, Hoxie J, Moreau L, Finan J (1985) The commonest chromosome change in 86 chronic B-cell or T-cell tumors: a 14q32 translocation. Cancer Genet Cytogenet, in press.

Rabbitts TH, Foster A, Hamlyn P, Baer R (1984) Effect of somatic mutation within translocated c-myc genes in Burkitt's lymphoma. Nature 309: 592.

Rowley JD (1984) Biological implications of consistent chromosome rearrangements in leukemia and lymphoma. Cancer Res 44: 3159-3168.

Sadmori N, Miyuki K, Nishino K, Tagawa M, Yao E, Yamada Y, Amagasaki T, Kinoshita K, Ichimaru M (1985) Abnormalities of chromosome 14 at band 14q11 in Japanese patients with chronic T-cell leukemia/lymphoma. Cancer Genet Cytogenet 17: 279.

Selden J, Emanuel B, Wang E, Cannizzaro L, Palumbo A, Erikson J, Nowell P, Rovera G, Croce C (1983) Amplified C-lambda and c-$\underline{abl}$ genes on the same marker chromosome in K562 leukemia cells. Proc Natl Acad Sci USA 80: 7289-7292.

Schwab M, Alitalo K, Klempnauer K-H, Varmus HE, Bishop JM, Gilbert F, Brodeur G, Goldstein M, Trent J (1983) Amplified DNA with limited homology to myc cellular oncogene is shared by neuroblastoma cell lines and a neuroblastoma tumor. Nature 305: 245.

Shtivelman E, Lifshitz B, Gale RP, Cananni E (1985) Fused transcript of $\underline{abl}$ and $\underline{bcr}$ genes in chronic myelogenous leukaemia. Nature 315: 550-554.

Tsujimoto Y, Jaffe E, Cossman J, Gorham J, Nowell PC, Croce CM (1985a) Clustering of breakpoints on chromosome 11 in human B-cell neoplasms with the t(11;14) chromosome translocation. Nature 315: 340-343.

Tsujimoto Y, Cossman J, Jaffe E, Croce CM (1985b) Involvement of the $\underline{bcl-2}$ gene in human follicular lymphoma. Science 28: 1440-1443.

Ueshima Y, Rowley JD, Variakojis D, Winter J, Gordon L (1984) Cytogenetic studies on patients with chronic T-cell leukemia/lymphoma. Blood 63: 1028.

Williams DL, Look AT, Melvin SL, Roberson OK, Dahl G, Flake T, Stass S (1984) New chromosome translocations correlate with specific immunophenotypes of childhood acute lymphoblastic leukemia. Cell 36: 101-109.

Wolman SR, Lanfrancone L, Dalla Favera R, Ripley S, Henderson AS (1985) Oncogene mobility in a human leukemia line HL-60. Cancer Genet Cytogenet 17: 133-141.

Yang-Feng TL, Francke U, Ullrich A (1985) Gene for human insulin receptor: localization to site on chromosome 19 involved in pre-B-cell leukemia. Science 228: 728-731.

Yunis J (1983) The chromosomal basis of human neoplasia. Science 221: 227.

BIOCHEMICAL CHANGES LEADING TO ONCOGENESIS

Herbert L. Cooper and Robert H. Bassin

Laboratory of Tumor Immunology and Biology
National Cancer Institute
Bethesda, Maryland 20205

INTRODUCTION

Retroviral oncogenes are segments of genetic information carried by a group of RNA viruses capable of rapidly transforming host cells to a neoplastic growth pattern. These genes, and the polypeptide sequences they encode, have been shown to be responsible for the oncogenic effect. The transforming DNAs arising from reverse transcription of retroviral genomes are homologous to, and thought to be derived from, proto-oncogenes carried in the genomes of normal cells which are presumed to have physiological functions in those cells when appropriately expressed (Bishop and Varmus, 1982). Recovery from human tumors of transforming DNAs which are identical to certain retroviral oncogenes has given added impetus to this field. Of particular relevance to this symposium is the accumulating evidence of involvement of some of the already described oncogenes in many neoplasms affecting various classes of leukocytes. These appear to arise through a common mechanism involving translocation of a proto-oncogene into the proximity of another genetic element, such as an immunoglobulin locus, which improperly enhances expression expression of the oncogene.

The accelerating pace of investigation in this field is yielding a wealth of information on the organization and primary nucleotide sequences of the various oncogenes; on their disposition in the cellular genetic architecture; on regulatory elements defined by their structure; on the proteins designated by the oncogenes and on the subcellular localization and biochemical activities associated with those proteins. Less data has accumulated, to date, on the biochemical events linking synthesis of an onc-protein to the set of derangements we recognize as neoplastic cell growth. In this presentation, I would like to present some of our work bearing on this question.

An intensively utilized cell system for studying oncogenes and their effects is the NIH3T3 mouse fibroblast line. These cells may be transformed by a large number of structurally unrelated oncogenes encoding different protein products. Nevertheless, the cells respond in a fairly uniform way when they express the various onc-proteins, exhibiting a growth pattern including loss of contact inhibition, multilayered growth pattern, loss of anchorage dependence of cell growth with emergence of the capacity for colonial growth in semisolid medium, and the ability to produce tumors in athymic (nude) mice. We have asked whether the common transformed phenotype induced by different oncogenes might be attributed to disturbance of a set of common cellular biochemical events involved in maintenance of the normal cell growth pattern.

Our approach to this question was based upon our previous experience with the effects of various growth-modifying agents on the synthesis of cellular proteins. These agents include lymphocyte and fibroblast mitogens, interferons, and tumor promoters. In every case, characteristic changes in the synthesis of groups of cell proteins were detected. Using two-dimensional gel electrophoresis of whole-cell proteins, we sought similar transformation-related changes in NIH3T3 cells expressing various oncogenes. Based on findings with this system, we have extended our investigations to include normal and neoplastic human lymphoid cells.

RESULTS AND DISCUSSION

Initially, we compared 2D patterns of newly synthesized proteins of NIH3T3 cells with those of a line transformed by the oncogene of Kirsten murine sarcoma virus (v-Ki-_ras_). Of the hundreds of proteins visualized in such gels, reproducible alterations in synthesis were detected in 27 cases. To eliminate changes due to _in vitro_ selection we examined synthesis of this set of proteins in

5 additional lines independently transformed by v-Ki-ras. Only 10 of these changes, all of them reductions from normal synthetic levels, were found in all lines transformed by this oncogene. We then screened this group of 10 proteins in cell lines transformed by a series of other related and unrelated oncogenes (v-Ha-ras, v-mos, v-fes, v-fms, and v-src) to determine whether production of any of these proteins might be affected as part of a mechanism common to the action of many oncogenes. Only 5 proteins of the original group were suppressed in lines transformed by all of the oncogenes studied, while 3 additional ones were suppressed in all but one case.

To clarify the relationship of synthesis of these proteins to the transformed growth pattern, we examined two lines derived from v-Ki-ras transformed cells which had been exposed to chemical mutagens. These cells had reverted to the non-transformed growth pattern and were no longer tumorigenic, nor did they form colonies in soft agar, despite evidence showing that they retained the intact oncogene and expressed its onc-protein. In these cells, of the 8 proteins under consideration, 5 showed restoration to normal synthetic levels in both revertant lines studied.

To focus our attention on events related to the onset of transformation, we examined a line of NIH3T3 cells that had been transfected with a genetic construction which placed the v-Ha-ras oncogene under the control of a corticosteroid sensitive promoter (line 433.3). When these cells shifted from the non-transformed to the transformed growth pattern in response to corticosteroid treatment, only two of the proteins under consideration (37kDa, pI 4.78, and 41kDa, pI 4.75) were suppressed during the initial stages of the transition (figure 1).

In subcellular localization studies these two proteins exhibited the resistance to detergent extraction typical of cytoskeletal components. Based on their MW, pI and cytoskeletal localization, we tentatively identified these proteins as tropomyosins, a group of highly conserved constituents of the actin microfilaments comprising as many as 10 closely related proteins. This identification was confirmed by demonstrating that p37 and p41 were heat stable, lacked tryptophan, and reacted with anti-tropomyosin antiserum.

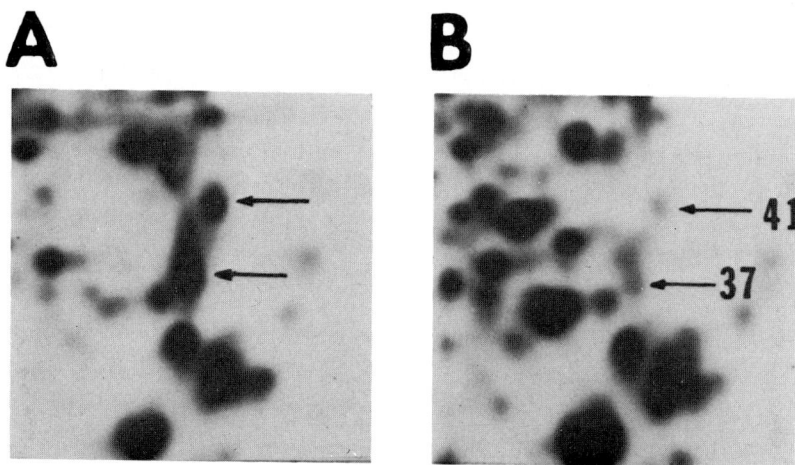

Figure 1. Suppression of synthesis of p37 and p41 tropomyosins during corticosteroid induced expression of the v-Ha-ras oncogene in 433.3 cells.

The 433.3 cell line contains a genetic construction placing transcription of the v-Ha-ras oncogene under control of a corticosteriod-responsive promoter derived from mouse mammary tumor virus. Portions of 2D gel analyses of newly synthesized (leucine labeled) proteins from cells cultivated in the absence and presence of corticosteroids are shown. (A) In the absence of corticosteroids, these cells grow with the non-transformed phenotype and show prominent synthesis of p37 and p41. (B) After 3 days of exposure to dexamethasone, the cells had assumed the transformed morphology and synthesis of p37 and p41 was markedly reduced. Other evident changes are related to response to corticosteroids and are not found in virally transformed cells.

To determine whether these tropomyosins were suppressed by oncogenic agents other than retroviral oncogenes, we examined cells transformed by the DNA tumor viruses, SV-40 and polyoma. In both cases synthesis of p37 and p41 tropomyosins was not inhibited, although the transformed growth pattern of these cells was virtually indistinguishable from that of cells transformed by retroviruses. In cells transformed by chemical mutagens, however, these tropomyosins were either completely or partially suppressed.

Summarizing our findings on the expression of retroviral oncogenes in NIH3T3 cells, we have found that, of the hundreds of newly synthesized proteins visualized by 2-dimensional analysis, only tropomyosins p37 and p41 displayed the following characteristics:

a. Their synthesis was markedly suppressed in cells transformed by a variety of related and unrelated retroviral oncogenes.
b. Their synthesis was closely correlated with expression of the normal or transformed growth pattern, being restored to normal levels in revertant cell lines.
c. Their synthesis was suppressed early in the course of transformation, during the onset of retroviral oncogene expression.

These observations support the hypothesis that expression of diverse retroviral oncogenes may initiate differing sequences of biochemical events which converge on the mechanism regulating synthesis of p37 and p41 tropomyosins. Suppression of these cytoskeletal components may contribute to disruption of the microfilament structures, which may be a crucial event in causing transformation. Since transformation by DNA tumor viruses did not suppress p37 and p41 tropomyosins, it is clear that transformation may also be imposed by mechanisms which do not involve such suppression. However, this finding also shows that tropomyosin suppression is not simply a secondary consequence of the transformed pattern of cell growth. Rather, it is associated particularly with the mechanism by which retroviral oncogenes transform cells. The uniqueness of suppression of synthesis of tropomyosin, among all proteins visualized, makes these cytoskeletal components an important focus for further study in unraveling the biochemical mechanisms underlying neoplastic transformation.

Since the NIH3T3 system utilizes cells already 'immortalized' and highly prone to transformation, it was of importance to determine whether altered synthesis of tropomyosins was relevant to human neoplasia. Human lymphoid cells offered an excellent experimental system, since controls (PBL), cultured neoplastic lines, and fresh clinical material were available for study. Moreover, evidence implicates a known oncogene (myc) in many B-cell lymphomas.

Our initial task was to identify the tropomyosins expressed by normal PBL and to determine their level of synthesis. This was done by identifying tryptophan deficient cytoskeletal proteins exhibiting the correct 2-dimensional electrophoretic mobility, followed by immunological confirmation. By this means, we determined that PBL expressed two tropomyosins of 35 kDa, but did not express the 37 and 41 kDa forms which were suppressed in transformed NIH3T3 cells (figure 2). NIH3T3 cells also express the 35 kDa tropomyosins, but these were unaffected by transformation. Not surprisingly, we found that cultured B- and T- cell lines, derived from lymphomas and lymphocytic leukemias, showed no suppression of tropomyosin synthesis.

However, in examining the proteins of various subcellular fractions of human PBL and lymphoma cell lines, we observed other significant alterations. One of these is a protein (21 kDa, pI 4.1, tentatively termed p21dr) which is found only in a cell fraction highly resistant to extraction with nonionic detergents, containing nuclear elements and certain cytoskeletal components. In resting PBL, synthesis of p21dr is virtually undetectable, but on mitogenic stimulation, its production usually becomes prominent within the first 24 hours of cell growth. Synthesis of p21dr was undetectable, however, in all B- and T- cell lymphoma and leukemia lines we have examined. Studies are in progress to determine whether p21dr is a nuclear protein or a cytoskeletal component tightly associated with the nucleus.

A second protein of interest was a 17 kDa, pI 5.5

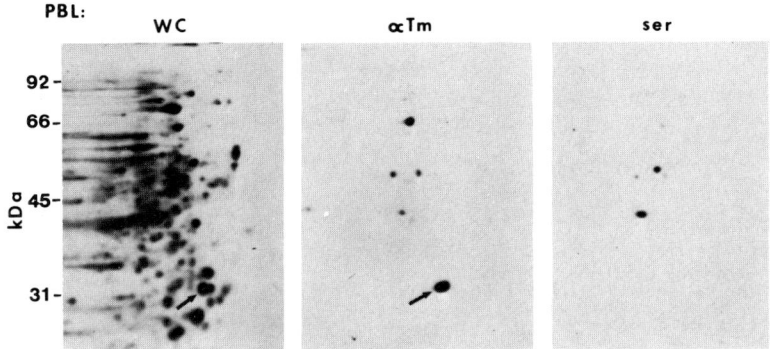

Figure 2. Identification of tropomyosins among newly synthesized proteins of human peripheral blood lymphocytes.

PBL were stimulated with phytohemagglutinin for 24 hrs, then labeled with (3-H) leucine for 4 hrs. Cytoplasmic extracts were prepared with high concentration of nonionic detergent. <u>Left</u>: portion of 2D gel pattern of complete extract. <u>Center</u>: 2D gel pattern of proteins recovered by immunoprecipitation with anti-tropomyosin antiserum. <u>Right</u>: Precipitation with control rabbit serum. <u>Arrow</u> indicates a pair of 35kDa proteins identified as tropomyosins. Resting PBL showed similar prominent synthesis of these tropomyosins. No synthesis of p37 and p41 tropomyosins was detected in PBL.

protein previously described in HL-60 promyelocytic leukemia and other neoplastic cell lines. Phosphorylation of this protein (pp17) is markedly and rapidly enhanced in HL-60 cells treated with phorbol ester (TPA), an event which may be crucial to cellular responses to these tumor promoters (Feuerstein and Cooper, 1983). We found both synthesis and phosphorylation of pp17 to be markedly elevated in neoplastic lymphoid cell lines when compared with resting or growing PBL. The finding that malignant lymphoid cells display a modification of pp17 similar to that associated with the action of TPA suggests, on the one hand, that the modification may indeed be related to tumorigenesis, and on the other, that pp17 modification may be a central event in effects, related to neoplasia, promoted by phorbol esters.

Subcellular fractionation revealed pp17, and its non-phosphorylated precursor, to be distributed between cytoskeletal and sol fractions. Such distribution is typical of cytoskeletal elements, where constituents occur both in the polymerized filamentous structures and free in the cytosol in a non-polymerized form. Thus, although our studies with lymphoid cells have not clarified the significance of tropomyosin suppression to human neoplasia, they have reinforced our interest in cytoskeletal and other structural proteins as ultimate targets of the action of oncogenic agents in tumorigenesis.

REFERENCES

Bishop JM, Varmus HE (1982). Functions and origins of retroviral transforming genes. In Weiss R, Teich N, Varmus HE, and Coffin JM (eds), "RNA Tumor Viruses." New York: Cold Spring Harbor Laboratories, pp 999-1108.
Feuerstein N, Cooper HL (1983). Rapid protein phosphorylation induced by phorbol ester in HL-60 cells: unique alkali stable phosphorylation of a 17000 Dalton protein detected by two dimensional gel electrophoresis. J. Biol. Chem. 258:10786-10793.

MODULATION OF IMMUNE RESPONSE IN THE ACQUIRED IMMUNO-DEFICIENCY DISEASE SYNDROME

Susanna Cunningham-Rundles, Bijan Safai, Craig E. Metroka and Michael Lange.
Departments of Medicine, Immunology and Dermatology, Memorial Sloan-Kettering Cancer Center, N.Y., N.Y. 10021 and St. Luke's-Roosevelt Hospital Center, N.Y., N.Y. 10025

INTRODUCTION

The sudden appearance of opportunistic infections and Kaposi's sarcoma in homosexual men in 1979 and 1980 has evolved into a well-defined syndrome, the Acquired Immunodeficiency Disease Syndrome, AIDS, affecting more than 9,000 persons including hemophiliacs, drug abusers, children of drug abusing mothers, and some blood transfusion recipients (1-6). The AIDS epidemic is now known to be closely associated with a retrovirus that specifically infects human T lymphocytes of the helper/inducer subset (7), OKT_4^+ or Leu 3^+, and is probably transmitted by infection by cell-free virus or virus in cells. The virus has been described and characterized by several groups as human T lymphotropic virus type III, HTLV-III, lymphadenopathy associated virus, LAV, AIDS related virus, ARV. The data obtained indicate that HTLV-III bears many similarities with HTLV-I and HTLV-II in infecting the human helper lymphocyte subset but is unique among HTLV viruses in causing cytolysis of the infected cell. Since profound lymphopenia and inverted ratio of helper/inducer to cytotoxic/suppressor lymphocyte subsets has been widely observed in AIDS patients, it has seemed logical to determine whether or not many or all of the immune dysfunctions found in AIDS might be ascribed to the selective destruction of this cellular population. Immunological assessment of AIDS patients prior to the discovery of the virus demonstrated a clear-cut lack of immune response in vitro that paralleled lack of host resistance in vivo. However, we and others did observe a high degree of variability in immune function in vitro in homosexual men with a generalized lymphadenopathy syndrome (LA), many of whom subsequently developed AIDS (8-10).

It was possible to show that a subgroup could be identified as having a distinct loss of B cell function in vitro and that 70% of the subgroup developed AIDS in contrast to 20% of the group as a whole. Greater than 80% of this population have antibodies to HTLV-III and thus are presumptive viral carriers. Similarly, among patients with KS, we found that impaired B cell function in vitro was significantly correlated with disease progression and survival (11), in such a way that it was possible to predict clinical outcome. These findings were striking in light of the fact that both groups showed highly reduced immune response in vitro compared to controls (12). The hypothesis that emerges from these findings is that modulation of viral infection may occur in ways which have positive as well as negative implications for the infected host.

Finding that B cell function may be a predictor of clinical outcome suggested to us that B cells might be able to harbor the retrovirus without being destroyed. Therefore, poor B cell function in vitro would imply B cell infection. We observed previously that B cell lines can be spontaneously derived from the peripheral blood of patients with lymphadenopathy or AIDS, and that these cells contain multiple copies of the EBV genome (13). In this circumstance, the second signal needed for active replication of HTLV-III would be in place.

The data presented here describe modulation of the immune response in HTLV-III associated lymphadenopathy and AIDS-KS, and the use of an in vitro model to explore possible mechanisms of host defense which might affect resistance to the effects of HTLV-III infection.

RESULTS AND DISCUSSION

Previous studies of immune function in patients with AIDS have shown that the disease is accompanied by loss of lymphocyte activation to T lymphocyte mitogens in vitro. Among patients with AIDS-KS, 75% of patients had responses 2 SD below the mean of control responses and 60% of patients with generalized lymphadenopathy, LA, also had abnormal response to mitogens. When peripheral blood mononuclear cells, PBM, from AIDS patients were activated by concanavalin A to induce suppressor cell generation, and these cells were added back as autologous suppressor cells, significant depression of an intrinsically low response was reduced even further (14). These findings suggested that the suppressor cell induction pathway was intact in AIDS and that response could be reduced as effectively as in controls. We then undertook to examine suppression of normal control cells by cells from AIDS patients used as a third party addition to an ongoing response to phytohemagglutinin, PHA. Data are shown in Figure 1.

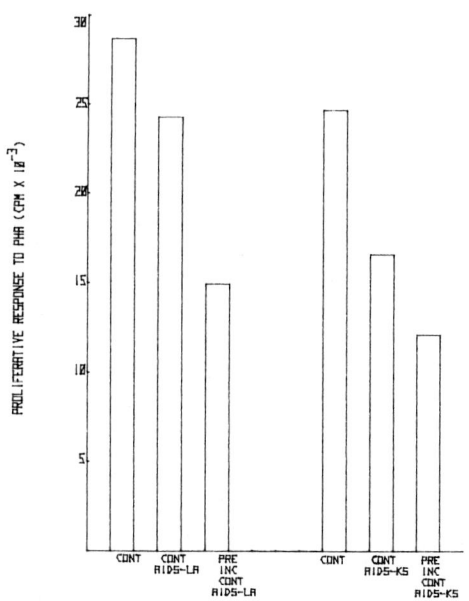

Figure 1. Effect of AIDS cells on normal PHA response. PBM from controls were cultured with PBM from patients with LA or KS. Mitogen was added either simultaneously or in delayed addition following coculture. Data are given as median net cpm of maximum response.

As shown when third party cells were cultured with responder cells, suppression occurred and this suppression was greater when AIDS and control cells were in contact for 12 hours before mitogen was added. Delaying addition of mitogen to cells in the absence of third party cells did not affect response. Related results were obtained when PBM from the same AIDS and LA patients were filtered through Sephadex G-10 columns. Following this procedure, the eluted cells were activated with PHA and results were compared with unfiltered cells. Data are shown in Figure 2.

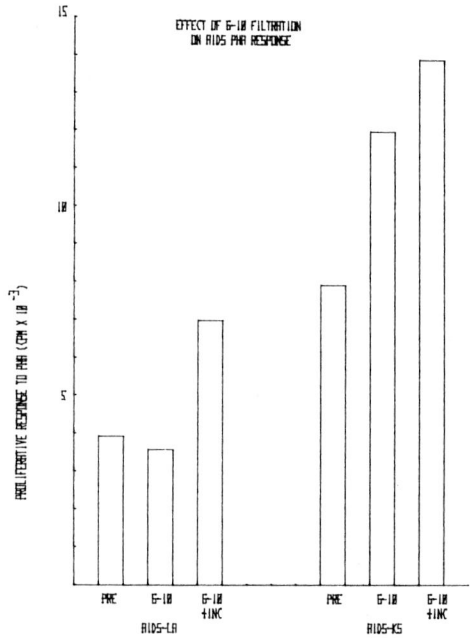

Figure 2. Effect of G-10 filtration on AIDS PHA response. Data show response to PHA of PBM pre G-10 filtration and post G-10 filtration, either with or without an additional incubation period prior to exposure to mitogen. Data are given as median net cpm of maximum response.

Since a post G-10 filtration incubation period and additional washing was noted to be more effective in restoring response in LA than direct culture of the eluted cells, the possibility of a soluble suppressor factor was suggested. Examination of T lymphocyte subpopulations eluted from the column and comparison of these with the unfiltered population by flow cytometry indicated no change in helper/inducer to suppressor/cytotoxic subsets. Quantitative removal of monocytes was achieved. Additional experiments in which indomethacin was added showed equal effectiveness in abrogating suppression. These data suggested that monocyte activation *in vivo* might have occurred, leading to prostaglandin production. Preliminary studies (Tartar *et al.*, manuscript submitted) indicate that prostaglandin is present in sufficient amounts in the serum of early stage AIDS patients to account for the results described.

Since natural killer, NK, activity has been widely recognized to be essential for host defense against viruses and tumors, we examined this function in AIDS and LA and compared the results with lymphocyte subpopulation analyses as an index of infective damage. We have previously reported that NK function may be quite strong or possibly elevated in individual patients with LA although as a group more than 50% of patients have abnormally low NK activity (13). In addition, in both LA and AIDS-KS, augmented NK activity response to interferons *in vitro* may be totally absent even when endogenous activity is normal. This observation had led us to suggest that NK function might be particularly important in host defense or modulation of viral infection in AIDS, and that loss of the interferon response might reflect either down regulation by a suppressive signal, possibly prostaglandin, or exhaustion of the precursor NK pool. Comparison of NK activity and lymphocyte subsets in LA patients is shown in Table 1.

As shown for patients LA 8 and 9, patients with nearly normal or normal lymphocyte subpopulations may have profoundly depressed NK activity or as in the cases of patients LA 5 and 6, normal NK function may be observed. In contrast, all patients with AIDS-KS studied to date have marked depression of the T4/T8 ratio. These data suggest that simple reduction of the T4 population by HTLV-III infection does not adequately account for the modulation of immune response observed.

In an effort to develop a model for studying a relevant immune mechanism in AIDS, we established cell lines from AIDS patients, usually AIDS-KS, and LA patients using PBM in the absence of exogenous growth factors, i.e., IL-2 or

TABLE 1. Comparison of T4/T8 Ratio and NK Activity in HTLV-III Infection

Patient	Endogenous NK^1			$T4^2$	$T8^3$	$Ratio^4$
	100:1	50:1	25:1			
LA-1	7.3	3.2	2.4	25.8	51.3	0.50
LA-2	7.5	2.7	1.2	18.7	50.7	0.36
LA-3	57.8	52.4	31.6	15.6	55.0	0.28
LA-4	27.3	26.2	22.8	15.1	50.3	0.30
LA-5	18.8	12.1	6.8	26.2	32.1	0.82
LA-6	32.9	24.1	10.6	32.1	44.6	0.72
LA-7	38.3	26.7	16.5	13.4	54.9	0.24
LA-8	6.2	2.5	2.4	33.6	35.2	0.95
LA-9	5.2	4.9	3.6	35.0	32.6	1.10

[1] Percent cytotoxicity directed against K562 in short term ^{51}Cr release assay; normal range 18.2% - 79.0%.
[2] Normal range 33.0% - 55.1%.
[3] Normal range 20.0% - 33.0%.
[4] Normal range 1.0% - 2.5%.

EBV, as previously published (13). The cell lines so derived are stable, rapidly growing, and contain multiple copies of the EBV genome as determined by DNA hybridization analysis. Recent preliminary work (Metroka et al., in preparation) suggests that under special conditions, presence of the HTLV-III virion may be demonstrated. The cell lines secrete large amounts of interferon, IFNα. These cell lines were found to serve as targets for cytotoxicity, as shown in Figure 3.

Control cells did not lyse this target when freshly exposed but could be induced by IFNα to a low level of killing. In contrast, AIDS patients could lyse the targets spontaneously and showed an additional augmentation of killing when IFNα was present. Cell surface marker characterization of the cell lines showed presence of B cell markers, the IL-2 receptors, the transferrin receptor, HLA-Dr, and the OKT-10 activation marker.

AIDS patients' PBM were then primed against an SLA cell or Raji cells, as a control EBV transformed cell, to determine specificity of the observed cytotoxicity. Data are shown in Figure 4.

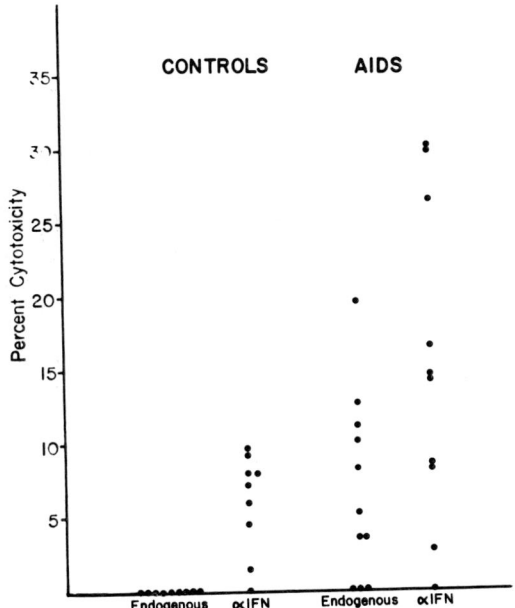

Figure 3. Lyses of an SLA cell line by AIDS patients and controls. Data are shown as percent specific release at an effector-target ratio of 100:1 following incubation with ^{51}Cr labeled target with or without addition of IFNα

Both patients were able to lyse the SLA target spontaneously in the absence of priming better than the Raji target. One patient showed enhanced lysis following priming that reflected the specificity of the priming cell. The other patient showed enhanced killing of the SLA target when primed with Raji and enhanced killing of Raji when primed with SLA, suggesting that the priming event affected the two responder cells differently.

Many of the functional disturbances in immunoregulation in AIDS can be interpreted to result from the interaction of HTLV-III with T4 lymphocytes since activation of T4 cells through the T cell antigen/MHC receptor complex is the first

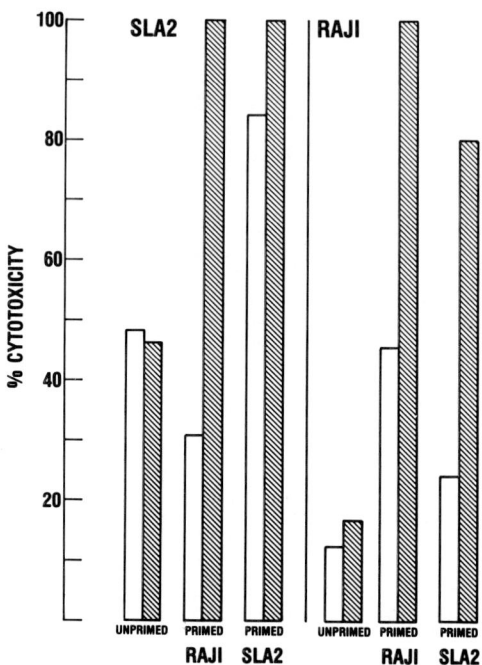

Figure 4. Effect of priming on lysis of SLA cell line and Raji cell line by AIDS patients following 6-day incubation with or without priming cells. Data is shown as percent lysis following incubation with ^{51}Cr labeled target post priming. Each bar type represents a different patient.

step in antigen specific triggering. Thus interleukin-2 receptor expression initiation of the regulatory program, and ultimately B lymphocyte activation, are all dependent upon the cell population destroyed by the retrovirus. However, our data support a role for EBV infected B cells in the pathogenesis of AIDS in 3 ways: 1) as T cell activators which insure the survival and replication of HTLV-III, 2) as producers of IFNα which is itself an inhibitor of cellular proliferation, and 3) as a safe harbor for HTLV-III virions.

Although NK cells may have the intrinsic capacity to destroy EBV transformed B cells from AIDS patients as described here in vitro, elevated serum prostaglandin may prevent this from occurring in vivo. Further study of the altered B cells on T lymphocyte subsets and monocytes may be critical for elucidating the mechanism of altered immunoregulation in AIDS.

ACKNOWLEDGMENTS

The authors are grateful for the excellent technical assistance of H. Campbell, R. Bedford, A. Hoppin. These studies were supported by NY AO-163, NIH NCI CA-34995 and G.M.H.C.

REFERENCES

1. Gottlieb MS, Schroff R, Schanker HM, Weisman JD, Fan PT, Wolf RA, Saxon A (1981). Pneumocystis carinii pneumonia and mucosal candiasis in previously healthy homosexual men: Evidence of a new acquired cellular immunodeficiency. New Engl J Med 305:1425-1431.
2. Masur H, Michelis MA, Greene JB, Onorato I, Vande Stouve RA, Holzman RS, Wormser G, Brettman L, Lange M, Cunningham-Rundles S (1981). A community acquired outbreak of Pneumocystis carinii pneumonia: initial manifestation of cellular immune dysfunction. New Engl J Med 305:1431-1438.
3. Siegal FP, Lopez C, Hammer GS, Brown AE, Kornfeld SJ, Gold J, Hassett J, Hirschman SZ, Cunningham-Rundles C, Adelsbert BR, Parham DM, Siegal M, Cunningham-Rundles S, Armstrong D (1981). Severe acquired immunodeficiency in male homosexuals manifested by chronic perianal ulcerative herpes simplex lesions. New Engl J Med 305: 1439-1444.
4. Masur H, Michelis MA, Wormser GP, Lewin S, Gold J, Tapper MA, Giron J, Lerner CW, Armstrong D, Setia U, Sender JA, Siebken RS, Nicholas P, Siegal FP, Cunningham-Rundles S (1983). Previously healthy women with opportunistic infection vs. the initial manifestation of a community acquired cellular immunodeficiency extension of an emerging syndrome. Ann Int Med 97:533-539.

5. Vieira J, Frank E, Spira RJ, Landesman SH (1983) Acquired immune deficiency in Haitians: opportunistic infections in previously healthy Haitians. New Engl J Med 308:125-129.
6. Elliott JH, Hoppes SL, Platt MS, Thomas JG, Patel IP, Gansar A (1983). The acquired immunodeficiency syndrome and Mycobacterium avium intracellular bacteremia in a patient with hemophilia. Ann Int Med 98:290-293.
7. Gallo RC, Sarin PS, Gelmann EP, Robert-Guroff M, Richardson E, Kalyanaraman VS, Mann D, Sidhu GD, Stahl RE, Zolla-Pazner S, Leibowitch J, Popovic M (1983). Isolation of human T-cell leukemia virus in acquired immune deficiency syndrome (AIDS). Science 220(4599):865-867.
8. Metroka CE, Cunningham-Rundles S, Pollack MS, Sonnabend JA, Davis JM, Gordon B, Fernandes RD, Mouradian J (1982). Generalized lymphadenopathy in homosexual men. Ann Int Med 99:585-591.
9. Zigler JL, Drew WL, Miner RC (1982) Outbreak of Burkitt's like lymphoma in homosexual men. Lancet 2:261-263.
10. Guarda LA, Butler JJ, Mansell P, Hersh EM, Reuben J, Newell GR (1983). Lymphadenopathy in homosexual men. Morbid anatomy with clinical and immunologic correlations. Am J Clin Pathol 79(5):559-568.
11. Vadhan SG, Real FX, Cunningham-Rundles S, Oettgen HF, Krown SE (1984). Lymphocyte proliferative response to phytohemagglutinin (PHA) in patients with Kaposi's sarcoma and acquired immunodeficiency. Proc Am Assoc Clin Res (in press).
12. Cunningham-Rundles S (1984) Analyses of altered immune function in the Acquired Immunodeficiency Syndrome. In Ma P, Armstrong D (eds): "The Acquired Immune Deficiency Syndrome and Infections of Homosexual Men," New York: Yorke Medical Books, pp. 331-340.
13. Cunningham-Rundles S, Metroka CE, Safai B, Krim M, Rubin BY, Hayward G (1985). Cytotoxic effector mechanisms in AIDS. In Gupta S (ed): "AIDS-Associated Syndromes," New York: Plenum, pp 97-110.
14. Cunningham-Rundles S, Safai B, Metroka C, Krown SE, Rubin BY, Stahl WE (1984). Lymphocyte effector function in vitro in the Acquired Immune Deficiency Syndrome. In Friedman-Kien AE, Laubenstein LJ (eds): "AIDS: The Epidemic of Kaposi's Sarcoma and Opportunistic Infections," USA: Masson, pp 153-159.

Section IV. Neuroendocrine-Immune Interactions

IMMUNOTRANSMITTERS: A NEW CLASS OF NEUROACTIVE PEPTIDES PRODUCED BY THE LYMPHOID SYSTEM THAT MODULATE BOTH IMMUNE AND NEUROENDOCRINE CIRCUITS

Nicholas R. Hall, Bryan L. Spangelo, John M. Farah, Jr.,*
Thomas L. O'Donohue* and Allan L. Goldstein.
Department of Biochemistry, The George Washington University School of Medicine and Health Sciences, Washington, D.C. 20037 and *Experimental Therapeutics Branch, NINCDS, Bethesda, MD. 20205.

INTRODUCTION

"He took her in his arms again and drew her to him, and suddenly she become small in his arms, small and nestling. It was gone, the resistance was gone, and she began to melt in a marvellous peace. And as she melted small and wonderful in his arms, she became infinitely desirable to him, all his blood-vessels seemed to scald with intense yet tender desire, for her, for her softness, for the penetrating beauty of her in his arms, passing into his blood. And softly, with that marvellous swoon-like caress of his hand in pure soft desire, softly he stroked the silky slope of her loins, down, down between her soft warm buttocks, coming nearer and nearer to the very quick of her. And she felt him like a flame of desire, yet tender, and she felt herself melting in the flame. She let herself go. She felt his penis rise against her with silent amazing force and assertion and she let herself go to him. She yielded with a quiver that was like death, she went all open to him. And oh, if he were not tender to her now, how cruel, for she was all open to him and helpless."

These immortal words of D.H. Lawrence (1928) have been incorporated into this introduction to illustrate the influence that just the written word can have upon our physiology. Mental images of past or fantasized experiences elicited by graphic verbal passages such as the quotation cited can profoundly influence physiological processes that are manifestations of a state of heightened sexual arousal. Is it, then, that far-fetched to propose that other types of mental activity may be capable of modulating other physiological processes such as host-defence? Indeed anectdotal reports and the results of a few preliminary studies suggest that mental processes may be capable of influencing the immune system (Sheikh, 1984). Furthermore, bidirectional neuroendocrine circuits have been found to exist between the central nervous system and the immune system. Thymosin and lymphokine peptides are able to regulate immunomodulatory neuroendocrine circuits at the level of the pituitary gland and/or the central nervous system in much the same way that gonadal steroids provide feedback signals as part of the reproductive axis.

At least two well-characterized hormonal systems are regulated in part by products of the activated immune system that are capable of transmitting information from this compartment to the central nervous system. These immunotransmitters include certain thymosin peptides as well as a variety of hormones previously thought to be neuro or pituitary peptides. (Hall et al. 1985a). The neuroendocrine circuits that they regulate include the hypothalamic-pituitary-gonadal axis and the hypothalamic-pituitary-adrenocortical axis.

THYMOSIN MODULATION OF REPRODUCTIVE HORMONES

We have previously reported that thymosin fraction 5 (TSN-5) and a component peptide, thymosin beta 4 (TSN β_4) were capable of stimulating luteinizing hormone releasing hormone (LHRH) from superfused sections of medial basal hypothalamus (Rebar et al. 1981). This resulted in a subsequent release of luteinizing hormone (LH) which was also observed when TSN-β_4 was injected directly into the lateral ventricle of chronically cannulated mice (Hall et al. 1985). Recently, we have found that prolactin can also be modulated by a component of TSN-5.

The GH3 pituitary tumor cell line which secretes prolactin and growth hormone was maintained as a monolayer culture and tested for responsiveness to TSN-5. After 72-96 hr in culture, medium was aspirated from each well and the cell monolayer washed two times with serum-free media. The cells were then treated with TSN-5 or media. As shown in Table 1 TSN-5 from 10 to 1000 µg stimulated prolactin release.

TABLE 1

THYMOSIN FRACTION-5-STIMULATES PROLACTIN RELEASE
FROM CULTURED GH3 PITUITARY CELLS.

TSN-5 (µg/ml)	PROLACTIN (ng/ml)
0	3.2 ± 0.28
1	2.1 ± 0.35
10	6.0 ± 0.84
100	14.4 ± 0.80
1,000	17.7 ± 0.98
10,000	2.9 ± 0.05

In a subsequent study the temporal kinetics of prolactin release were examined. As shown in Table 2 TSN-5 at 50 µg/ml caused an approximate 7-fold increase in prolactin in the supernatant fluids from cultures incubated for 15 minutes.

TABLE 2

TEMPORAL KINETICS OF THYMOSIN STIMULATION OF
PROLACTIN FROM GH3 PITUITARY CELLS

Incubation Time (min)	Media	TSN-5 (50 µg/mL)
15	0.77 ± 0.21*	5.47 ± 0.43
30	1.66 ± 0.22	8.87 ± 0.51
60	5.22 ± 0.65	16.7 ± 1.49
120	15.0 ± 1.15	37.0 ± 4.27

* ng/ml of released prolactin

The correlation coefficients for both thymosin-stimulated and media controls were greater than 0.99 for accumulation of prolactin in the wells. Studies are in progress to determine if growth hormone is also modulated by thymosin.

In summary, two important hormonal systems that regulate reproductive function can be directly stimulated by thymosin peptides. These include LH which is stimulated subsequent to the release of LHRH at the level of hypothalamus and prolactin which appears to be stimulated by a direct action of thymosin at the level of the pituitary gland. Both hormones have been found to modulate the immune system (Hall and Goldstein, 1984, Spangelo et al. 1985).

THYMOSIN MODULATION OF THE PITUITARY-ADRENAL AXIS

On the basis of prior studies in which it was observed that during the course of an immune response there was a significant elevation in serum corticosterone (Besedovsky and Sorkin, 1977) it was hypothesized that a product of the immune system might be responsible for this elevation. To test the possibility that a component of TSN-5 might be responsible, prepubertal female macaque monkeys were fitted with mobile tether assemblies that enabled the femoral vein to be cannulated with minimal constraints upon the animals (Healy et al. 1983). Test materials were injected and blood samples withdrawn without disturbing the subjects. TSN-5 as well as the component peptides, TSN- α_1, α_7, β_4, were injected at either 1 or 10 milligrams per killogram for TSN-5 or 75 micrograms per killogram for the purified peptides. Two control conditions were included. In one, animals were treated with saline which was the vehicle used to dissolve the thymosin peptides. In the second, monkeys were treated with 10 milligrams per killogram of bovine serum albumin (BSA). The latter control was included to rule out the possibility that any measured changes were not due to the immunogenicity of the bovine TSN-5.

Of all the treatments, only TSN-5 proved corticogenic. In a dose dependent manner, cortisol was increased 145 percent over control values. ACTH and beta endorphin were 210 and 165 percent, respectively, suggesting that the observed effects were subsequent to stimulation of the brain and/or pituitary gland. Further evidence of a cause-effect relationship between the ACTH and cortisol values was the observation that peak levels of ACTH were detected at 30 minutes while peak levels of cortisol followed at 90 minutes. (Healy et al. 1983).

In a subsequent study, 8 thymectomized monkeys were cannulated and their ACTH, beta endorphin and cortisol profiles were compared with age matched, intact animals. ACTH and beta endorphin were significantly lower in the athymic monkeys (ACTH: athymic, 39.6±5.7 pg/ml versus intact, 90.7±26.6 pg/ml; β-endorphin: athymic, 85.8±11.3 pg/ml versus intact, 147.1±24.0 pg/ml). Although it did not achieve statistical significance ($p > 0.05$) the level of cortisol showed the same trend with levels of 33.1±4.0 µg/dl in the athymic group compared with 46.5±7.6 µg/dl in the control animals.

The corticogenic effect of TSN-5 was subsequently verified and extended to rodents (McGillis et al., 1985). In this series of studies, TSN-5 was found to elevate levels of corticosterone in a dose dependent manner with a maximum effect being observed at 1 hour after injection. These studies conducted using mice incorporated three control conditions:1. non-injected:2. vehicle injected and 3. BSA injected groups. Only mice treated with the thymosin preparation exhibited a significant incease in corticosterone (TSN-5, 71.8±14.5 ng/ml; vehicle, 38.3±3.6; BSA, 33.1±3.8). Comparable findings were observed in an experiment in which rats were treated with 20 mg/kg of TSN-5. Highest levels were observed at 2 hours following treatment compared with noninjected and vehicle treated animals. (TSN-5, 136.1±38.0 ng/ml; noninjected, 55.3±15; vehicle, 45.4±11.2). The levels of corticosterone were comparable to those observed 2 hours following the injection of 5 units of ACTH (115±31.7 ng/ml).

The observed changes in adrenal glucocorticoids could have been due to an action of thymosin at three potential sites:1. a direct action at the level of the adrenal cortex 2. stimulation of ACTH producing cells in the anterior pituitary gland and/or 3. stimulation of corticotrophin releasing hormone (CRF) pathways at the level of the central nervous system. Each of these has been systematically evaluated with the following results.

Direct stimulation of isolated adrenal fasciculata cells was evaluated by treating cultured cells with varying concentrations of a variety of thymosin peptides (Vahouny et al., 1983). Both cAMP and corticosterone were measured in the supernatant fluids of cells treated with from 0.002 to 200 µg of TSN-5, but neither was affected using this in vitro model system. The possibility was then considered that the TSN might act synergistically with a suboptimal dose of ACTH. This possibility was subsequently tested, but again with no evidence that the thymosin was acting directly upon the adrenal fasciculata cell (Vahouny et al. 1983).

The second site of action that was considered was the anterior pituitary gland, especially since both ACTH and beta endorphin were found to be elevated following infusion of TSN-5 into primates. Monolayers of cultured rat pituitary cells were initially tested (Vale et al. 1981).

Using this system, it was found that there was a

significant increase in ACTH release at doses of 250 µg/ml and higher, however, a significant depression in ACTH release was observed when the cells were treated with doses between 7.8 and 31.3 µg/ml (McGillis, 1985). Subsequent studies revealed that the stimulatory effect was optimal following a 4 hour incubation period. It was also found that in addition to direct stimulation of ACTH release, there was also a synergistic effect when a suboptimal dose of thymosin (20 µg) was incubated with 10^{-11} M CRF.

These studies have been extended using the AtT20/D16-16 pituitary cell line (Farah et al. 1985). Five days prior to the experiment, the cell cultures were supplemented with charcoal-stripped fetal calf serum. Treatment of the serum with charcoal was carried out to remove endogenous steroid that might have interferred with normal release of ACTH through feedback mechanisms. Beta endorphin was measured in the supernatant fluid as well as in the cells at the end of the incubation. The results are summarized in Table 3.

While the previously discussed data clearly identify the pituitary gland as at least one site of action where TSN-5 is capable of activating the pituitary-adrenal axis, these data do not preclude

TABLE 3

EFFECTS OF TSN-5 ± CRF ON ACUTE RELEASE AND INTRACELLULAR CONATENT OF IMMUNOREACTIVE BETA ENDORPHIN IN AtT 20 CELLS

	RELEASE		CELL CONTENT
	4 h. ng/ml	24 h. ng/ml	24 ng/mg protein
VEHICLE	16.1±1.0	130.4±9.4	417.1±17.8
TSN-5 (600 µg/ml)	37.9±2.0 (235%)	218.8±11.8 (168%)	401.1±27.4 (96%)
CRF (0.1 µM)	42.1±5.7 (261%)	191.0±17.5 (146%)	401.1±27.4 (56%)
TSN-5 + CRF	96.2±6.2 (598%)	336.5±15.2 (258%)	181.3±11.6 (43%)

a central nervous system site of action as well. Indeed, a dual site of action would be consistent with the mechanism by which a number of hormones are able to ultimately regulate their own levels via feedback circuits.

Several types of evidence suggest that TSN-α_1 may have a neurendocrine function at the level of the central nervous system. First, TSN-α_1 is present within discrete brain nuclei and in regions that have been implicated in regulating the release of ACTH and beta-endorphin. These include the arcuate nucleus and median eminence of the hypothalamus as well as the posterior lobe of the pituitary gland (Hall et al. 1982, Palaszynski et al. 1983). In addition, TSN-α_1 is corticogenic when injected directly into the lateral cerebroventricle of the brain (Hall et al. 1985b). Mice fitted with polyethylene guide tubes were used to establish this effect. The tubes were secured in the calvarium overlying the lateral ventricle and were precisely measured so that the tip protruded slightly into the cerebrospinal fluid. At the time of the experiment, a microsyringe was inserted into the guide tube and the peptide injected in a volume of 2 microliters. Three control groups were included. One remained untreated, a second received an injection of the saline vehicle while a third group received an intracerebroventricular injection of the control thymosin peptide, TSN-β_4. The only preparation that stimulated a significant rise in corticosterone was TSN-α_1 which was injected at a concentration of 1 µg (TSN-α_1, 225.6±57.5 ng/ml; TSN-β_4 82.6±19.6; Vehicle, 92.2±13.2; Noninjected, 118.1±31.3). In another study, TSN-5 was injected into the third ventricle of similarly cannulated rats. The thymosin was injected at a concentration of 10 µg per animal and on 5 consecutive days. Adrenal weight was determined at the conclusion of the experiment. Control groups included untreated rats, or animals that were treated with either vehicle, kidney fraction 5, or TSN-5 injected intraperitoneally. Only those animals that received brain injections of the TSN-5 had a significant change ($p<0.025$) in their combined adrenal weight. (TSN-5, brain, 114±8 mg; TSN-5 ip, 74±5; Kidney fraction-5, 81±9; noninjected, 70±4). The fact that TSN α_1 was not corticogenic when injected systemically in rodents and monkeys may have been due to inadequate dosage.

DISCUSSION

If the central nervous system provides efferent signals via neuroendocrine circuits and the autonomic nervous system to the central and peripheral tissues of the immune system compartment, one would have to postulate a mechanism by which these signals would be coordinated so as to maintain homeostatic balance. Based upon the mechanism by which this is accomplished within other endocrine circuits, it would not be unreasonable to propose that a product of the activated immune system provides a feedback signal that either initiates or terminates the message from the brain, depending upon which is required. In the example of reproductive physiology, this signal is provided by gonadal steroids. With respect to the immune system, the signal(s) appears to exist within the thymosin peptides and in this capacity, could be considered as an immunotransmitter (Hall et al. 1985a).

In view of the high degree of specificity that is inherent in a typical reponse against an immunogen, it is unlikely that the relatively non-specific signals originating from the central nervous system constitute a mechanism for fine tuning of the immune response. However, it is plausible that these signals provide an adjunct role in concert with the autoregulatory mechanisms that have evolved within the immune system compartment. A degree of specificity could exist as a function of the responsiveness of the lymphocyte or phagocytic cell to the hormonal system. For example, it has been established that responsiviness to glucocorticoids diminishes as the T-lymphocyte undergoes further differentiation. Catecholaminergic receptors also undergo a change in density during lymphocyte differentiation (Bourne et al. 1974). Preliminary evidence also suggests that prolactin may act differentially depending upon the state of lymphocyte activation (unpublished observation).

The biological relevance of thymosin activated neuroendocrine circuits is at best highly speculative. It has been proposed that elevated glucocorticoids might function to downregulate lymphocytes with low affinity for the sensitizing immunogen (Besedovsky and Sorkin, 1977). These cells would be expected to be more steroid sensitive than higher affinity cells that had differentiated to a stage at which the density of glucocorticoid receptors would be less. Exactly how beta-endorphin and prolactin might function in this scenario is not known, however, each of these hormones has immunomodulatory capabilities. Regardless of the precise role played by these systems during the course of immunogenesis, the fact remains that gonadotropins and adrenal steroids can be stimulated by thymosin peptides. Since each class of hormones has well documented effects upon immunity, the possibility that their release by immunotransmitters is part of a regulatory circuit has to be considered.

REFERENCES

Besedovsky, H.O., and Sorkin, E. (1977). Network of immune-neuroendocine interactions. Clin. Exp. Immunol. 27:1-12.

Bourne, H.R., Lichtenstein, L.M., Melmon, K.L., Henney, C.S., Weinstein, Y. and Shearer, G.M. (1974). Modulation of inflammation and immunity by Cyclic AMP. Science 184:19-28.

Farah, J.M., Bishop, J.F., McGillis, J.P., Hall, N.R., Goldstein, A.L. and O'Donohue, T.L. (1985). Thymosin stimulates hormone secretion from AtT20 mouse corticotropic tumor cells. Society For Neuroscience Abstracts, 886.

Hall, N.R., and Goldstein, A.L. (1984). Endocrine regulation of host immunity: The role of steroids and thymosins. IN: Immune Modulation Agents and Their Mechanisms (R.L. Fenichel and M.A. Chirigos, eds.) Marcel Dekker, New York, pp. 533-563.

Hall, N.R., McGillis, J.P., Spangelo, B.L., Palaszynski, E., Moody, T.W. and Goldstein, A.L. (1982). Evidence for a neuroendocrine-thymus axis mediated by thymosin polypeptides. IN: Current Concepts in Human Immunology and Cancer Immunomodulation. (B. Serrou, C. Rosenfeld, J.C. Daniels and J.P. Saunders, eds). Elsevier/North Holland, New York, pp. 853-660.

Hall, N.R., McGillis, J.P., Spangelo, B.L. and Goldstein, A.L. (1985a). Evidence that thymosins and other biological response modifiers can function as immunotransmitters. J. of Immunology, 135:806-811.

Hall, N.R., McGillis, J.P., Spangelo, B.L., Healy, D.L., Chrousos, G.P., Schulte, H.M., and Goldstein, A.L. (1985b). Immunomodulatory peptides and the central nervous system. IN: Seminars in Immunopathology, 8:153-164.

Healy, D.L., Hodgen, G.D., Schulte, H.M., Chrousos, A.L., Loriaux, D.L., Hall, N.R. and Goldstein, A.L. (1983). The thymus-adrenal connection: Thymosin has corticotropin releasing activity in primates. Science, 222:1353-1355.

Lawrence, D.H. (1928). Lady Chatterley's Lover. (New American Library edition, New York).

McGillis, J.P. (1985). Doctoral dissertation submitted to The George Washington University, College of Arts and Sciences.

McGillis, J.P., Hall, N.R., Vahouny, G.V., and Goldstein, A.L. (1985). Thymosin fraction 5 causes increased serum corticosterone in rodents in vivo. J. of Immunology, 134:3592-2955.

Palaszynski, E.W., Moody, T.W., O'Donohue, T.L. and Goldstein, A.L. (1983). Thymosin alpha-1 like peptides: localization and biochemical characterization in the rat brain and pituitary gland. Peptides, 4:463.

Rebar, R.W., Miyake, A., Low, T.L.K. and Goldstein, A.L. (1981). Thymosin stimulates secretion of luteinizing hormone-releasing factor. Science 214:669.

Sheikh, A.A. (1984) (ed.) Imagination and Healing, Baywood Publishing Co., Inc. Farmingdale, N.Y. 291.

Spangelo, B.L., Hall, N.R. and Goldstein, A.L. (1985). Evidence that prolactin is an immunodulatory hormone. IN: Prolactin: Basic and Clinical Correlates. (R.M. MacLeod, M.O. Thorner, U. Scapagnini, eds.) Liviana Press, Padova, Italy, pp. 343-349.

Vahouny, G.V., Kyeyune-Nyombi, E., McGillis, J.P., Tare, N.S., Huang, K-Y., Tombes, R., Goldstein, A.L. and Hall, N.R. (1983). Thymosin peptides and lymphokines do not directly stimulate adrenal corticosteroid production in vitro. J. Immunology, 30:791-794.

Vale, W., Spiess, J., Rivier, C. and Rivier, J. (1981). Characterization of a 41 residue ovine hypothalamic peptide that stimulates secretion of corticotropin and beta-endorphin. Science 213:1394.

INTEGRATION OF ACTIVATED IMMUNE CELL PRODUCTS IN IMMUNE-
ENDOCRINE FEED-BACK CIRCUITS

Hugo O. Besedovsky, A. del Rey, and E. Sorkin

Schweiz. Forschungsinstitut
Medizinische Abteilung
CH-7270 Davos
Switzerland

In this paper, we summarize evidence showing that activated immune cell products can affect endocrine functions resulting in immunoregulatory signals mediated by hormones. We shall especially emphazise the mechanisms underlying a glucocorticoid-associated circuit. Evidence suggesting the existence of other immune-endocrine circuits involving hormones such as thyroxine, insulin, prolactin and sexual steroids will also be discussed.

Hormones and neurotransmitters are known to influence immune processes. This information on potential extrinsic immunoregulatory agencies is, however, not sufficient to prove neuro-endocrine immunoregulation. Such evidence must be based on identification of information channels between immunological cells and the neuro-endocrine system. Since the immune response is a phasic phenomenon, it is a prerequisite that its extrinsic regulation should also be reflected in phasic neural and endocrine changes. Such changes are thought to be mediated by hormone-like agents and other messengers derived from the immune system which continually informs the central nervous system about its functional state. The brain or brain related mechanisms may then respond by emitting regulatory signals, capable of interacting or interfering with autoregulatory immunological signals.

IMMUNOREGULATION BY HYPOTHALAMUS-PITUITARY-ADRENAL AXIS

a. ENDOGENOUS GLUCOCORTICOID BLOOD LEVELS CONTROL IMMUNE
   CELL FUNCTIONS.

Glucocorticoid hormones exert well-known multifaceted effects on immunity, but it has remained unclear whether these hormones are relevant for immunoregulation under physiological conditions. We have shown that fluctuations in endogenous levels of blood glucocorticoids are relevant for the continuous endocrine surveillance of the immune cell network (del Rey et al., 1984). Thus we have studied in non-overtly immunized mice the relationship between endogenous corticosterone blood levels and the number of immunoglobulin secreting cells (Ig-SC). Corticosterone blood levels were reduced by adrenalectomy (Ax) and a clear-cut increase in the number of total Ig-SC was found in Ax animals when compared with sham-operated controls. The opposite situation was observed in stressed animals. This event resulted in a five-fold increase in corticosterone levels and in a five-fold decrease in the number of Ig-SC. Taken together these experiments show that an approximately 10- to 15fold variation in glucocorticoid blood levels was paralleled by oscillations of the same magnitude in the number of Ig-SC. Changes in lymphoid cell mass can not be the only explanation for variations in the number of Ig-SC. This evidence suggests that endogenous corticosterone blood levels strongly influence the overall activity of the immune system and consequently the degree of autoregulatory interactions of immune cells. In the following we describe how the hypothalamus-pituitary-adrenal axis reacts when previous steady-state conditions are disturbed by an acute immune response.

b. CHANGES IN GLUCOCORTICOID BLOOD LEVELS DURING THE IMMUNE RESPONSE

Following injection of three different antigens in two species we have observed increased glucocorticoid blood levels at about the time of the peak of the immune response (Besedovsky et al., 1975). This increase occurred only in animals showing a strong immune response suggesting that a threshold needs to be reached to elicit the glucocorticoid response. Other authors (Shek and Sabiston, 1983), using the Biozzi immunologically high and low responder mice, found increased glucocorticoid blood levels only in high responder animals. The hormone levels thus reached are known to be immunosuppressive. In fact, prevention of this hormone increase by adrenalectomy (Besedovsky et al., 1979) or hypophysectomy (Tokuda et al., 1984) can overcome sequential antigenic competition. Increased glucocorticoid blood levels, however, do not seem to be a general reaction caused by all types of immune responses, since the opposite effect, namely a decrease in the levels of this hormone during skin graft rejection has been observed (Besedovsky et al., 1978).

c. ACTIVATED IMMUNE CELL PRODUCTS (AICP) MEDIATE THE IN-
CREASE IN GLUCOCORTICOID BLOOD LEVELS.

What is the mechanism of increase in corticosterone levels observed during the immune response? One methodological approach consisted of a search for soluble messengers released in vitro by activated immune cells which, upon injection into normal animals, may increase glucocorticoid blood levels. We detected such activity using products obtained from human peripheral blood leukocytes (HPBL) in mixed lymphocyte culture (MLC) stimulated with phytohemagglutinin (PHA) (MLC+PHA sup.) Administration of such supernatants to rats produced about a 4fold corticosterone increase when compared with different control supernatants. Injection of supernatants prepared from human MLC alone resulted only in a moderate though significant 2fold increase in glucocorticoid levels (Besedovsky et al., 1981, 1985). The supernatants used were obtained from cultures of an almost pure population of human peripheral blood lymphocytes containing less than 0,1% monocytes. This fact practically proves the lymphoid cell origin of the factor which increases corticosterone blood levels. We have named this activity glucocorticoid increasing factor (GIF). The existence of GIF has recently been confirmed by other authors (Pulley et al., 1982; Bindon et al., 1983). Its potency is indicated by the fact that quantities produced by less than 5×10^5 stimulated lymphoid cells can increase severalfold the corticosterone blood level in an adult rat. The MLC+PHA sup. used was endotoxin- and pyrogen-free and it contained no detectable or only marginal amounts of IL-1. Treatment of these supernatants with anti-IL-1 serum did not abrogate GIF activity. Also removal of gamma-interferon from such supernatants did not result in reduced GIF activity. Since MLC+PHA sup. contain IL-2, we injected recombinant IL-2 or purified IL-2 into rats. The quantities injected were similar or severalfold higher than those present in the supernatants. No changes in corticosterone blood levels were observed (unpublished results).

What is the site of action of GIF? Experimental evidence shows that it does not act directly on the adrenal cortex. Pituitary gland involvement is attested by increased ACTH blood levels following GIF injection and by the fact that blockade of ACTH output prior to injection of GIF led to abrogation of the GIF effect (Besedovsky et al., 1985). Preliminary experiments, showing that intracerebro-ventricular injection of supernatants containing GIF produces increased glucocorticoid blood levels, strongly suggest that at least one pathway of action of this factor is via the hypothalamus, presumably by increasing CRF production (unpublished results). Preliminary studies indicate that human GIF has a molecular weight of 10'000-25'000 daltons.

We investigated also in collaboration with Dr. K. Bienz, Basel, the mechanism of increase in glucocorticoid blood levels during certain viral infections. Newcastle Disease Virus (NDV) was inoculated into mice because this virus does not replicate in this species and causes only a transitory disease. Already a few hours after virus inoculation a remarkable severalfold increase in corticosteroid and ACTH blood levels was noted. To clarify whether the virus itself causes the increase of corticosterone blood levels or whether AICP mediate this phenomenon, we have injected into rats supernatants from HPBL co-cultured in vitro with NDV. Virus depleted supernatants induced a 3-4fold increase in corticosterone and ACTH blood levels when compared with appropriate controls. Also in this model a functional pituitary is required since the corticosterone increase was abrogated by blockade of ACTH release from the pituitary. When supernatants of HPBL co-cultured with NDV were treated with anti-IL-1 antiserum and then injected into rats, a complete disappearance of glucocorticoid increasing activity resulted (Medium + anti-IL-1: $11,13 \pm 3,53$ µg/100 ml plasma (n=6), HPBL+ NDV: $36,97 \pm 11,03$ µg/100 ml (n=6), HPBL+NDV anti IL-1: $7,68 \pm 2,24$ µg/100 ml (n=6). This contrasts with persistent GIF activity of MLC+PHA supernatants after treatment with IL-1 antiserum. These data led us to study in collaboration with Dr. Ch. Dinarello the effect of IL-1 administration on corticosterone blood levels. When highly purified IL-1 was injected i.p. in non-pyrogenic doses (mouse-test) into endotoxin resistant C3H/HeJ mice, a remarkable increase in corticosterone blood levels was detected (control: $1,20 \pm 0,31$ µg/100 ml serum; IL-1: $8,10 \pm 1,73$ µg/100 ml serum, $p < 0,005$). (Manuscript submitted).

In summary, messengers of lymphoid origin (GIF) and of monocyte origin (IL-1) were able to increase glucocorticoid blood levels. Other authors (see N. Hall, this volume) have now shown that also thymosine fraction V can increase glucocorticoid blood levels.

d. GLUCOCORTICOID-ASSOCIATED IMMUNOREGULATORY CIRCUIT

Our data led us to postulate the first immunoregulatory circuit linking neuro-endocrine structures and the immune system. Activated immune cells release factors which increase the blood glucocorticoid level via the hypothalamus-pituitary axis to a level known to affect the functions of several types of immunological cells.

What could be the regulatory meaning of this circuit? It is known that glucocorticoids at increased but still physiological concentrations inhibit amongst others IL-1 and IL-2 production and/or action (Gillis et al., 1979; Snyder and Unanue, 1982; Kelso and Munck, 1984). In this way, increased glucocorticoid levels can control the clonal expansion of committed cells with high affinity for the antigen. On the other hand, since resting immunological cells are much more sensitive to glucocorticoids than activated cells, we propose that this circuit may have the function of preventing the excessive expansion of cells with low affinity for the antigen or of those cells which are recruited under the polyclonal influence of lymphokines. It is conceivable that this circuit, by impeding a cumulative excessive expansion of lymphoid and accessory cells, plays a role in preventing autoimmune and lymphoproliferative diseases.

The glucocorticoid response may also contribute to pathological states. A massive release e.g. of IL-1, causing an increase in the glucocorticoid blood level may be a contributing factor to the immunosuppression observed during the acute phase of several infectious diseases thus favouring superinfection. Nevertheless other mechanisms such as the one mediated by a macrophage-derived factor capable of inhibiting ACTH-induced steroidogenesis as described by Mathison et al. (1983) may counteract the effect of AICP.

II. EVIDENCE SUGGESTING PARTICIPATION OF OTHER IMMUNE-ENDOCRINE CIRCUITS IN IMMUNOREGULATION

a. CHANGES IN THYROXINE BLOOD LEVELS DURING THE IMMUNE RESPONSE

During the course of the immune response of rats to SRBC or to TNP-haemocyanin we have observed decreased blood levels of thyroxine (Besedovsky et al., 1975). These changes were correlated in time with the appearance of plaque-forming cells (PFC) in the spleen. Animals injected with homologous erythrocytes showed no changes in thyroxine blood levels. Supernatants from Con A stimulated rat spleen cells or HPBL, which increased glucocorticoid blood levels, failed however to induce the decrease in thyroxine, indicating that the decrease in thyroxine during the immune response is not an effect secondary to the increased corticosterone blood levels. Further investigations will be necessary to identify the factor(s) mediating this thyroxine decrease.

b. DECREASE IN INSULIN BLOOD LEVELS AFTER ADMINISTRATION OF AICP

Administration of human MLC+PHA sups. to rats causes a significant decrease in insulin levels when compared with supernatants from non-stimulated human cells from individual donors or from HPBL in MLC only (control: $1155,18 \pm 83,03$ pg/ml plasma (n=17), MLC sup.: $1116,00 \pm 81,17$ pg/ml (n=17), MLC+PHA sup: $855,35 \pm 80,70$ pg/ml (n=17), $p < 0,02$). This activity was observed in 5 out of 7 batches of MLC+PHA sup. tested. All the batches used had powerful glucocorticoid increasing activity including those in which no insulin decreasing activity was detected. Furthermore, in supernatants inducing the insulin decrease, this decrease was not correlated with the increase in corticosterone blood levels. These facts suggest that the factor causing the insulin decrease is different from GIF.

c. HORMONAL CHANGES FOLLOWING TUMOR CELL INOCULATION: POSSIBLE MEDIATION BY AICP

Within the theoretical framework of immune-neuro-endocrine circuits, we studied whether injection of neoplastic cells can also elicit neuro-endocrine changes in the host. Male DA rats were inoculated with $1-2 \times 10^6$ syngeneic but immunogenic tumor cells induced by DMBA or MCA. 1-5 days after tumor cell inoculation and before the tumor became palpable a decrease in insulin, thyroxine and testosterone and a pronounced severalfold increase in prolactin and corticosterone were noticed. All these changes were transient with the exception of thyroxine which showed a progressively decreasing level throughout tumor development. Insulin and testosterone were decreased again in a late phase. Inoculation of normal liver cells did not evoke an endocrine response (Besedovsky et al., 1985). It seems a remarkable coincidence that both during the early phase of tumor growth and during the immune response to antigens or after administration of AICP an increase in corticosterone and decrease in thyroxin and insulin occurred. This suggests that immune cells may mediate at least the early endocrine changes during tumor growth.

OVERVIEW

Evidence was provided that the immune response itself can bring about neuro-endocrine responses with immunoregulatory consequences. Some of these responses can be attributed to soluble messengers derived from activated immune cells (AICP) Although these messengers are not yet characterized, we believe that, in contrast to locally operating factors, they fulfill requirements which confer on them the characteristics of true immunologic cell-derived hormones. GIF and IL-1 are first examples of immunohormones acting through the hypothalamus-pituitary-adrenal axis, they are thus integrated in the network of neuro-endocrine homeostatic mechanisms. It is likely that these immunohormones, aside from their immunologic effects may influence other nonimmunologic mechanisms.

REFERENCES

Besedovsky HO, del Rey A, Schardt M, Sorkin E, Normann S, Baumann J, Girard J (1985). Changes in plasma hormone profiles after tumor transplantation into syngeneic and allogeneic rats. Int J Cancer, in press.

Besedovsky HO, del Rey A, Sorkin E (1979). Antigenic competition between horse and sheep red blood cells as a hormone-dependent phenomenon. Clin Exp Immunol 37:106-113.

Besedovsky HO, del Rey A, Sorkin E (1981). Lymphokine containing supernatants from Con A-stimulated cells increase corticosterone blood levels. J Immunol 126:385-387.

Besedovsky HO, del Rey A, Sorkin E, Lotz W, Schwulera U (1985). Lymphoid cells produce an immunoregulatory glucocorticoid increasing factor (GIF) acting through the pituitary gland. Clin Exp Immunol 59:622-628.

Besedovsky HO, Sorkin E, Keller M (1978). Changes in the concentration of corticosterone in the blood during skin graft rejection in the rat. J Endocrinol 76:175-176.

Besedovsky HO, Sorkin E, Keller M, Müller J (1975). Changes in blood hormone levels during the immune response. Proc Soc Exp Biol Med 150:466-470.

Bindon C, Czerniecki M, Ruell P, Edwards A, McCarthy WH, Harris R, Hersey P (1983). Clearance rates and systemic effects of intravenously administered interleukin 2 (IL-2) containing preparations in human subjects. Br J Cancer 47:123-133.

del Rey A, Besedovsky HO, Sorkin E (1984). Endogenous blood levels of corticosterone control the immunological cell mass and B cell activity in mice. J Immunol 133:572-575.

Gillis S, Crabtree GR, Smith K (1979). Glucocorticoid-induced inhibition of T cell growth factor production. I. The effect on mitogen-induced lymphocyte proliferation. J Immunol 123:1624-1631.

Kelso A, Munck A (1984). Glucocorticoid inhibition of lymphokine secretion by alloreactive T lymphocyte clones. J Immunol 133:784-791.

Mathison JC, Schreiber RD, La Forest AC, Ulevitch RJ (1983). Suppression of ACTH-induced steroidogenesis by supernatants from LPS-treated peritoneal exudate macrophages. J Immunol 130:2757-2762.

Pulley MS, Dumonde DC, Carter G, Muller B, Fleck A, Southcott BM, den Hollander F (1982). Hormonal, haematological and acute phase protein responses of advanced cancer patients to the intravenous injection of lymphoid-cell lymphokine (LCL-LK). In Kahn A, Hill NO (eds.): "Human Lymphokines", New York: Academic Press, pp 651-664.

Shek PN, Sabiston BH (1983). Neuroendocrine regulation of immune processes: Change in circulating corticosterone levels induced by the primary antibody response in mice. Internat J Immunopharmacol 5:23-33.

Snyder DS, Unanue ER (1982). Corticosteroids inhibit murine macrophage Ia expression and interleukin-1 production. J Immunol 129:1803-1805.

Tokuda S, Trujillo LC, Nofchissey RA (1984). Hormonal regulation of the immune response. In Cooper EL (ed.): "Stress, Immunity and Aging", Marcel Dekker, Inc., pp 141-155.

This work was supported by the Swiss National Science Foundation Grant Nr. 3.399.0.83 SR and the Swiss Cancer Ligue.

SOME IMMUNOLOGICAL EFFECTS OF METHIONIN-ENKEPHALIN IN MAN : POTENTIAL THERAPEUTICAL USE

Joseph Wybran and Liliane Schandene

Department of Immunology, Hematology and Transfusion, Erasme Hospital, Université Libre de Bruxelles, 1070 Brussels, Belgium

INTRODUCTION

In the recent years, a new stream of investigations emerged which tightens more narrowly the relations existing between the central nervous system, the endocrine system and more recently the immune system. It appears that one of the links between these systems are the endogenous opioid peptides.

The endogenous opioid peptides are constituted by three groups of various peptides : the endorphins, the enkephalins and the dinorphin group. The endogenous opioids play a major role as chemical messengers of inhibitory signalling systems like the opening of K^+ channels and the depression of transmitter release. This explains their action on pain inhibition. They are essentially released after various stimuli including shock and stress.

The endorphins are small peptides composed of 16 amino acids (AA) for α endorphin, 31 A.A. for β endorphin and 17 A.A. for γ endorphin. The precursor of endorphins is pro-piomelanocortine composed of 264 A.A.. Proenkephalin A, the precursor of the enkephalins, is composed of 236 A.A.. It is localized in the chromatoffin cells of the medulla of the adrenals. Two enkephalins are known : Met-Enkephalin (Met-Enk) and Leu-Enkephalin (Leu-Enk). They are both composed by 5 A.A. and their structure is the following : Tyr-Gly-Gly-Phe-Met for Met-Enk and Tyr-Gly-Gly-Phe-Leu for Leu-Enk. The last group of endogenous opioids is composed by dinorphin (17 AA), α and β neoendorphin and peptide E;

their precursor is prodynorphin (265 AA). Interestingly enough the five first A.A. of β and γ endorphins correspond to Met-Enk and the five first A.A. of Dynorphin correspond to Leu-Enk. The opioid peptides, once released, are localized in the central nervous system (endorphins, enkephalins) as well as the peripheral nervous system (enkephalins). This localization is due to the presence of various opioid receptors like μ, δ, K and σ on the nervous cells. Naloxone is a specific antagonist of the opioid functions of the endogenous opioids (as well as of morphine which is an exogenous opioid). Naloxone will bind to μ receptors at low concentrations and to other receptors at high concentrations. It may, itself, have some slight agonist activities. It acts at the NH_2 side of the opioids. The enkephalins are rapidly destroyed in the blood by serum enkephalinases so that normally Met-Enk is not present, or only at trace amounts difficult to detect, in the blood.

RECEPTORS FOR MET-ENK ON LYMPHOCYTES

In 1979, Wybran et al. demonstrated suggestive evidence for the presence of Met-Enk receptors on human T lymphocytes (Wybran et al., 1979). This work was based on the following observations : when peripheral blood lymphocytes were incubated in presence of various concentrations of Met-Enk, they showed an enhanced property of binding to sheep red blood cells using the active rosette test (Wybran and Dupont, 1982). This enhancement was fully inhibited by the preincubation or the simultaneous incubation with Naloxone showing thus that this effect was opioid specific. Relevant to this receptor problem is the finding of Merishi et al. who showed the presence of morphine and nalaxone receptors on human lymphocytes and platelets using direct labeling (Merishi and Mills, 1983). Also, Johnson et al. have demonstrated, by direct radiolabeling, the presence of Met-Enk receptors on mice spleen cells (Johnson et al., 1983). The property of Met-Enk to increase, in vitro, active T rosettes has been confirmed using both the blood lymphocytes of healthy subjects or of lymphoma patients (Miller et al., 1984; Miller et al., 1983). All these data can thus be interpreted as evidences for the presence of Met-Enk receptor on both human and animal lymphocytes. Furthermore since both specific antigens (to which the subject is sensitive) as T cell immunomodulatory agents like isoprinosine and thymosin 5 can enhance active T cell rosette formation (Wybran et al., 1978; Wybran et al., 1975), it can also be suggested that Met-Enk possesses enhancing T cell properties both in normal subjects as well as in patients with malignant or other diseases (Wybran, 1985; Plotnikoff and Miller, 1983).

NATURAL KILLER ACTIVITY

Various investigators have shown that Met-Enk can enhance, in vitro, the natural killer (NK) activity of human cells isolated from peripheral blood (Mathews et al., 1983; Faith et al., 1984; Wybran, 1985). The increase is consistent but may vary between 10 % to 60 % according the experiments. Usually an increase of about 25 % is obtained around 10^{-7} Mol of Met-Enk. The effect is observed between 10^{-12} Mol and 10^{-5} Mol. This can be abolished by the simultaneous incubation with naloxone suggesting that Met-Enk acts through opiate specific (receptor ?) mechanisms. Interestingly and perhaps due to the fact that naloxone has some agonist properties, naloxone itself produces a slight increase in NK activity.

In order to unravel the mechanisms by which NK activity is enhanced, we have incubated blood mononuclear cells with Met-Enk for 20 hours, washed the cells, incubated them in fresh culture medium for 24 hours and remove this medium to incubate it with fresh blood monocuclear cells. These cells were then used in a NK assay. It can be shown, by this indirect procedure, that the supernatant of Met-Enk treated cells also enhances by approximatively 25 % the NK activity (Wybran, 1985). This indicates that Met-Enk induces the release of factor(s) able to enhance NK activity. Preliminary experiments do not indicate that such factor(s) are linked to interferons. However, as we will discuss later, interleukin 2 may play a role in such findings. Finally as also indicated later Met-Enk enhances the mononuclear cells bearing the Leu 11 phenotype which is related to large granular lymphocytes and NK cells.

MET ENK AND SURFACE MASKERS

In these series of experiments, we have investigated whether Met-Enk can influence various surface antigens of human lymphocytes. We have used the following monoclonal antibodies OKT9 (transferrin receptor), OKT10 (activated T cells, immature T cells, NK cells, monocytes), OKIA1 (DR antigens), Leu 11 (NK cells belonging to the large granular lymphocytes) and Tac antiserum which recognizes the interleukin 2 receptor.

Blood mononuclear cells were incubated with various concentrations of Met-Enk, the cells were then washed and the surface antigens were detected with the monoclonal antibodies using secondary antibodies labelled with colloidal gold followed by silver sensitization and counterstained with a Giemsa stain (Romasco et al., 1985). The positive cells can be recognized by the presence of black granules on the cells. Met-Enk did not modify the percentages of OKT9 or Ia positive cells. However, very consistenly between 10^{-12} and 10^{-7} Mol, Met-Enk enhanced the percentages of OKT10, Leu 11 and Tac positive cells (e.g. for OKT10 from 27 % to 38 %, for Leu 11 from 13 % to 20 % and for Tac from 15 % to 22 %). These results are highly significant (from $p < 0.05$ to $p < 0.001$). When naloxone is incubated simultaneously with Met-Enk, the enhancing effect is completely inhibited for OKT10 and Leu 11 and almost completely for Tac. Here too, these results indicate that the induction of surface markers by Met-Enk is probably due to the opiate activities of Met-Enk.

Purified populations of blood B and T cells by monocyte removal still show the enhancing effect of Met-Enk on OKT10, Leu 11 and the interleukin 2 receptor indicating that monocytes are not necessary for this effect. In contrast, isolated T cell populations showed only an enhancement of OKT10 positive cells.

These findings indicate that Met-Enk acts directly on T cells. Furthermore, since T10 positive cells are also found in the NK population, these results indicate that the T10 increments were not due to NK cells since the Leu 11 cells were not increased using a pure T cell population. Finally since cells with Leu 11 phenotype were not increased in the T cell population, it is suggested that Met-Enk probably recruits non T pre NK cells rather than T pre NK cells.

Finally, the increases in Leu 11 positive cells have to be put in correlation with the enhancement of NK activity described above in the previous section. We have also performed indirect experiments using the supernatants of blood mononuclear cells incubated with various concentrations of Met-Enk as described in the previous section. The supernatant still enhances the percentages of OKT10 and Leu 11 positive cells as it has been observed with the NK activity.

INTERLEUKIN 2 PRODUCTION

We have investigated the influence of Met-Enk upon the production of interleukin 2 according the following experimental procedure. Human peripheral blood mononuclear cells are incubated with PHA and various concentrations of Met-Enk for 3 days. The supernatants are then tested on the mouse $CTLL_2$ IL_2 dependent T cell line by measuring thymidine incorporation.

The results indicate that Met-Enk at concentrations between 10^{-9} and 10^{-6} Mol increase the thymidine uptake (e.g. from 15,780 c.p.m. to 22,539 c.p.m. for 10^{-9} Mol of Met-Enk). Thus, Met-Enk enhances the production of interleukin 2.

IN VIVO EFFECTS OF MET-ENK IN HUMANO

1. LUNG CANCER PATIENTS

Met-Enk was administred intravenously at the dose of 50 µg/Kg or 100 µg/Kg to seven patients with lung cancer. These patients were newly diagnosed without prior surgery, chemotherapy, radiotherapy or immunotherapy. Some immunological tests were performed before and after Met-Enk administration (2 h, 24 h and day 6 post injection) (Wybran et al., 1985). The results can be summarized as follows : no toxic effects were observed. Out of seven patients, 4 showed an increase in the percentage of blood active T rosettes, 5 in the percentage of OKT10 blood lymphocytes, 7 in the percentage of the Leu 11 blood positive cells (in 4 more than twice the initial value). In these 7 patients, 5 showed an enhancement in NK activity (in 3, the NK activity increased by 100 %).

These effects were usually observed 24 h after Met-Enk injection and were usually no more seen at day 6.

The results of this study indicate that Met-Enk induces, in vivo, the same immunological changes as the ones observed in vitro.

2. AIDS PATIENT

One AIDS patient received a single injection of 20 µg/Kg of Met-Enk. Two hours after the injection, a slight increase in NK activity was seen as well as an enhancement of PHA response (4,300 c.p.m. to 14,000 c.p.m.) (Wybran and Schandené, 1985).

3. PRE AIDS PATIENT

One pre AIDS (ARC patient) patient was injected with Met-Enk. He received 3 injections weekly during 2 weeks of Met-Enk at 20 µg/Kg for the first week and at 50 µg/Kg for the second week (Nimeh et al., 1985; Wybran and Schandené, 1985). No toxic effect were seen. The following data were observed at day 11 : increase in leucocyte count from 2,300 to 3,800 per µl and lymphocytes counts from 700 to 1900 per µl. The following lymphocyte subpopulations were also increased : active T rosettes (182 to 541/µl), T 11 (604 to 1682), T4 (22 to 240), T3 (393 to 1402), T10 (437 to 1302) and Leu 11 (65 to 360). Natural killer activity against K 562 cells line augmented from 48 % to 69 % and PHA response increased from 590 c.p.m. to 14,963 c.p.m..

MECHANISMS OF ACTION OF MET-ENK

When taking into account both the in vitro and the in vivo data, one can postulate that Met-Enk is able to influence the immune system through a chain of events. Met-Enk is recognized by T lymphocytes through a specific opiate sensitive surface receptor. Such recognition leads to an induction of various T cell receptors like the sheep red blood cell receptors (active E rosette), the T10 receptors and the interleukin 2 receptors. In presence of a T cell mitogen like PHA, interleukin 2 production is enhanced. Met-Enk per se augments NK function probably by recruiting non T pre NK cells and acting directly on NK cells. All these mechanisms are observed in vitro and appear operative in vivo. They suggest that Met-Enk may act as molecules of lymphocyto activation (Wybran, 1985).

CONCLUSIONS : POTENTIAL ROLES FOR MET-ENK

1. Met-Enk, at very low concentrations, is able to trigger multiple mechanisms related to T cell activation as well as to NK function : does Met-Enk play a physiological role in the immune response ?

2. In patients with cancer, pre AIDS and perhaps AIDS, Met-Enk appears to be able to trigger mechanisms related to T cell and NK cell activation.

Can Met-Enk be used as therapeutical agent (immunomodulator, modifier of the biological response) in diseases with primary or secondary immunodeficiencies ? (Wybran, 1985).

3. Since stress induces the release of a variety of hormones with opposito immunological activities like cortisol (which suppresses some immune responses) and Met-Enk (which enhances some immune functions), can immune mechanisms be responsible (pathophysiology) for stress related diseases including psychosomatic medicine ?

4. Finally, Met-Enk provides a new humoral link by which the endocrine system, the nervous system and the immune system communicate. It appears that Met-Enk may be an integral part of a network system necessary to the communications between the three major systems (Wybran et al., 1979).

REFERENCES

Faith RE, Liang JH, Murgo AJ, Plotnikoff NP (1984). Neuroimmunomodulator with enkephalins : enhancement of human natural killer (NK) cell activity in vitro. Clin Immunol Immunopathol 31 : 412-418.
Johnson HM, Smith EM, Torres BA, Blalock JE (1983). Regulation of the in vitro antibody response by neuroendocrine hormones. Proceedings of the National Academy of Sciences 79 : 4171-4174.
Mehrishi JN, Mills IH (1983). Opiate receptors on lymphocytes and platelets in man. Clin Immunol Immunopathol 27, 240-249.

Mathews PM, Froelich CJ, Sibbit WL Jr, Bankhurst AD (1983). Enhancement of natural cytotoxicity by β-endorphin. J Immunol 130 : 1658-1662.

Miller GC, Murgo AJ, Plotnikoff NP (1983). Enkephalin-enhancement of active T-cell rosettes from lymphoma patients. Clin Immunol Immunopathol 26 : 446-451.

Miller GC, Murgo AJ, Plotnikoff NP (1984). Enkephalins : enhancement of active T cell rosettes from normal volunteers. Clin Immunol Immunopathol 31 : 132-137.

Nimeh NF, Plotnikoff NP, Miller GC, De Bruyere M, Latinne D, Sonnet J, Wybran J (1985). In preparation.

Plotnikoff NP, Miller GC (1983). Enkephalins as immunomodulators. Int J Immunopharmacol 5 : 437-441.

Romasco F, Rosenberg J, Wybran J (1985). An immunogold silver staining method for the light microscopical analysis of blood lymphocyte subsets with monoclonal antibodies. Amer J Clin Pathol (in press).

Wybran J, Levin AS, Fudenberg HH, Goldstein AL (1975). Thymosin : effects on normal human blood T cells. Ann N Y Acad Sci 249 : 300-307.

Wybran J, Appelboom T, Govaerts A (1978). Inosiplex, a stimulating agent for normal human T cells and human leucocytes. J Immunol 121 : 1184-1187.

Wybran J, Appelboom T, Famaey JP, Govaerts A (1979). Suggestive evidence for morphine and methionine-enkephalin receptors-like on normal blood T lymphocytes. J Immunol 123 : 1068-1070.

Wybran J, Dupont E (1982). The active T rosette : an early marker for T-cell activation. Ann Immunol (Paris) 133 : 211-218.

Wybran J (1985). Enkephalins and endorphins as modifiers of the immune system : present and future. Fed Proc 44 : 92-94.

Wybran J (1985). Enkephalins and endorphins : activation molecules for the immune system and natural killer activity ? Neuropeptides 5 : 371-374.

Wybran J (1985). Enkephalins as molecules of lymphocyte activation and modifiers of the biological response. In Plotnikoff NP, Murgo AJ, Faith RE (eds) : "Enkephalins-Endorphins : Stress and the Immune System", Plenum Press, New York (in press).

Wybran J, Schandené L (1985). In preparation.

Wybran J, Vandermoten G, Plotnikoff NP (1985). In preparation.

INHIBITION OF MACROPHAGE IN VIVO ACTIVATION BY PHARMACOLOGIC BLOCKADE OF PROLACTIN RELEASE.

Edward Bernton, Dan Hartmann*, Micheal Gilbreath, John Holaday, and Monte S. Meltzer

Walter Reed Army Institute of Research, Washington, D.C. 20307-5100 and Dept. of Pathology, Georgetown Univ. School of Medicine, Washington, D.C. 20007.*

Reports over several decades suggest that personality structure, life events, and behavioral stress alter the course of auto-immune disease, infection, and cancer (review, see Schindler 1985). Recent findings document these interactions between the immune and central nervous systems (CNS). One group of potential mediators for such interactions are anterior pituitary hormones: the synthesis and secretion of ACTH, beta-endorphin, TSH, and possibly gonadotropin by lymphocytes has been demonstrated (Blalock 1984); beta-endorphin and ACTH can modify lymphocyte function (Johnson 1983, Kay 1984, Johnson 1982).

We examined the role of prolactin in the immune response. Primarily regarded as a lactogenic stimulus, prolactin release is also a graded and sensitive response to stress. The target tissues for stress-induced prolactin release, however, are not known. Lymphocytes and monocytes have prolactin receptors (Russell 1984), and prolactin induces ornithine decarboxylase, an enzyme necessary for cell proliferation. Studies in rats (Nagy 1983) show that hypophysectomy or treatment with bromocryptine (a dopamine D_2 agonist that inhibits pituitary prolactin release) inhibits certain in vivo immunopathologic responses: adjuvant arthritis, experimental allergic encephalitis, and delayed cutaneous hypersensitivity. Simultaneous treatment with exogenous prolactin reverses this inhibition. However, the cellular locus of action within the immune system for these in vivo effects of bromocryptine or of prolactin are not known.

Tumoricidal activation of macrophages occurs following exposure, in vivo or in vitro, to lymphokines secreted by T-lymphocytes. Resident or elicited macrophages do not kill tumor cells unless activated by lymphokines. We examined effects of bromocryptine and pergolide (another D_2 agonist) treatment on in vivo activation of peritoneal macrophages 8 to 10 days following ip injection of 200ug killed Propriobacterium acnes.

Male C3H/HeN mice (6/group) were treated ip with 0.25 mg of bromocryptine, 0.1mg of pergolide mesylate, or vehicle, for 5 days beginning 1 day prior to injection of P.acnes. On day 8 to 10, peritoneal exudate cells (PEC) were harvested by sterile lavage. Pooled PEC from each group of mice were adjusted to equal numbers of macrophages, and cultured in 48 well plates. After washing to remove non-adherent cells, 5 x 10^4 ^{3}H-thymidine-labelled TU-5 tumor cells were added. Tumoricidal activity was estimated by measuring radiolabel released into culture fluids at 48 hrs and expressed as a percentage of total counts. Both bromocryptine and pergolide treatment diminished macrophage tumoricidal activity to levels comparable to resident macrophage controls (Table 1). Thus, mice treated with D_2 agonists fail to develop tumoricidal macrophages.

Table-1. The effect of bromocryptine and pergolide treatment on induction of tumoricidal macrophages in P.acnes-treated mice.

Macrophages/well:	Tumor Cytotoxicity		
	4×10^5	2×10^5	1×10^5
Mice treated with:			
nothing	10%	10%	10%
P.acnes + saline	85%	65%	20%
P.acnes + bromocryptine	20%	20%	10%
P.acnes + pergolide	15%	10%	10%

The first step for induction of tumoricidal PEC in P.acnes-treated mice is an inflamatory response. Total numbers of PEC per mouse and cell differentials were not significantly different 10 days following P.acnes in mice treated with bromocryptine, pergolide, or saline (Table 2). Thus, these drugs did not inhibit peritoneal inflammatory responses.

Table-2. The effects of bromocryptine and pergolide treatment on peritoneal inflamatory cells in P.acnes-treated mice.

	PEC/Mouse	Macros	Lymphs	Polys
resident cells	1.5×10^6	78%	18%	4%
P.acnes/saline	6.3×10^6	77%	12%	11%
P.acnes/bromocryptine	5.1×10^6	65%	17%	18%
P.acnes/bromocryptine + prolactin	4.2×10^6	71%	6%	23%

Consistent with this observation, we also found that macrophages from bromocryptine- or pergolide-treated mice can be fully activated in vitro: macrophage tumoricidal activity was evident in cells from both saline and P.acnes-treated mice after exposure to LK in vitro. That inflammatory responses and in vitro responses to LK were normal in bromocryptine-treated mice suggests the defect may be secondary to LK production by T cells in vivo.

Treatment with D_2-agonists may inhibit prolactin release, prevent a change in serum prolactin levels associated with antigen recognition, and thereby modulate the ensuing immune response. We examined prolactin levels 4 and 20 hours after injection of killed P.acnes or saline with and without treatment 2 hrs prior with 0.25mg bromocryptine (Table 3). Bromocryptine suppressed prolactin to nearly unmeasurable levels in both groups at 2 and 20 hrs. A significant decrease in serum prolactin also occurred after injection of P.acnes in mice not pretreated with bromocryptine, and was evident as early as 2 hrs following inoculation. Injection of another antigen, sheep red blood cells, caused a similar decrease in prolactin levels. Bromocryptine, which dramatically lowers serum prolactin, suppresses in vivo induction of tumoricidal macrophages. This suppression is prevented (Table 3) by simultaneous treatment with exogenous prolactin. Yet injection of P.acnes also results in lesser but significant decrease in prolactin. The response to P.acnes may be biphasic, an early decrease followed by a later increase. Alternately, macrophage induction may depend on non-pituitary secretion of prolactin into the immune cell micro-environment, undetectable in serum, with changes in serum levels being causally unrelated to macrophage activation.

Table-3. Changes in serum prolactin (ng/ml±SEM) at 4 and 20 hrs following bromocryptine treatment or injection with P.acnes.

TREATMENT:	4 HRS	20 HRS
saline / saline	22.0 ± 6.0	17.0 ± 3.0
saline / bromocryptine	.3 ± 0.1	.2 ± 0.1
P.acnes / saline	7.0 ± 3.0	11.0 ± 4.0
P.acnes / bromocryptine	.2 ± 0.1	.3 ± 0.1

The effect of pergolide treatment days 1-5 on induction of tumoricidal macrophages in P.acnes-injected mice was compared to effects of treatment on days 1 and 2 only, and days 4-7. (Table 4). Treatment days 1-2 only or on days 4-7 was not sufficient to inhibit macrophage activation. Thus, an early step in the pathway of macrophage activation may be blocked by pergolide, and several days of sustained treatment is required. It also argues against a direct toxic effect of pergolide on macrophages, as treatment on days 4-7 allows less time for recovery from drug exposure before harvest of macrophages.

Table-4. Treatment time requirements for inhibition of macrophage activation by pergolide.

TREATMENT:		Tumor Cytotoxicity
nothing		25%
P.acnes		45%
P.acnes + pergolide:		
	Days 1-5	25% *
	Days 1,2	50%
	Days 4-7	50%

We also examined whether pergolide or prolactin could directly affect tumoricidal effector mechanisms or the in vitro activation of starch-elicited peritoneal macrophages by lymphokines from PPD-stimulated spleen cells (Table 5). Pergolide, even at doses in excess of those achieved in vivo, does not inhibit activation of macrophages by lymphokines, nor does prolactin potentiate activation. In other experiments, prolactin could not substitute for lymphokines in activating macrophages, nor did pergolide added in vitro inhibit tumor killing in macrophages activated in vivo by P.acnes.

Table-5. In vitro effects of addition of lymphokines, pergolide, and prolactin to tumoricidal assays using starch-elicited PEC.

Starch-elicited MO:	Tumor Cytotoxicity
+ Media	5%
+ Lymphokines	30%
+ Lymphokines +PERG 6 ug/ml	30%
+ Lymphokines + PERG 30 ug/ml	25%
+ Prolactin 200ng/ml	10%
+ Lymphokines + Prolactin 200ng/ml	25%

The data above suggest that D_2-agonists inhibit macrophage activation in vivo, probably by a mechanism which decreases production of lymphokines. This mechanism might not necessarily involve the action of bromocryptine on pituitary prolactin release. The postranslational processing and release of proopiomelanocortin derivatives such as beta-endorphin in the rodent pars intermedia is also under dopaminergic control. Lymphocytes themselves could express D_2 receptors. Therefore we determined if treatment with exogenous prolactin would reverse the effects of bromocryptine. Mice (5/group) received i.p. injections of vehicle, bromocryptine 0.25 mg/day , or bromocryptine and ovine prolactin 100 ug/day, for the same 5 day treatment period used in prior experiments. Simultaneous prolactin treatment prevented the inhibition of macrophage tumor cytotoxicity seen in bromocryptine- treated mice (Table-6). While the inhibition of tumoricidal activity by bromocryptine and its restoration by prolactin could be effected via different mechanisms, this experiment strongly suggests that the effects of bromocryptine depend on its ability to inhibit prolactin release.

Table-6. Simultaneous administration of ovine prolactin prevents inhibition of macrophage tumoricidal activation by bromocryptine injections on days 1-5.

Mice Treated With:	Tumor Cytotoxicity
nothing	5%
P.acnes and:	
saline	45%
bromocryptine	20%
bromocryptine + prolactin	40% *

In sum, our results demonstrate that bromocryptine treatment severely inhibits the in vivo tumoricidal activation of peritoneal macrophages. The treatment time requirements of this effect, its reversibility in vitro by lymphokines, and the lack of in vitro inhibition by bromocryptine or pergolide of macrophage activation by lymphokines or of tumoricidal effector mechanisms all suggest that these drugs interfere with the production of macrophage activating factors by lymphocytes following stimulation by antigen. Supporting this hypothesis, preliminary data show that splenocytes from bromocryptine-treated mice made subnormal quantities of macrophage-activating factors following 48 hr incubation with concanavalin A (Con A) in serum-free medium. Simultaneous in vivo treatment with prolactin prevented this inhibition. Furthermore, under certain conditions, prolactin dramatically increases the proliferation of mouse splenocytes in response to Con A.

While D_2 agonists have many CNS actions, our data suggests their ability to alter patterns of prolactin release are critical to their immunomodulatory effects. Our results also suggest that antigen-recognizing or responding cells may convey information to the anterior pituitary, resulting in decreases in serum prolactin. Specific increases in serum gonadotropin levels occurring within hours after innoculation of mice with sheep red blood cells or allogenic but not syngeneic lymphocytes have been reported (Pierpaoli and Maestroni 1977). Since prolactin and gonadotropin levels vary reciprocally in response to most pharmacologic and physiologic stimuli (i.e. opiates, estrogens, lactation), these findings are consistent with our results. It was also demonstrated that drug treatment to block pituitary hormone release could block primary antibody response and subsequent amnestic response to T-dependent antigens administered during the treatment period (Pierpaoli and Maestroni 1977). Our findings indicate that T-lymphocyte responses involving the production of lymphokines, or perhaps earlier and more critical proliferative events, may be affected in vivo by a regulatory network including the neuroendocrine axis. Further studies should provide insight into the mechanisms by which immune cell products can modulate anterior pituitary hormone release, and by which lactogenic hormones may regulate lymphocyte proliferation and secretion.

REFERENCES

Blalock JE (1984). The immune system as a sensory organ. J. Immunol. 132(3):1067-1070.

Johnson HM, Torres BA, Smith EM, Dion LD, Blalock JE (1983). Regulation of lymphokine (gamma-interferon) production by corticotropin. J. Immmunol. 132(3):1067-1070.

Johnson HM, Smith EM, Torres BA, Blalock JE. (1982). Regulation of in vitro antibody response by neuro-endocrine hormones. Proc Natl Acad Sci. 79:4171-4174.

Kay N, Allen J, Morley J (1984). Endorphins stimulate normal peripheral blood lymphocyte NK activity. Life Sci. 35:53-59.

Nagy E, Berczi I, Wren G, Asa S, Kovacs K (1983). Immunomodulation by bromocryptine. Immunopharmacology 6(3):231-243.

Pierpaoli W, Maestroni G (1977). Pharmacologic control of the immune response by blockade of early hormonal changes following antigen injection. Cell. Immunol. 31:355-363.

Russell DH, Matrigian L, Kilber R, Larson D, Magun B (1984). Prolactin receptors on human lymphocytes and their modulation by cyclosporine. BBRC 121(3):899-906.

Schindler BA (1985). Stress, affective disorders and immune function. Med Clin of N Amer. 69(3):585-597.

IMMUNOREGULATORY MOLECULES MODULATE GLIAL CELL GROWTH

Etty N. Benveniste, Sally Kutsunai, and
Jean E. Merrill

Department of Neurology, University of California,
Los Angeles, California 90024

INTRODUCTION

The traditional role of the interleukins (IL1, IL2, IL3) is in the initiation, propagation, and regulation of the immune response (Gillis et al., 1978). IL1 released by a variety of cells including monocytes stimulates cells to produce IL2 (Larsson and Coutinho, 1979) which induces expansion of T cells. IL2 has recently been shown to induce differentiation (Kishi et al., 1985) and proliferation of B cells (Boyd et al., 1985), indicating that its action is not restricted to T cells. There is now evidence for regulation of growth of glial cells by monokines and lymphokines. Both astrocytes and oligodendrocytes proliferate in the presence of mitogen-induced T cell factors or supernatants from human T cell leukemia virus (HTLV) transformed T cells (Fontana et al., 1980, 1981; Merrill et al., 1984). Immature astrocytes proliferate in response to IL1 (Giulian and Lachman, 1985).

In addition Fontana et al. have shown astrocytes and glioma cell lines produce prostaglandin E (PGE) and an IL1-like factor (Fontana et al., 1982, 1984) which have effects on lymphoid cells, thus expanding the potential for an immune response in the central nervous system. We now have examined the role of immunoregulatory molecules in modulating glial cell growth.

MATERIALS AND METHODS

Primary glial cell cultures were established from 1-2 day old rat cerebral hemispheres (Merrill et al., 1984); a single cell suspension was plated in 75 cm^2 tissue culture flasks. On day seven, oligodendrocytes were separated from the astroglial cell monolayer by mechanical dislodgement and seeded at 2×10^4 cells/well in a Falcon Microtest II plate. On day 10, astrocytes were trypsinized and plated at 2×10^3 cells per well. After a 3-day exposure to immunoregulatory or astrocyte-conditioned medium (ACM), cells were pulsed with 1 µCi ^{3}H-thymidine and harvested on day 4. Purified IL1 was purchased from Cistron and Genzyme and used at 0.25-25 U/ml. Recombinant IL2 was obtained from AM-GEN and Genetics Institute and was used at 5-200 U/ml.

Astrocyte-conditioned media (ACM) was generated by incubating astrocytes for 7 days. ACM generated in the presence of indomethacin was produced from astroglial monolayers incubated for 3 days. Assessment of ACM for IL1 was by exposure of supernatants to the LBRM 33 mouse cell line for 24 hours. LBRM supernatants were then incubated on CTLL-2 cells (Linker-Israeli et al., 1983) and IL1 activity was expressed as IL2 U/ml.

RESULTS

As shown in Table 1, astrocytes in logarithmic growth produce IL1; as the cultures reach confluency, the cells stop producing IL1. PGE is also produced in early cultures and reaches a peak as the cells reach confluency. In contrast, ACM inducing oligodendrocyte proliferation is optimally derived from 4 to 5 week old cultures when astrocytes are confluent and PGE is no longer being produced. The production of PGE by astrocytes in culture inhibits concomitant production of astrocyte-derived IL1 and ACM (Table 2). While endogenous PGE inhibits astrocyte growth as evidenced by an increased proliferation in the presence of indomethacin, astrocytes are less sensitive to the inhibitory effects of PGE than are oligodendrocytes (Table 3).

Neither astrocytes nor oligodendrocytes produce IL2 (Table 1), but oligodendrocytes respond to recombinant IL2 at an optimal concentration of 50 U/ml (Fig. 1). Astrocytes do not proliferate to IL2 but show a modest increase (2-fold) in response to 10-20 units of IL1.

TABLE 1. Astroglial Secretion of Immunoregulatory Molecules

Conditions of Astroglial Monolayers	IL1 2-3 D†	PGE 3 D	ACM* 7 D	IL2 2-3 D
1. Log Growth Monolayer				
AGE: 2 weeks	N.D.	N.D.	++	–
3 weeks	+++	N.D.	+++	–
2. Confluent Monolayer				
AGE: 2 weeks	++	+++	±	–
3 weeks	+	+	±	–
4 weeks	±	±	+++	–

* ACM = Astroglial conditioned media
† Number of days of incubation
N.D. = Not done

TABLE 2. Indomethacin Regulation of Astroglial Immunoregulatory Molecules

Conditions	Conc. of Indo.	IL1 (units)	Oligo* Prolif. (cpm)
Conditioned media from astroglial monolayer (day 13-17) 3 day incubation	...	183 (–)	1749
	3×10^{-10} M	260 (+)	3537
	3×10^{-9} M	351 (++)	4185
	3×10^{-8} M	355 (++)	2105
Control media only: no cells present 3 day incubation	...	N.D.	2271
	3×10^{-10} M	N.D.	2851
	3×10^{-9} M	N.D.	1808
	3×10^{-8} M	N.D.	1902

* Induced by astroglial-conditioned media
N.D. – Not done

TABLE 3. Exogenous PGE Regulation of Glial Cells

Concentration of PGE	Oligo Proliferation (cpm)*	Astrocyte Proliferation (cpm)*
None	2087 ± 409	27,148 ± 708
3×10^{-5} M	215 ± 23	14,079 ± 1641
3×10^{-6} M	1495 ± 218	22,415 ± 751
		$p < 0.01$
3×10^{-7} M	1397 ± 294	25,200 ± 1042
	$p < 0.04$	N.S.
3×10^{-8} M	2225 ± 293	21,279 ± 2180
	N.S.	

* Mean ± Standard Error
N.S. = Not significant

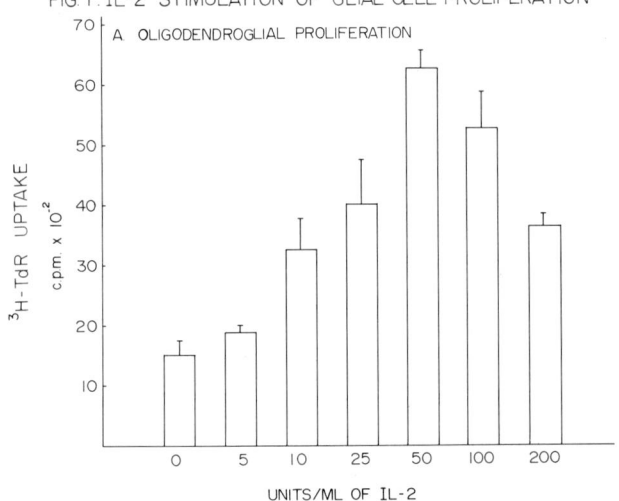

FIG. I. IL-2 STIMULATION OF GLIAL CELL PROLIFERATION
A. OLIGODENDROGLIAL PROLIFERATION

CONCLUSIONS

Our results demonstrate two new findings: (1) that recombinant IL2, previously shown to influence the growth of T and B cells is also capable of inducing proliferation of rat oligodendrocytes in vitro. To our knowledge, this is the first observation of IL2 stimulating a nonleukocytic cell and provides further evidence that cells of the central nervous system can be influenced by cells of the immune response. This could have major relevance in demyelinating diseases caused by chronic inflammatory infiltrates such as multiple sclerosis; (2) that astrocytes produce the regulatory molecules IL1, ACM, and PGE, which provide internal positive and negative signals for induction of proliferation of both glial cell types. This suggests that the central nervous system may influence both the immune component of a chronic inflammation as well as wound healing repair mechanisms of the brain itself.

REFERENCES

Boyd AW, Fischer DC, Fox DA, Schlossman SF, Nadler LM (1985). Structural and functional characterization of IL2 receptors on activated human B cells. J Immunol 134: 2387-2392.

Fontana A, Grieder A, Arrenbrecht ST, Grob PJ (1980). In vitro stimulation of glial cells by a lymphocyte-produced factor. J Neurol Sci 46:55-62.

Fontana A, Hengartner H, de Tribolet N, Weber EJ (1984). Glioblastoma cells release interleukin 1 and factors inhibiting interleukin 2-mediated effects. J Immunol 132: 1837-1844.

Fontana A, Kristensen F, Dubs R, Gemsa D, Weber E (1982). Production of prostaglandin E and an interleukin-1 like factor by cultured astrocytes and C_6 glioma cells. J. Immunol 129:2413-2419.

Fontana A, Otz U, DeWeck AL, Grob JJ (1981). Glial cell stimulating factor (GSF): A new lymphokine. J Neuroimmunol 2:73-81.

Gillis S, Ferm MM, Ou W, Smith KA (1978). T cell growth factor: Parameters of production and a quantitative microassay for activity. J Immunol 120:2027-2032.

Giulian D, Lachman LB (1985). Interleukin-1 stimulation of astroglial proliferation after brain injury. Science 228: 497-499.

Kishi H, Inui S, Muraguchi A, Hirano T, Yamamura Y, Kishimoto T (1985). Induction of IgG secretion in a human B cell clone with recombinant IL2. J Immunol 134: 3104-3107.

Larsson EL, Coutinho A (1979). The role of mitogenic lectins in T-cell triggering. Nature 280:239-241.

Linker-Israeli M, Bakke AC, Kitridrou RC, Gendler S, Gillis S (1983). Defective production of interleukin 1 and interleukin 2 in patients with systemic lupus erythematosus (SLE). J Immunol 130:2651-2655.

Merrill JE, Kutsunai S, Mohlstrom C, Hofman F, Groopman J, Golde DW (1984). Proliferation of astroglia and oligodendroglia in response to human T cell-derived factors. Science 224:1428-1430.

THE ASSOCIATION OF NERVES AND PLASMA CELLS IN A TEAR GLAND

Benjamin Walcott, Kent T. Keyser and Patrick A. Sibony

Departments of Anatomical Sciences (BW), Psychiatry (KTK), Ophthalmology and Neurology (PAS), School of Medicine, State University of New York, Stony Brook, New York 11794

INTRODUCTION

There is considerable evidence that suggests that the autonomic nervous system can modulate the activity of the immune system. This evidence includes the identification of neurotransmitter receptors on lymphocytes (eg. Loveland et al 1981), the effect of putative neurotransmitters such as substance P on lymphocyte activity (eg. Payan et al 1983), the location of nerves in lymphoid tissues (eg. Bulloch 1985) and the effect of the sympathetic nervous system on the immune response (eg Besedovsky et al 1979). We have been studying the secretory immune system and have developed a model system in which many aspects of the problem can be examined.

Immunoglobins are a major constituent of tears and are produced by plasma cells in the lacrimal glands (Albini et al 1974). The Harderian gland is a major lacrimal gland of birds and consists of a secretory epithelium which produces serous fluid and an interstitial cell population, most of which are plasma cells, that produces the immunoglobins. The lymphoid cells are numerous and are grouped among the secretory tubules and along the ducts. The gland is known to be densely innervated by the autonomic nervous system (Stammer 1964) although the distribution of the nerves within the gland was not clear. This paper summarizes our work to date on the nature and pattern of the innervation of the gland.

RESULTS

The avian Harderian gland is lobular with each lobe consisting of a cortical tubular secretory epithelium which drains into a central canal. The medullary region of each lobe consists of masses of interstitial cells most of which are plasma cells (Fig 1). The gland is highly vascularized although there are no muscular walled vessels within the stroma of the gland. Ultrastructural examination

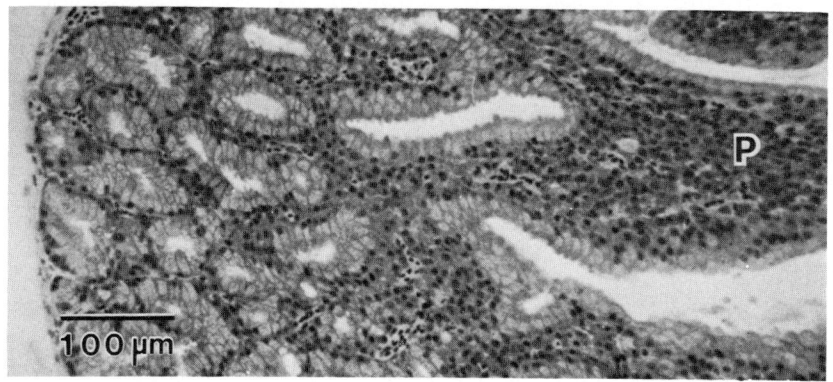

Fig. 1. Light micrograph of the structure of the Harderian gland. Note the large number of plasma cells (P) in the medulla.

of the medulla showed many large bundles of nerves among the plasma cells (Fig 2).

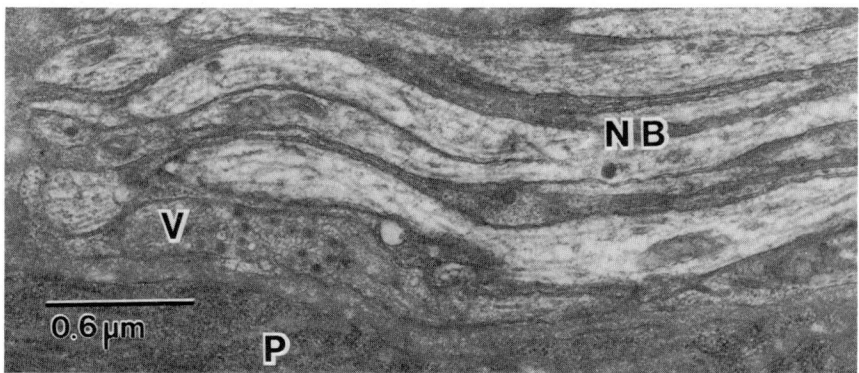

Fig. 2. Electron micrograph showing a nerve bundle (NB), varicosity (V) and plasma cell (P).

In some cases, vesicle filled varicosities were observed,

suggestive of autonomic transmitter release sites. Histochemistry and immunocytochemistry were used to characterize the nature of the neurotransmitters present in these nerves.

We used a modification of the Coupland and Holmes method (Walcott and McLean 1985) to reveal the acetylcholinesterase (AChE) positive fibers. There is a network of these fibers which is particularly dense in the medulla of the gland (Fig 3). This staining is blocked by

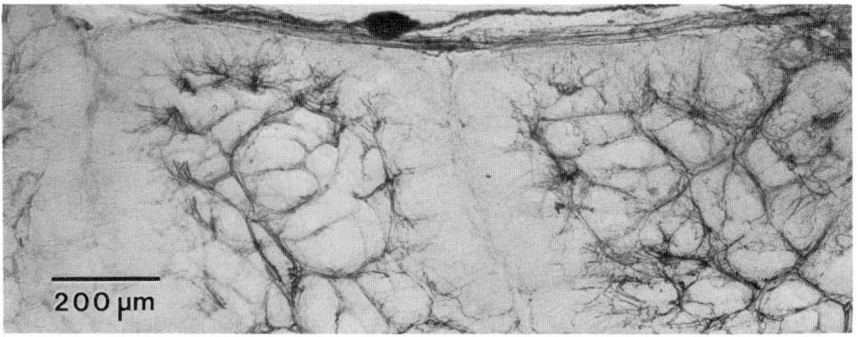

Fig. 3 Histochemistry of a thick frozen section of the gland showing AChE positive fibers.

the specific inhibitor, BW 284 C51. The adjacent pterygopalatine ganglion which is thought to provide innervation to the gland is also positive for AChE. The

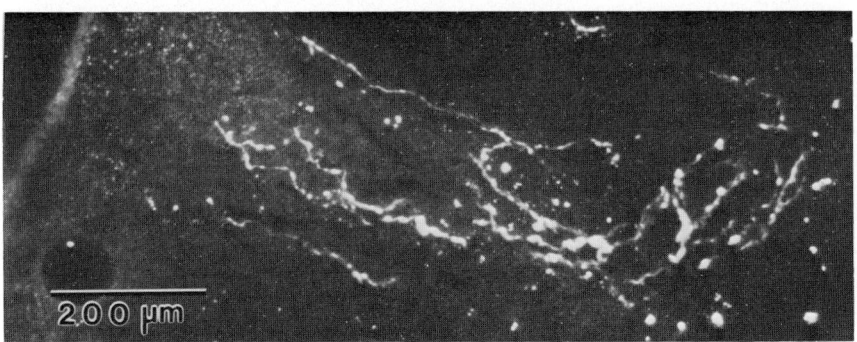

Fig. 4 Glyoxylic acid histochemical staining of a 12 um frozen section revealing the catecholamine fibers within the medulla of the gland.

Falck-Hillarp and glyoxylic acid histochemical methods showed many positive catecholamine fibers which ramified extensively and gave rise to varicosities among the interstitial cells (Fig 4). This was confirmed using an ultrastructural chromaffin method to reveal dense-cored amine containing vesicles.

Immunohistochemistry was used to determine the presence of some putative small peptide neurotransmitters/ modulators in the gland. Commercial antisera were used with a conventional indirect immunoflourescent method. Controls for selectivity were carried out by pre-absorbing the antisera with an excess of pure peptide. There was consistent and extensive substance p-like (SPL) (Fig 5) and vasoactive intestinal polypeptide-like (VIPL) (Fig 6) immunoreactivity within the gland. Again, as with the

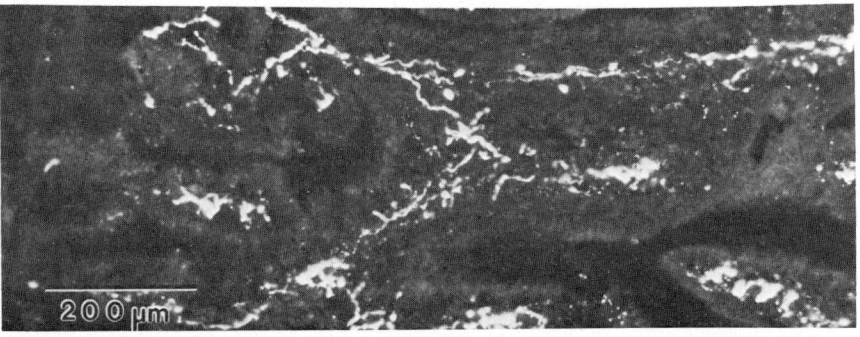

Fig. 5 Indirect immunoflourescence showing substance P-like immunoreacitivity.

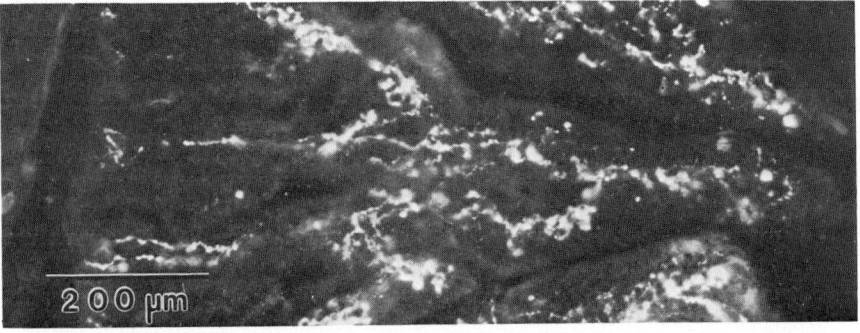

Fig. 6 Indirect immunoflourescence showing vasoactive intestinal polypeptide-like immunoreactivity in the medulla of the gland.

catecholamine fibers, the small peptide staining was predominantly within the medulla of the gland.

Most of the neurons in the pterygopalatine ganglion as well showed VIPL immunoreactivity. The source of the SPL immunoreactive fibers is not known.

At the time of hatching, the gland is formed but does not contain lymphocytes. At this time there were AChE positive fibers and weak SPL and VIPL immunoreactivity but no catecholamine fibers could be detected within the gland. As the chicks aged, the gland grew and became populated with plasma cells until the adult size was reached at about 50-60 days after hatching. During this time, the amount of small peptide immunoreactivity increased and catecholamine positive fibers appeared. The adult levels of catecholamines were not observed histochemically until after the birds are 60 days old.

DISCUSSION

Our results confirmed previous studies which show that the avian Harderian gland is extensively innervated by fibers of the autonomic nervous system that are positive for both catecholamines and AChE. However, we have also showed the presence of substance P-like and vasoactive intestinal polypeptide-like immunoreactivity. We have also shown that the distribution of the innervation is mainly to those regions of the gland rich in lymphocytes and ultrastructurally, we have observed vesicle filled varicosities near plasma cells (Walcott and McLean 1985). These anatomic data suggest that there may be neuro-modulation of the secretory immune response in this system.

The avian Harderian gland differs from mammalian lacrimal glands in that it contains a larger number of lymphocytes although the concentration of immunoglobins in the tears is similar. Mammalian lacrimal glands also have AChE and catecholamine fibers (eg Huhtal et al 1977) and there is VIP-like immunoreactivity (Dartt et al 1984). In these mammalian systems, however, the density of the amine and neuropeptide fibers is much less than that seen in the bird. It is tempting to correlate this observation with the differing quantity of interstial cells.

Functional studies have shown that acetylcholine and VIP have a stimulatory effect on the secretion of mammalian lacrimal glands (eg Dartt et al 1984) and substance P has been reported to stimulate rat salivary glands (Kudo 1983). Thus it is possible that these transmitters could serve two roles in the avian gland, one to stimulate the secretion of tear fluid and the other to increase the rate of release of immunoglobins by activated plasma cells. Functional studies currently underway on the effect of transmitters on gland fragments directly address this possibility.

Acknowledgements:

We are grateful to Cissy McKeon for her expert help and to Chris Laverach and Jane Blanchard for technical assistance. Supported by NIH NS 19350 (to BW).

REFERENCES

Albini B., Wick G., Rose E., Orlans E. (1974) Immunoglobin production in chicken Harderian glands.
Int. Arch. Allergy 47: 23

Besedovsky, H.O., del Ray, A., Sarkin, E., DePrada M., Keller, H.H. (1979) Immunoregulation mediated by the sympathetic nervous system.
Cell Immunol. 48: 346-355

Bulloch, K. (1985) Neuroanatomy of lymphoid tissue: a review. in "Neural Modulation of Immunity" ed. R. Guillemin et al Raven Press
New York pp. 111-141

Dartt, D.A., Baker, A.K., Vaillant C., Rose, P.E. (1984) Vasoactive intestinal polypeptide stimulation of protein secretion from rat lacrimal gland ascini.
Am. J. Physiol. 247: G502-509

Huhatala, A., Huikuri, K.T., Palkama, A.,Tervo, T. (1977) Innervation of the rat Harderian gland by adrenergic and cholinergic nerve fibers.
Anat. Rec. 188: 263-272

Kudo, T., Inoki, R., Nishimoto, T., Akai, M., Shiosaka, S., Tohyama, M. (1983) A possible role of substance P in the salivary secretion in rats.
Adv. Exptl. Med. Biol. 156: 681-692

Loveland, B.E., Jarrott, B., McKenzie, I.F.C. (1981) The detection of beta-adrenoceptors on murine lymphocytes.
J. Immunopharm. 3: 45-55

Payan, D.G., Brewster, D.R., Goetzl, E.J. (1983) Specific stimulation of human T lymphocytes by substance P.
J. Immunol. 131: 1613-1615

Stammer, A. (1964) Ein Beitrag zur Struktur un mikroskopischen Innervation der Harderschen Druse der Vogel. Acta Univ. Szegedinsis 10: 99

Walcott, B., McLean, J.R. (1985) Catecholamine containing neurons and lymphoid cells in a lacrimal gland of the pigeon. (1985) Brain Res. 328: 129-137

Section V. Development and Differentiation of Macrophages

REGULATION OF THE PRODUCTION, CLONING OF THE COMPLEMENTARY (cDNA), AND FUNCTIONS OF HUMAN MACROPHAGE GROWTH FACTOR, CSF-1

Peter Ralph

Department of Cell Biology, Cetus Corporation, Emeryville, California 94608

INTRODUCTION

Mature blood cells are derived from precursors in the bone marrow. This hemopoietic development originates from a totipotent stem cell whose progeny are progressively more restricted in their development. The generation of the different types of blood cell is regulated by a number of growth and differentiation factors. Some, such as the pleuripoietins or murine IL-3, are growth factors for the very immature precursor cells and can cause complete differentiation of some lineages of blood cells. Other factors are restricted to one or two lineages of blood cells and promote the growth and subsequent differentiation of the respective progenitor cell. Thus, NM-CSF (GM-CSF) is the factor for the production of mature neutrophils and macrophages, N-CSF (G-CSF) for neutrophils and CSF-1 (M-CSF) for macrophages. They are called colony-stimulating factors (CSF) because the convenient assay is the formation of a colony of mature cells from a single precursor cell in semi-solid culture (Metcalf, 1984).

Although most of the CSF's have been partially purified, the small quantities available from natural sources have hindered their biochemical and biological characterization. Recently, the complementary DNA (cDNA) for murine IL-3 (Fung et al., 1984; Yokota et al., 1984), and murine (Gough et al., 1984) and human NM-CSF (Wong et al., 1985) have been cloned. The large amount of these growth factors that will thus be made available through recombinant DNA technology will greatly aid our understanding of the physiological and pharmacological mechanisms of hemopoiesis. I will now describe the production, amino acid sequence, and cloning and characterization of the cDNA for human CSF-1, the macrophage growth factor.

RESULTS

Human CSF-1 is a glycoprotein of dimer structure found in urine and serum (Das et al., 1981). Human CSF-1 has about one-fifth the activity as a colony-stimulating factor for human bone marrow cells compared with NM-CSF, when the two preparations are nomalized to their activity on mouse bone marrow cells. However, the colonies produced in semi-solid media are almost all macrophage type with either assay species (Das et al., 1981; Ralph et al., 1985; P. Greenberg and H. E. Broxmeyer, personal communications).

Induced Production of CSF-1

CSF-1 as well as a small amount of NM-CSF is produced constitutively by the human pancreatic carcinomas MIA-PaCa-2 and Panc-1 when grown in 10% fetal bovine serum (FBS) (Wu et al., 1979). In order to produce CSF-1 in a low protein medium for ease of purification, serum-free formulations were tested. As the serum concentration was lowered, the CSF-1 levels in the supernatants of MIA-PaCA and Panc dropped, and in serum-free media including HB-104 (Hana Biologics) and Iscove's with insulin, human transferrin and human albumin CSF-1 was practically undetectable. Addition of phorbol myristic acetate (PMA) reinduced CSF-1 production to levels similar to that in 10% FBS (Ralph et al., 1985).

Amino Acid Sequences of Human Murine CSF-1

Examination of murine CSF-1 purified from L929 cells yielded an N-terminal 39 amino acid sequence and a 25 amino acid sequence from an internal cyanogen bromide fragment. Human urinary CSF-1 was also purified and the sequence of the first 12 amino acids was determined. This sequence was highly homologous to the N-terminus of murine CSF-1, differing at only two positions (Boosman et al., 1985).

Isolation of Human CSF-1 Genomic Clones

Using the oligonucleotides probes based on the amino acid sequence data, a human genomic library was screened and several CSF-1 genomic clones were isolated. Nine separate phage isolates shared a common 3.8 kilobase (kb) fragment that contained an exon coding for the N-terminus of the mature protein, an intron, and a second coding region corresponding to the N-terminal 39 amino acid sequence obtained from the murine CSF-1. A 32 base oligonucleotide probe (Exon II probe) was derived for screening a cDNA bank (Kawasaki et al., 1985). The frequency of the active mRNA in MIA-PaCa cells is estimated at one in a million.

Isolation of Human CSF-1 cDNA Clones

Messenger RNA was isolated from the MIA-PaCA line cultured serum-free and induced for CSF-1 production by PMA. To partially enrich for CSF-1 RNA sequences, mRNA was fractionated on a sucrose gradient. Aliquots of the size fractions were injected in Xenopus frog oocytes and the supernatants tested in a mouse bone marrow proliferation assay (Moore and Rouse, 1983). Aliquots were also dot blotted and probed with the exon II oligonucleotide. The biological activity and probe-positive peaks were pooled for construction of a DNA bank by the Okayama Berg method. Approximately 300,000 cDNA clones were screened with the exon II probe. Ten colonies were picked, colony purified, and plasmid DNA prepared. The purified DNAs were screened by a transient expression assay in primate COS-7 cells. Only one clone, clone 17, expressed CSF-1 bioactivity. The other nine clones were inactive in this assay (Kawasaki et al., 1985).

Characterization of CSF-1 Produced in COS-7 cells.

Clone 17 transfected into COS-7 produced about 2000 U/ml CSF-1 by the mouse proliferation and specific radioreceptor assays. As shown in Table 1, the bone marrow colony cells generated by the clone 17 transfection were 85% macrophage type and a specific rabbit antiserum that neutralizes native CSF-1 completely blocked colony formation. As a control, another source of CSF, GCT that contains mainly NM-CSF, generated mostly neutrophil-macrophage mixed colonies. One of the negative cDNA clones, clone 12 is shown to have no detectable CSF-1 or other CSF.

Structure of the CSF-1 cDNA Clones and Predicted Amino Acid Sequence of CSF-1

Sequence analysis of clone 17 indicated that there was only one methionine codon upstream of the start of the presumptive mature protein, yielding a presumed leader sequence of 32 amino acids. The sequence following the leader matches exactly the predicted amino acid sequence obtained from the N-terminus of human urinary CSF-1, extending a total length of 224 amino acids. There are two potential N-linked glycosylation sites (Asn-X-Ser/Thr) in the mature protein.

Analysis of the inactive clones, revealed several anomalies, including the presence of 115 bases of an intron that apparently was not spliced out accurately. These clones are inactive in the COS-7 cell assay because there is a stop codon immediately after the beginning of the intron sequence resulting in a very short protein of only 23 amino acids excluding the leader peptide (Kawasaki et al, 1985).

Analysis of CSF-1 mRNA and Its Gene

Northern analysis of the mRNA from MIA-PaCa cells showed several species of mRNA ranging in size from 1.5 to 4.5 kb. Because there were so many species of CSF-1 mRNAs, the possibility existed that they were transcribed from a family of CSF-1 genes. However, Southern analysis using four restriction endonucleases suggest that CSF-1 is encoded by a unique gene. If two or more closely related genes exist, their sequences would have to be highly homologous over many kilobases to give the simple restriction pattern obtained here. The restriction pattern of the genomic clone also suggested the existence of only one CSF-1 gene.

A computer screen of the amino sequence of CSF-1 with the sequences recorded in the National Protein Information Resource data base showed no significant homology. In addition, the recently published sequences for other hemopoietic factors, including human GM-CSF, erythropoietin (Jacobs et al., 1985), erythroid-potentiating activity (Gasson et al., 1985), interluekin-1 alpha and beta (March et al., 1985) and interleukin-3 showed no obvious homology.

DISCUSSION

CSF-1 has direct stimulating effects on the mature monocyte and macrophage, in addition to being a growth and differentiation factor for bone marrow precursors (Table 2). It stimulates the production of prostaglandin, interleukin-1 (IL-1), and the neutral protease, plasminogen activator. It is a cofactor for production of interferon and a separate tumor toxic factor. Other experiments suggest that CSF-1 stimulates macrophages to kill tumor cells and increases the phagocytosis and intracellular killing of the yeast microorganism Candida. Our preliminary results and the research by Metcalf and Nicola (1985) and by Motoyoshi et al., (1982) also indicated that CSF-1 will induce the production of N or NM-CSF by monocytes and macrophages. We therefore anticipate (Table 3) that pharmacological effects of CSF-1 may find clinical utility in restoring monocyte and neutrophil numbers that have been reduced by myelosuppressive chemotherapy or gamma irradiation for cancer treatment or bone marrow transplantation, and in naturally occurring leukopenias. CSF-1 may also have direct promoting effects on mononuclear phagocytes that will improve the body's resistance to infectious diseases - viral, bacterial and fungal - and that will stimulate the macrophages within tumors to destroy the neoplastic cells. The recent finding that the CSF-1 receptor is identical or closely related to the proto-oncogene c-fms (Sherr et al, 1985) suggests that this growth factor-receptor system may also be involved in oncogenesis.

TABLE 1. Expression of CSF-1 cDNA In COS-7 Cells

Sample	RRA	BM Prolif. Assay	BM Colony Assay	Colony Morphology
Clone 17	+	+	+	85% M
Clone 17 + NR	ND	+	+	
Clone 17 + a CSF-1	ND	-	-	
Clone 12	-	-	ND	
CSF-1	+	+	+	94% M
GCT	(-)	ND	+	15% M/85% NM

Supernatants of COS-7 cells tranfected with cDNA clone 17 or clone 12 were assayed for CSF-1 by the CSF-1 specific radioreceptor assay (RRA), and mouse bone marrow proliferation and colony assays. Normal rabbit (NR) and specific anti-CSF-1 antibody (a CSF-1) were tested for neutralizing the activity. Partially purified CSF-1 from MIA-PaCa cells and a predominately neutrophil-macrophage (NM)-CSF (GCT, GIBCO) preparations were used as controls.

TABLE 2. Stimulation of Mature Macrophage and Monocyte Functions by CSF-1

Function	Reference
Plasminogen activator production	Lin and Gordon 1979
PGE production	Ralph 1984
IL-1 production	Moore et al., 1980
pIC-induced IFN production	Ralph 1984 Warren 1985
Intracellular killing of candida	Ralph 1984
Tumor cytotoxicity	Wing et al., 1982
Tumor cytotoxin	Warren 1985

Table 3. Expected Pharmacologic Effects of CSF-1 In Vivo

o Restore monocyte and neutrophil numbers reduced during:

  Myelosuppressive chemotherapy for cancer
  Gamma irradiation for bone marrow transplantation

o Improve resistance to infection in patients at risk:

  Cancer, bone marrow transplantation
  Immunodeficiencies and leukopenias
  Elderly
  During major surgery

o Anti-cancer therapy via stimulation of macrophages

REFERENCES

Boosman A, Strickler JE, Wilson KJ, Stanley ER (1985). Partial amino acid sequences of human and murine mononuclear phagocyte growth factor, CSF-1. Submitted for publication.

Das SK, Stanley ER, Guilbert LJ, Forman LW (1981). Human colony-stimulating factor (CSF-1) radioimmunoassay: Resolution of three subclasses of human colony-stimulating factors. Blood 58: 630-641.

Fung MC, Hapel AJ, Ymer S, Cohen DR, Johnson RM, Campbell HD, Young IG (1984). Molecular cloning of cDNA for murine interleukin-3. Nature 307: 233-237.

Gasson JC, Golde DW, Kaufman SE, Westbrook CA, Hewick RM, Kaufman RJ, Wong GG, Temple PA, Leary AC, Brown EL, Orr EC, Clark SC (1985). Molecular characterization and expression of the gene encoding human erythroid-potentiating activity. Nature 315: 768-771.

Gough NM, Gough J, Metcalf D, Kelso A, Grail D, Nicola NA, Burgess AW, Dunn AR (1984). Molecular cloning of cDNA encoding a murine haematopoietic growth regulator, granulocyte-macrophage colony stimulating factor. Nature 309: 763-767.

Jacobs K, Shoemaker C, Rudersdorf R, Neill SD, Kaufman RJ, Mufson A, Seehra J, Jones SS, Hewick R, Fritsch EF, Kawakita M, Shimizu T, Miyake T (1985). Isolation and characterization of genomic and cDNA clones of human erythropoietin. Nature 313: 806-810.

Kawasaki ES, Ladner MB, Wang AM et al. Molecular cloning of a cDNA encoding human macrophage-specific colony stimulating factor (CSF-1). Science In press.

Lin H-S, Gordon S (1979). Secretion of plasminogen activator by bone marrow-derived mononuclear phagocytes and its enhancement by colony-stimulating factor. J Exp Med 150: 231-245.

March CJ, Mosley B, Larsen A, Douglas PC, Braedt G, Price V, Gillis S, Henney CS, Kronheim SR, Grabstein K, Conlon PJ, Hopp TP, Cosman D (1985). Cloning, sequence and expression of two distinct human interleukin-1 complementary DNAs. Nature 315: 641-647.

Metcalf D (1984). The Haemopoietic Colony Stimulating Factors (Elsevier, Amsterdam).

Metcalf D, Nicola NA (1985). Synthesis by mouse peritoneal cells of G-CSF: Stimulation by endotoxin, M-CSF and multi-CSF. Leuk Res 9: 35-50.

Moore RN, Oppenheim JJ, Farrar JJ, Carter CS jr, Waheed A, Shadduck RK (1980). Production of lymphocyte-activating factors (interleukin 1) by macrophages activated with colony-stimulating factors. J Immunol 125: 1302-1305.

Moore RN, Rouse BT (1983). Enchanced responsiveness of

committed macrophage precursors to macrophage-type colony stimulating factor (CSF-1) induced in vitro by interferons $\alpha+\beta$. J. Immunol 131: 2374-2379.

Motoyoshi K, Suda T, Kusumoto K, Takaku F, Miura Y (1982). Granulocyte-macrophage colony-stimulating and binding activities of purified human urinary colony-stimulating factor to murine and human bone marrow cells. Blood 60: 1378-1386.

Ralph P (1984). Activating factors for nonspecific and antibody-dependent cytotoxicity by human and murine mononuclear phagocytes. Lymphokine Res 3: 153-161.

Ralph P, Warren MK, Lee MT, Csejtey J, Weaver J, Kawasaki ES (1985). Inducible production of human macrophage growth factor, CSF-1. Submitted for publication.

Warren, MK (1985). Increased production of interferon, colony stimulation factor and tumor toxin by human monocytes treated with CSF-1. Manuscript in preparation.

Wing EJ, Waheed A, Shadduck RK, Nagle LS, Stephenson K (1982). Effect of colony stimulation factor on murine macrophages. J Clin Invest 69: 270-276.

Wong GG, Witek JS, Temple PA, Wilkens KM, Leary AC, Luxenberg DP, Jones SS, Brown EL, Kay RM, Orr EC, Shoemaker C, Golde DW, Kaufman RJ, Hewick RM, Wang EA, Clark SC (1985). Human GM-CSF: Molecular cloning of the complementary DNA and purification of the natural and recombinant proteins. Science 228: 810-815.

Wu M-C, Cini JK, Yunis AA (1979). Purification of a colony-stimulating factor from cultured pancreatic carcinoma cells J Biol Chem 254: 6226-6235.

Yokota T, Lee F, Rennick D, Hall C, Arai N, Mosmann T, Nabel G, Cantor H, Arai K-I (1984). Isolation and characterization of a mouse cDNA clone that expresses mast-cell growth-factor activity in monkey cells. Proc Natl Acad Scie 81: 1070-1074.

ACKNOWLEDGMENTS

I thank Drs. A. Boosman, E. S. Kawasaki, M. B. Ladner, E. R. Stanley, K. Warren and T. White for their unpublished data and help.

Leukocytes and Host Defense, pages 243-251
© 1986 Alan R. Liss, Inc.

BIOCHEMICAL MECHANISM OF SIGNAL TRANSMITTANCE BY Fc RECEPTORS FOR IgG2a AT THE SURFACE OF A MURINE MACROPHAGE-LIKE CELL LINE, P388D1: ACTIVATION OF ADENYLATE CYCLASE BY IgG2a-BINDING PROTEINS.

Tsuneo Suzuki and Rafael Fernandez-Botran

Department of Microbiology, University of Kansas Medical Center, Kansas City, Kansas 66103

Introduction

Murine macrophages and macrophage-like cell line such as P388D1 carry on their surface at least two biochemically distinct Fc receptors, one specific for IgG2a (Fcγ2aR) and another for IgG2b (Fcγ2bR) (Walker, 1976; Anderson & Grey, 1978; Suzuki et al, 1982a). FcγR plays an essential role in antibody-dependent cell-mediated cytotoxicity (Perlman et al, 1972), suppression of humoral immune response or B cell differentiation by circulating immune complexes (Uhr & Moller, 1968; Kolsch et al, 1980), or triggering of prostaglandin synthesis by macrophages (Bonney et al, 1979). Two different FcγRs should therefore transmit, upon binding of specific ligands, signals unique to each type which lead to the regulation of cellular functions. Indeed, we have shown that FcγR which triggers the arachidonic acid metabolic cascade upon binding of immune complex (IC) on the surface of P388D1 cells is the one specific for IgG2b but not that for IgG2a (Nitta & Suzuki, 1982b), by activating phospholipase A2 associated with Fcγ2bR within the lipid bilayer (Suzuki et al, 1982a). Prostaglandins, whose synthesis is triggered by Fcγ2bR, then activate the membrane adenylate cyclase via prostaglandin receptors. The binding of IC2a to Fcγ2aR leads to the intracellular accumulation of cAMP by the mechanism which differs from a classical hormone sensitive pathway (Nitta & Suzuki, 1982c).

In this paper, we briefly summarize our recent works which showed that Fcγ2aR activates, upon binding of IC2a, the catalytic subunit of the adenylate cyclase system through cooperation with second protein components copurified with them by the mechanism independent of stimulatory G/F protein.

Results

Our previous works (Nitta & Suzuki, 1982c) raised a question of whether or not Fcγ2aR confers its effect directly on the catalytic subunit of adenylate cyclase, because Fcγ2aR-mediated increase of intracellular cAMP was not affected by a stimulator of G/F protein. We have examined this question by testing the ability of IgG2a-binding proteins isolated from the detergent lysate of P388D1 cells and inserted into liposomes to activate, upon fusion, adenylate cyclase activity of G/F protein-dificient cyc⁻ cell membrane, particularly because cyc⁻ cells are found by EA rosetting technique not to carry Fcγ2aR on their surface, as follows.

1. Isolation and fractionation of IgG-binding (IgG-B) proteins. IgG-B proteins and phosphatidylcholine (PC)-binding proteins were extracted from the detergent lysate of 5×10^9 P388D1 cells (containing the cells biosynthetically radiolabeled with ^{14}C-leucine and also externally radiolabeled with ^{125}I) by affinity chromatography over the columns of Fab-, PC- and IgG-Sepharose connected in tandem in this order as described (Suzuki et al, 1982a). Subsequent Sephadex G-100 gel filtration of IgG-B proteins in the presence of 6 M urea yielded about 55% of the material as a sharp peak in the void volume and about 45% as a broad shoulder material that followed the first peak. They were denoted as IgG-B1 and IgG-B2, respectively. IgG-B1 and PC-B proteins were further purified by isoelectric focusing as described.

2. Insertion of IgG-B1, IgG-B2 and PC-B proteins into liposomes. IgG-B1, IgG-B2, and PC-B proteins (24 to 14 ug) were then inserted into liposomes consisting of phosphatidylcholine and phosphatidylethanolamine (1/1, w/w) by the method of Cerione et al, (1983). Liposomes containing 10 ug of IgG-B1 inhibited about 43% of EA2a but none of EA2b rosetting by S49 cells, whereas those containing 10 ug of PC-B proteins inhibited about 32% of EA2b, but none of EA2a rosetting by S49 cells. Thus, at least portion of the IgG-B1 and PC-B proteins inserted into liposomes are oriented themselves in a proper fashion.

Table 1. Changes in adenylate cyclase activity of cyc⁻ membranes upon fusion with liposome preparations in the presence or absence of NaF, IC2a, or IC2b.

Proteins in Liposomes	NaF[1]	IC2a[2]	IC2b	AC activity (pmol/mg/30 min)	% Change in AC Activity
None	−	−	−	43.1±18.5	
	+	−	−	50.6±15.1	
	−	+	−	34.1± 9.9	
	−	−	+	36.5±10.0	
IgG-B1	−	−	−	48.8±14.2	+ 13.2
	+	−	−	64.0±10.2	+ 26.5
	−	+	−	42.9±15.3	+ 25.8
	−	−	+	46.9± 9.4	+ 28.5
IgG-B2	−	−	−	50.6±21.8	+ 17.4
	+	−	−	36.6± 6.5	− 27.7
	−	+	−	37.3± 7.6	+ 9.4
	−	−	+	37.6±11.9	+ 3.0
IgG-B1 & IgG-B2	−	−	−	50.4±13.2	+ 16.9
	+	−	−	44.7±14.2	− 11.7
	−	+	−	125.3±30.8	+267.4**
	−	−	+	43.5± 7.0	+ 19.2
PC-B	−	−	−	49.3±16.6	+ 14.4
	+	−	−	28.6±14.2	− 45.5
	−	+	−	19.9± 6.5	− 58.4*
	−	−	+	7.2± 3.1	− 80.3**

1. NaF (10 mM)
2. IC2a & IC2b (10 ug/ml)
* $p<0.05$
** $p<0.02$

3. **Activation of adenylate cyclase of cyc⁻ cells with liposome-inserted IgG-B proteins.** Liposomes containing IgG-B1, IgG-B2, or PC-B proteins were fused separately with cyc⁻ cells by the method of Schramm (1979). The adenylate cyclase assays of hybrid membranes performed by the method of Salomon (1979) gave results summarized by Table 1. Thus, the fusion of cyc⁻ cells with liposomes containing either IgG-B1 or -B2 proteins alone did not significantly affect adenylate cyclase of cyc⁻ membrane in the presence or absence of NaF or ICs. However, the fusion of cyc⁻ cells with the 1 to 1 mixturre (w/w) of the liposomes containing IgG-B1 and those containing IgG-B2 proteins was found to result in about 3.7 fold enhancement in the enzymatic activity over the control, when assayed in the presence of IC2a ($p<0.02$). Neither NaF nor IC2b stimulated the enzymatic activity of this hybrid membrane. The prior boiling for 2 min or pronase treatment for 3 hr at 37°C of liposome preparations totally eliminated the capability of IgG-B1 and -B2 proteins to stimulate cyc⁻ membrane adenylate cyclase. The fusion of PC-B protein-containing liposomes with cyc⁻ cells resulted, on the other hand, in a significant suppression of the enzymatic activity, particularly in the presence of IC2b ($p<0.02$).

4. **Effects of soluble IgG-B proteins on cyc⁻ membrane adenylate cyclase.** Since adenylate cyclase of cyc⁻ cells has been shown to be reconstituted by cholate extracts of S49 cells (Sternweiss & Gilman, 1979), the effects of IgG-B1 and of cyc⁻ membrane was also investigated. As shown in Table 2, the enzymatic activity of cyc⁻ membranes were, in two separate experiments, about 2.4 to 2.3 fold increased by the mixtures of IgG-B1 and -B2 proteins in the presence of IC2a over the buffer control ($p<0.02$). The activating effects of the mixtures were again not augmented by NaF (10 mM).

5. **Other factors affecting IgG-B protein-mediated activation of adenylate cyclase.**

   A. **Effects of IC2a concentration.** The increase in the activating effect of IgG-B proteins on cyc⁻ membrane adenylate cyclase is dependent on the concentration of IC2a and approaches to the maximum at 10 ug/ml.

   B. **Effects of EGTA.** Simultaneous addition of 0.1 mM EGTA caused about 40% reduction in the IgG-B protein-mediated activation of the enzyme. Addition of 1 mM EGTA to the system further reduced the enzymatic activity to about 60% of the control value, although the inhibitory effects of two different concentrations of EGTA were not significantly different. Since the assay was performed in the presence of the excess Mg^{2+} (10 mM), the noted inhibitory effect of EGTA is probably not due to depletion of Mg^{2+}, but of some other divalent cation such as Ca^{2+}, which may be associated with cyc^- membranes.

Table 2. Effects of cholate-soluble IgG-B proteins on adenylate cyclase of cyc^- membrane.*

Samples	IC2a	AC activity pmol/mg/30 min	% change
Buffer	-	60.0±10.3	
	+	60.8±11.2	
IgG-B1 & B2	-	84.9±20.0	+ 41.5
	+	146.5±31.0	+ 141.0**
IgG-B1 & B2	-	85.0±16.5	+ 41.7
	+	141.9±33.5	+ 133.4**

*IgG-B1 and -B2 proteins (∼10 ug) were incubated with cyc^- membrane (∼100 ug) for 60 min at 10°C at pH 8. Adenylate cyclase activities of the mixtures were assayed in triplicates in the presence or absence of IC2a (10 ug/ml).
**p<0.02

C. Effects of calmodulin.
Since calmodulin has been implicated in the activation of adenylate cyclase of some cell types (Westcott et al, 1979; Wolff et al, 1980), the above results prompted us to investigate next the potential effect of calmodulin on IgG-B protein-mediated activation of cyc^- membrane adenylate cyclase. Inclusion of low concentration of calmodulin (0.1 ug/ml) in the assay mixtures enhanced the enzymatic activities of the mixtures in the presence of IC2a. Further increase in calmodulin concentration to 1.0 ug/ml resulted in no enhancement of the enzymatic activity.

6. Association of protein kinase activity with IgG-B2 protein. A potential association of protein kinase activity with IgG-B proteins was then investigated, since: (1) calmodulin has been shown to activate a number of protein kinases such as myosin light chain kinase (Silver & Stull, 1983) and (2) the involvement of protein kinase C in β-adrenergic activation of pineal gland adenylate cyclase has

been recently reported (Sugden et al, 1985). Results showed, as summarized by Table 3, the association of protein kinase activity (175 pmol/mg/min) with IgG-B2 proteins. This activity was found to be only slightly reduced when the assay was carried out in the presence of 0.5 mM EGTA. IgG-B1 proteins also showed some protein kinase activity but their specific activity was only 7.2 pmol/mg/min. PC-B proteins which were included as a control showed no detectable protein kinase activity, as in the case of the buffer control.

Table 3. Protein kinase activity of IgG-B1, -B2, and PC-B proteins.*

Samples	Ca^{2+}	EGTA	$^{32}PO_4$ cpm/250 ug histone	Activity pmol/mg/min
Buffer	+	-	0	0
	-	+	0	0
IgG-B1	+	-	276	7.2
	-	+	160	5.3
IgG-B2	+	-	4689	175
	-	+	4187	157
PC-B	+	-	0	0
	-	+	0	0

*IgG-B1, IgG-B2 or PC-B proteins (10 ug) were incubated for 30 min at 30°C with (γ-^{32}P) ATP as substrate and calf thymus histone as phosphate acceptor in the presence or absence of 0.5 mM Ca^{2+} or EGTA. After the incubation period, the incorporation of ^{32}P into TCA (25%)-precipitated proteins was measured.

Since IgG-B1 and -B2 proteins copurify during the affinity chromatography step of the isolation of IgG-B proteins and can be only poorly separated by Sephadex G-100 gel filtration in the presence of 6 M deionized urea, they are probably tightly associated with each other. It follows that IgG-B1 proteins may serve as substrate for protein kinase present in IgG-B2 proteins. By assaying the protein kinase activity of IgG-B2 proteins using IgG-B1 proteins as phosphate acceptor, IgG-B2 proteins were indeed found to promote the phosphorylation of IgG-B1 proteins although the specific activity (56.5 pmol/mg/min) was about one third of that obtained with histone as phosphate acceptor.

Discussion

The data presented in this paper demonstrate that IgG2a-binding (IgG-B1) proteins copurify with the second protein component(s) (IgG-B2) during the affinity chromatography of the detergent lysate of P388D1 cells over a column of IgG-Sepharose, which can be separated, although poorly, by Sephadex G-100 gel filtration in the presence of 6 M urea. Both IgG-B1 and -B2 proteins can be effectively inserted into liposome in a proper orientation. Simultaneous fusion of the liposomes containing IgG-B1 and -B2 proteins with G/F protein-deficient cyc⁻ cells results in the formation of the hybrid whose adenylate cyclase responds to IC2a by about 3.7 fold increase in the activity over the control. IgG-B1 and -B2 proteins together can confer their effects on adenylate cyclase of cyc⁻ membrane in their cholate-solubilized form as well. The latter activation is dependent on the concentration of IC2a, suppressed exogeneously-added EGTA, and significantly enhanced by low concentration of exogeneously-added calmodulin. Furthermore, IgG-B2 proteins are associated with protein kinase activity which catalyzes phosphorylation of not only exogenously-added histone but also IgG-B1.

Since either IgG-B1 or -B2 proteins alone or their mixture did not possess GTPase activity or cholera toxin sensitive ADP-ribosylation site, and since activation of adenylate cyclase of G/F protein-deficient cyc⁻ membrane by either cholate-solubilized or liposome-inserted IgG-B proteins is not enhanced by NaF, the noted effects of IgG-B proteins may be not due to supplementation of G/F protein, but rather due to direct interaction between the catalytic subunit of the enzyme and exogeneously-added IgG-B proteins. Our data suggest that the activation may be initiated by specific binding of IC2a to Fcγ2aR (obtained as IgG-B1 proteins) which promotes the interaction of Fcγ2aR with the protein components tightly associated with the receptor and obtained as IgG-B2 proteins. Such interaction may activate protein kinase associated with IgG-B2 proteins and results in the phosphorylation of Fcγ2aR proteins, which in turn activate the catalytic subunit of membrane adenylate cyclase. Alternatively, calmodulin which may be associated with IgG-B2 proteins may directly activate adenylate cyclase as shown in bovine brain cortex (Westcott et al, 1979) or in prokaryotic system (Wolff et al, 1980), irrespective of phosphorylation of Fcγ2aR. The latter hypothesis cannot explain, however, the requirement of IC2a as well as simultaneous presence of both IgG-B1 and -B2 proteins in medating the enhancing effect on cyc⁻ membrane adenylate cyclase. However, the nature of protein kinase activity associated with IgG-B2 proteins and its role in the activation of the catalytic subunit of adenylate cyclase is still unclear at present.

Acknowledgement

Studies described in this paper were supported in part by a grant from the National Cancer Institute (CA 35977).

Reference

Anderson CL, Grey HM (1978). Physicochemical separation of two distinct Fc receptors on murine macrophage-like cell lines. J. Immunol. 121:648.
Bonney RJ, Nuruns P, Davies P, Humes JL (1979). Antigen-antibody complexes stimulate the synthesis and release of prostaglandins by mouse peritoneal macrophages. Prostaglandins. 18:605.
Cassel D, Selinger Z (1976). Catecholamine-stimulated GTPase activity in turkey erythrocytes membranes. Biochim. Biophys. Acta. 452:538.
Cassel D, Selinger Z (1977). Mechanism of adenylate cyclase activation by cholera toxin: Inhibition of GTP hydrolysis at the regulatory site. Proc. Nat'l. Acad. Sci. USA. 74:3307.
Cerione RA, Strulovic B, Benovic JL, Strader CD, Caron MG, Lefkowitz RJ (1983). Reconstitution of β-adrenergic receptors in lipid vesicles: Affinity chromatography-purified receptors confer catecholamine responsiveness on a heterologous adenylate cyclase system. Proc. Nat'l. Acad. Sci. USA. 80:4899.
Kolsch E, Oberbannscheidt J, Bruner K, Heuer J (1980). The Fc receptor; it's role in the transmission of differentiation signals. Immunol. Rev. 49:61.
Nitta T, Suzuki T (1982b). Fcγ2b receptor-mediated prostaglandin synthesis by a murine macrophage cell line (P388D1). J. Immunol. 128:2527.
Nitta T, Suzuki T (1982c). Biochemical signals transmitted by Fcγ receptors: Triggering mechanisms of the increased synthesis of adenosine-3', 5'-cyclic monophosphate mediated by Fcγ2a- and Fcγ2b-receptors of a murine macrophage-like cell line (P388D1). J. Immunol. 129:2708.

Perlman P, Perlman J, Wigzell H (1972). Lymphocyte-mediated cytotoxicity in vitro. Induction and inhibition by humoral antibody and nature of effector cells. Transplant. Rev. 13:91.
Ross EM, Gilman AG (1977). Reconstitution of catecholamine-sensitive adenylate cyclase activity: Interaction of solubilized components with receptor-replete membranes. Proc. Nat'l. Acad. Sci. USA. 74:3175.
Salomon Y (1979). Adenylate cyclase assay. Adv. Cyclic Nucleotide Res. 10:35.
Schramm M (1979). Transfer of glucagon receptor from liver membranes to a foreign adenylate cyclase by a membrane fusion procedure. Proc. Nat'l. Acad. Sci. USA. 76:1174.
Silver P, Stull J (1983). Myosin light chain phosphorylation in smooth muscle cell and non-muscle cells as a probe of calmodulin function. In Methods in Enzymology. Vol. 102. eds. AP Means and BW O'Malley. Acad. Press, N.Y., p. 62.
Sugden D, Vauccek J, Klein D-C, Thomas TP, Anderson WB (1985). Activation of protein kinase C potentiates isoprenaline-induced cyclic AMP accumulation in rat pinealocytes. Nature. 314:359.
Suzuki T, Saito-Taki T, Sadasivan R, Nitta T (1982a). Biochemical signal transmitted by Fcγ receptors: phospholipase A2 activity of Fcγ2b receptor of murine macrophage cell line P388D1. Proc. Nat'l. Acad. Sci. USA. 79:591.
Uhr JW, Moller G (1968). Regulatory effect of antibody on the immune response. In Adv. Immunol. Vol. 8. eds. FJ Dixon and HG Kunkel. Acad. Press, N.Y., p. 81.
Walker WS (1976). Separate Fc-receptor for immunoglobulins IgG2a and IgG2b on an established cell line of mouse macrophages. J. Immunol. 116:911.
Westcott KR, LaPorte DC, Storm DR (1979). Resolution of adenylate cyclase sensitive and insensitive to Ca^{2+} and calcium-dependent regulatory protein (CDR) by CDR-Sepharose affinity chromatography. Proc. Nat'l. Acad. Sci. USA. 76:204.
Wolff J, Cook GH, Goldmanner AR, Berkowitz SA (1980). Calomodulin activates prokaryotic adenylate cyclase. Proc. Nat'l. Acad. Sci. USA. 77:3841.

MOLECULAR BASES FOR ACTIVATION OF CYTOTOXIC MACROPHAGES

Luigi Varesio[1], Michael A. Clayton[1], Elisabetta Blasi[1], Ezio Bonvini[2] and Danuta Radzioch[1]
[1]Laboratory of Molecular Immunoregulation, BRMP, DCT, NCI-FCRF, Frederick, MD 21701
[2]Laboratory of Cell Biology, Center for Drugs and Biologics, FDA, Bethesda, MD 20892

INTRODUCTION

Macrophages (Mø) can be activated in vivo or in vitro to exert cytotoxic activity (Varesio, 1985a). We have previously shown that two major changes in RNA metabolism occurred in Mø expressing tumoricidal activity. Downregulation of total RNA synthesis was evident in Mø-activated in vitro by poly I:C (Varesio et al., 1984a), crude lymphokine-containing supernatants (Varesio et al., 1984b) or in vivo by P.acnes (Varesio, 1984). Moreover, in P.acnes or lymphokine-activated Mø, an altered metabolism of ribosomal RNA (rRNA) was observed characterized by reduced accumulation of mature 28S rRNA and normal maturation of 18S rRNA (Varesio, 1985b). We address here two questions: 1) whether the above changes in rRNA metabolism are common features of Mø-activated to a cytotoxic stage and 2) whether the changes in mature rRNA involve the processing of precursor rRNA. A model which connects cytolytic activity and ribosomal RNA metabolism is proposed.

MATERIALS AND METHODS

In vivo or in vitro activation of peritoneal murine Mø and assay for cytotoxic activity have been detailed elsewhere (Varesio et al., 1984). Moreover, the following published techniques have been utilized: a) evaluation of total RNA synthesis by ^{3}H-uridine uptake into acid precipitable material (Varesio et al, 1981); b) agarose gel analysis of radiolabelled RNA (Varesio, 1985b); c) northern blot analysis of macrophage RNA (Maniatis et al., 1982).

RESULTS

Mø were activated either in vitro for 18 hr or in vivo with the agents indicated in Table 1. After activation, the Mø monolayers were pulsed for 3 hr with ^{3}H-uridine or tested for tumoricidal activity in an 18 hr ^{111}Indium release assay. The ^{3}H-uridine labelled cultures were assayed for total RNA synthesis (TCA precipitable radioactivity) or the RNA was extracted, separated on agarose gels in order to determine the distribution of radioactivity among the different molecular species of RNA. Table 1 summarizes the results of various experiments. The changes depicted are relative to control Mø cultured in the absence of activating agents for the in vitro activation, or to proteose peptone-elicited peritoneal Mø for the in vivo activation. A complete correlation exists between down regulation of RNA synthesis and expression of cytotoxic activity (Table 1). Both phenomena are evident upon in vivo or in vitro activation of macrophages from a responder stain of mice (C57BL/6) whereas they are absent in macrophages from non-responder mice (C3H-HeJ). Cytotoxicity and inhibition of RNA synthesis were induced by similar concentrations of activating agent and followed similar kinetics (data not shown).

TABLE 1. Altered RNA Metabolism in Tumoricidal Mø

Mouse Strain	Activator	Cyto-toxicity[c]	RNA Synthesis[d]	28/18S[e] ratio
C57BL/6				
LK+LPS 10 ng/ml[a]	(in vitro)	+	↓	↓
LPS 10 ng/ml	(in vitro)	–	↔	↔
Poly I:C	(in vitro)	+	↓	↓
IFN- α, β, γ	(in vitro)	+	↓	↓
CSF[b]	(in vitro)	–	↔	ND
IL 2	(in vitro)	–	↔	ND
P.acnes	(in vivo)	+	↓	↓
LPS	(in vivo)	+	↓	↓
C3H/HeJ				
LK+LPS 10 ng/ml[a]	(in vitro)	–	↔	↔
IFN-γ	(in vitro)	–	↔	↔

a LK = lymphokine containing supernatants generated by stimulation of spleen cells with Concanavalin A (Varesio et al., 1984).
b CSF = colony stimulating factor containing supernatants from L-cell fibroblast or WEHI cell line.
c Cytotoxicity is indicated as "+" when statistically significant and above 20% or as "-" when non significant or less than 20%, relative to control Mø.
d RNA synthesis was measuraed by ^{3}H-uridine uptake and it is indicated "↓" when statistically lower than the control; when unchanged it is indicated as ↔.
e 28/18S ratio indicates the relative accumulation of 28S or 18S mature ribosomal RNA species evaluated by size fractionation of ^{3}H-uridine labelled Mø RNA on agarose gels. 28/18S ratio was calculated by dividing the radioactivity in the 28S peak by that of the 18S peak. In control Mø the 28/18S ratios is >1 (more labelled 28S that 18S). The symbol "↓" indicates a decrease in the 28S/18S ratio. In all of the above cases the 18S was unchanged and the decreased ratio was caused by reduction of 28S.

In addition to the decrease of total RNA synthesis a second alteration of RNA metabolism (indicated in Table 1 as a decrease in 28/18S ratio) correlated with the expression of cytotoxicity. Electrophoresis analysis of the labelled RNA from cytotoxic macrophages showed a marked decrease in the 28S peak but normal 18S peak resulting in a decrease of the 28/18S peak ratio relative to controls. The decrease in 28S/18S rRNA ratio correlated, in every situation, with the expression of cytolytic activity by activated Mø.

28S and 18S are the most prominent species of mature rRNA which are derived from a high molecular weight rRNA precursor (45S) through sequential processing. The selective down-regulation of labelled 28S rRNA in cytotoxic macrophages suggests that correct processing of de novo synthesized rRNA may not proceed. To test this hypothesis, total unlabelled RNA was extracted from control or activated macrophages, separated on agarose gels, blotted onto nitrocellulose membranes and hybridized with ^{32}P-labelled DNA probes specific for ribosomal RNA precursors (Northern blot analysis). Under these conditions the extent of hybridization to the various rRNA species was proportional to their absolute amount. The data relative to control Mø or Mø activated in vitro for 24 hr with poly I:C, IFN-α, β or γ are summarized in Table 2.

TABLE 2

	rRNA Precursors[a]		
Activator	45S	41S	36-32S
IFN-α	↑↑[b]	↑	↑↑
IFN-β	↑↑	↑	↑↑
IFN-γ	↑↑	↑	↑↑
Poly I:C	↑↑	↑	↑↑

[a] rRNA precursors were identified using specific DNA probes that were subcloned in our laboratory.

[b] Each arrow (↑) indicates a two-fold increase in the intensity of the specific band relative to RNA from control cultures of Mø.

Activation to a cytotoxic stage by IFN or poly I:C resulted significant accumulation of rRNA precursors. No major difference in the pattern of rRNA precursor accumulation were seen by comparing the effects of the different activating agents.

DISCUSSION

The results presented here clearly show that activation of macrophage for cytotoxicity is associated with major changes in rRNA metabolism and processing. Inhibition of total RNA synthesis and inhibition of 28S rRNA maturation are induced by every in vivo or in vitro stimulus tested that renders macrophages tumoricidal. Interestingly, a normal pattern of RNA synthesis was found in noncytotoxic macrophage populations although at a different stages of activation. For example, comparable RNA profiles were observed in resident, thioglycollate- or peptone-elicited macrophages (Varesio, 1984) which differ in their secretory activity and in their susceptibility to activation by lymphokines (Morahan et al., 1980 and Johnson et al., 1983). Thus it appears that the down-regulation of RNA synthesis and the selective decrease of 28S rRNA are functional markers of selective for cytotoxic activity. This conclusion was strengthened by the fact that similar decrease in 28S rRNA was found in macrophages activated to

a cytolytic stage by IFN-γ or IFN-β, which have a
differential requirement for protein synthesis for activation (Blasi et al., 1984), and by poly I:C and LK that also
differ in their mechanisms of macrophage activation
(Taramelli et al., 1981). Thus, irrespectively of the
activation pathway followed by different agents to stimulate macrophages, the imbalance in the 28S/18S rRNA accumulation appears to be a common step associated with expression of cytotoxic activity.

The analysis metabolically labelled RNAs provides
information regarding synthesis, processing and degradation
of <u>de novo</u> sintesized RNA. By Northern Blotting analysis
we have found accumulation of precursor rRNA in cytotoxic
Mϕ. This finding, together with the decreased accumulation
of 28S rRNA found in tha same cells, is compatible with the
hypothesis that the metabolic changes occurring during the
activation process lead to inhibition of the processing
of rRNA precursor. If the processing is reduced, the
precursors of rRNA will tend to accumulate, as shown by
increased amounts of 45S, 41S, 36S and 32S rRNA in cytotoxic macrophages. Accumulation of rRNA precursors could
inhibit synthesis of rRNA in a feed-back loop, thus accunting for the reduced ^{3}H-uridine uptake into activated
macrophages. Moreover, the processing of 28S rRNA is more
complex and involves more intermediates than that of 18S
rRNA. In fact, the 36S and 32S precursors do not contain
any longer the 18S but only the 28S. Therefore, as we
observed, inhibition of rRNA processing may effect mainly
the maturation of 28S rRNA. Selective down regulation of
28S rRNA accumulation has been shown also in resting
leukocytes and in growth inhibited cells (Abelson et al.,
1974, Cooper, 1973, Emerson, 1971, and Weber, 1972).

Our result provide the firs indication that IFNs can
modulate gene expression at post-transcriptional level
by affecting the processing of RNA.

Computer analysis showed that rRNA precursors may
fold in very stable double stranded secondary structures.
We propose that the rRNA precursors represent an endogenous
source of double stranded RNA able to activate double
stranded RNA-dependent enzymes, constitutively present in
many cell types including macrophages and whose synthesis
is augmented by IFN. One enzyme, which needs double

stranded RNA for its activity, is a protein kinase which could initiate a cascade of phosphorylation reactions involved for the expression of cytotoxic activity. This enzyme has been found also in the nucleous where rRNA processing occurs.

This model contains a number of major and novel implications on the regulation of cell functions by RNA.

1. rRNA can regulate cell functions not only indirectly through ribosome formation but also through rRNA precursors which directly activate double stranded RNA-dependent enzymes.

2. rRNA precursors are the physiological donors of double stranded RNA, capable of activating double stranded RNA-dependent enzymes, and possibly involved in the biological effects of IFN, including induction of cytotoxic macrophages.

REFERENCES

Varesio L (1985a). Induction and expression of tumoricidal activity by macrophages. In R.T. Dean and W. Jessup (Eds.), Mononuclear Phagocytes: Physiology and Pathology. Elsevier Science Publishers, B. U. (Biomedical Division) Amsterdam, in press.

Varesio L, Issaq HJ, Taramelli D (1984a). RNA synthesis in activated macrophages. I. Poly I:C induced triggering of cytolytic activity is associated with decrease in RNA synthesis. Eur J Immunol 13:959.

Varesio L, Issaq HJ, Kowal R, Bonvini E, Tarmelli D (1984b). Lymphokines inhibit macrophage RNA synthesis. Cell Immunol 84:51.

Varesio L (1984). Down-regulation of RNA labeling as a selective marker for cytotoxic but not suppressor macrophage. J Immunol 132:2683.

Varesio L (1985b). Activation of macrophages: Altered metabolism of ribosomal RNA in macrophages activated in vivo or in vitro to a cytolytic stage. J Immunol 134:1262.

Varesio L, Naglich J, Brunda MJ, Taramelli D, Eva A (1981). Microsystem to evaluate the incorporation of ^{3}H-urdine in macrophage RNA. Immunol Commun 10:577.

Maniatis T, Fritsch EF, Sambrook J (1982). Molecular cloning: A laboratory manual. New York, Cold Spring Harbor Laboratory.

Morahan PS, Endleson PJ, Gass K (1980). Changes in the macrophae ectoeuzymes associated with anti tumor activity. J Immunol 125:1313.

Johnson WJ, Marino PA, Schreiber RD, Adams DO (1983). Sequential activation of murine mononuclear phagocytes for tumor cytolysis: Differential expression of markers by macrophages in the several stages of development. J Immunol 131:1038.

Blasi E, Herberman RB, Varesio L (1984). Requirement for protein synthesis for induction of macrophage tumoricidal activity by IFN-α and IFN-β but not IFN-γ. J Immunol 132:3226.

Taramelli D, Varesio L (1981). Activation of murine macrophages: I. Different pattern of activation by poly I:C than by lymphokine or LPS. J Immunol 127:58.

Abelson HT, Johnson LF, Penman S, Green H (1974). Changes in RNA in relation to growth of the fibroblast. II. The lifetime of mRNA rRNA and tRNA in resting and growing cells. Cell 1:161.

Cooper L (1973). Degradation of 28S RNA pate in ribosomal RNA maturation in non-growing lymphocytes and its reversal after growth stimulation. J Cell Biol 59:250.

Emerson CP (1971). Regulation of the synthesis and the stability of ribosomal RNA during contact inhibition of growth. Nature New Biol 232:101.

Weber MJ (1972). Ribosomal RNA turnover in contace inhibited cells. Nature New Biol 235:58.

ACTIVATED MACROPHAGE MEDIATED IRON REMOVAL FROM ENZYMES WITH IRON-SULFUR CLUSTERS IN TUMOR TARGET CELLS: A POSSIBLE MECHANISM FOR SELECTIVE INHIBITION OF METABOLIC PATHWAYS[1]

John B. Hibbs, Jr. and Jean Claude Drapier

VA Medical Center and Department of Medicine
Division of Infectious Diseases
University of Utah School of Medicine,
Salt Lake City, Utah 84148

CYTOTOXIC ACTIVATED MACROPHAGES CAUSE A HIGHLY REPRODUCIBLE PATTERN OF METABOLIC INHIBITION IN ALL TUMOR TARGET CELLS BUT THIS PATTERN OF METABOLIC INHIBITION DOES NOT ALWAYS RESULT IN CYTOLYSIS

Cytotoxic activated macrophages do not cause rapid or global metabolic disorganization in tumor target cells. The metabolic dysfunction induced by cytotoxic activated macrophages in tumor target cells develops slowly, is quite discrete, and in many cases is fully reversible. For example, we have demonstrated that cytotoxic activated macrophages inhibit DNA synthesis and mitochondrial respiration while certain other metabolic pathways such as glycolysis remain functional (Granger et al., 1980; Hibbs et al., 1984). This pattern of selective inhibition of metabolic pathways in transformed target cells appears to be a universal response to cytotoxic activated macrophages. However, two transformed cell phenotypic responses to the activated macrophage induced cytotoxic reaction exist (Granger et al., 1980; Cook et al., 1980; Cook et al., 1982; Hibbs and Granger, 1982). Both transformed cell phenotypes develop inhibition of mitochondrial respiration and inhibition of DNA replication, but their ultimate fate in response to cocultivation with activated macrophages is different. The nonlytic phenotype (L1210 mouse lymphoblastic leukemia cells are an example) responds with prolonged cytostasis but eventually recover if glucose is available for glycolytic ATP production. Target cells with the lytic

[1]Supported by the Veterans Administration, Washington, D.C.

phenotype (TCMK SV40 transformed mouse kidney cells are an example) progress to cytolysis in the presence or absence of glucose. Target cells with the nonlytic phenotype are most useful for studying bioenergetic and biochemical effects induced by cytotoxic activated macrophages, because tumor cells with this phenotype do not undergo significant lysis during cocultivation with or after removal from activated macrophages.

ENDOCYTOSIS OF ERYTHROCYTES, IRON CONTAINING MOLECULES, OR ELEMENTAL IRON BY ACTIVATED MACROPHAGES INHIBITS THEIR CYTOTOXIC EFFECT FOR TUMOR CELLS

A number of years ago, we published experiments showing that exogenously added iron inhibited the cytotoxic mechanism of activated macrophages (Weinberg and Hibbs, 1977). Activated macrophages that had phagocytized glutaraldehyde treated or antibody opsonized erythrocytes were unable to express a cytotoxic effect for tumorigenic mouse 3T12 cells (Figure 1). Erythrocytes that were added to the activated macrophage-tumor cell cocultures but were not phagocytized, had no inhibitory effect. Other experiments showed that erythrocyte lysates, hemoglobin, methemoglobin, iron dextran, $FeSO_4$ and $FeCl_3$ all inhibited the activated macrophage cytotoxic effect for tumor cells. This study showed that iron or iron containing molecules, when added to cocultures of activated macrophages and tumor target cells, could inhibit the cytotoxic effect of activated macrophages for tumor target cells.

TUMOR CELLS COCULTIVATED WITH CYTOTOXIC ACTIVATED MACROPHAGES LOSE A SIGNIFICANT PORTION OF THEIR INTRACELLULAR IRON-59 LABEL

More recent experiments provide further evidence for a role for iron in the development of activated macrophage cytotoxicity for tumor cells (Hibbs et al., 1984). L1210 cells were labeled with iron-59 citrate (^{59}Fe) for 24 hours, washed, and added to monolayers of cytotoxic activated macrophages for a 24 hour cocultivation period.

There was 64% specific release of ^{59}Fe from prelabeled fully viable L1210 cells cocultivated with cytotoxic activated macrophages. Pronase treatment of L1210 cells

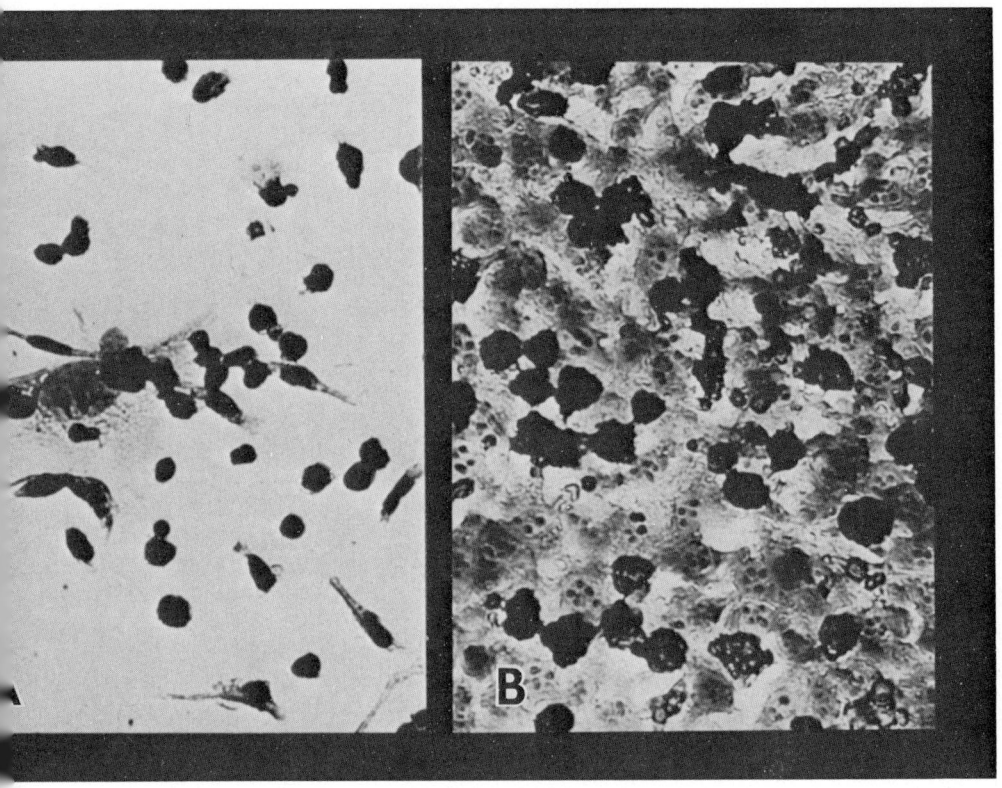

Figure 1. Phagocytosis of red blood cells (RBC's) by activated macrophages inhibits their cytotoxic effect. Photomicrographs of giemsa-stained cytotoxic activated macrophages plus mouse 3T12 sarcoma cells following 60 hours of cocultivation. Cytotoxic activated macrophages were harvested from the peritoneal cavity of mice that had been infected intraperitoneally two weeks earlier with Mycobacterium bovis, strain Bacillus Calmette Guerin and the cytotoxicity assay prepared as previously described (Weinberg and Hibbs, 1977). (A) Cytotoxic activated macrophages without added RBC's have destroyed the majority of 3T12 cells. This typical field shows one residual tumor cell among the cytotoxic activated macrophages. (B) The activated macrophages with phagocytosed RBC did not cause cytostasis or cytolysis of 3T12 cells. This typical field shows numerous 3T12 cells with their prominent nucleoli among the RBC-laden activated macrophages.

following cocultivation did not significantly increase ^{59}Fe release (68% specific release). Also, L1210 cells prelabeled with [^{3}H] TdR or [^{3}H] L-leu do not release either isotope when cultivated with cytotoxic activated macrophages and pronase treatment does not increase release. The same group of cocultivated L1210 cells developed a requirement for glucose to remain viable during a second 24 hour incubation which is a result of cytotoxic activated macrophage induced inhibition of mitochondrial respiration. There was 100% cell death during a second 24 hour incubation in DMEM-glucose (G). However, only 11% of the same cocultivated L1210 cells died in DMEM+G. L1210 cells prelabeled with ^{59}Fe and heated to 70°C for 30 minutes were 100% trypan blue positive after heat treatment and were unable to resume proliferation upon further cultivation. The heat killed L1210 cells released 69% of ^{59}Fe label and that ^{59}Fe release was moderately increased by pronase treatment. However, unlike viable cocultivated L1210 cells, heat killed L1210 cells released significant amounts of [^{3}H] L-leu and [^{3}H] TdR after pronase treatment. These experiments demonstrate that a 24 hour cocultivation with cytotoxic activated macrophages induces depletion of ^{59}Fe label from viable L1210, which remain viable in DMEM+G during a second 24 hour incubation but die when transferred to DMEM-G (Hibbs et al., 1984).

KINETICS OF ^{59}FE SPECIFIC RELEASE FROM L1210 CELLS COCULTIVATED WITH CYTOTOXIC ACTIVATED MACROPHAGES

Figure 2A shows that the first detectable release of ^{59}Fe from cytotoxic activated macrophage cocultivated L1210 cells occurs between four and five hours after initiation of cocultivation (7% specific release). Specific release of ^{59}Fe progressively increased during the first 10 hours and at the termination of the 24 hour cocultivation period reached 72%. Figure 2B shows there was 12% cell death in DMEM+G and 100% cell death in DMEM-G during a second 24 hour incubation after removal from cytotoxic activated macrophage monolayers. These results demonstrate that ^{59}Fe release from L1210 cells is a relatively early event in the development of activated macrophage induced cytotoxicity (Hibbs et al., 1984).

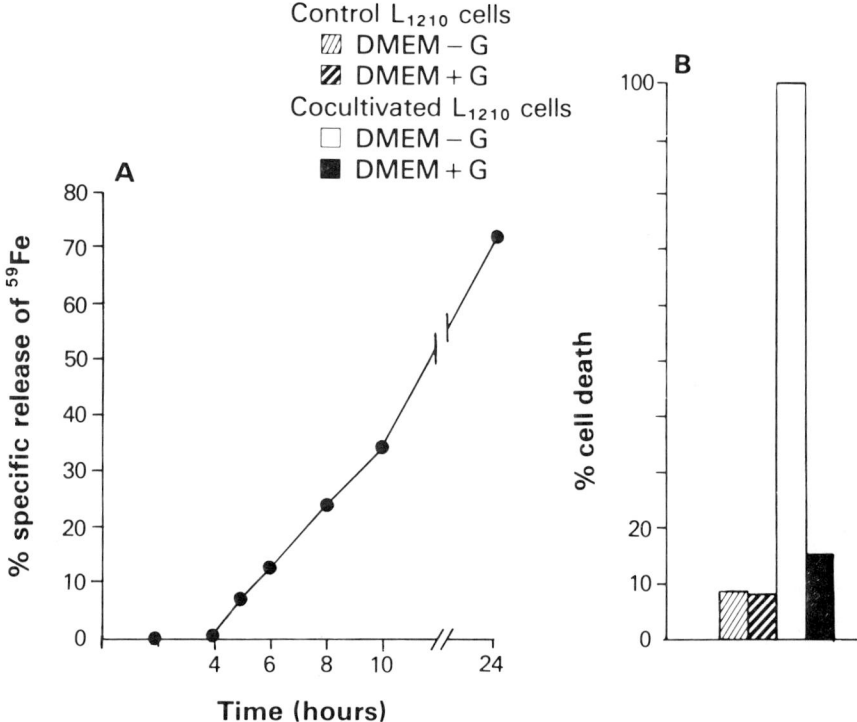

Figure 2. (A) Kinetics of ^{59}Fe specific release from L1210 cells cocultivated with AM. (B) L1210 cells from the same experiment develop inhibition of mitochondrial respiration which is detected by a requirement for glucose to remain viable during a second 24 hour incubation after removal from the AM monolayers. (From Hibbs et al., 1984, with permission of the publisher.)

CYTOTOXIC ACTIVATED MACROPHAGE INDUCED SUPPRESSION OF TARGET CELL MITOCHONDRIAL RESPIRATION IS DUE TO INHIBITION OF NADH-COENZYME Q REDUCTASE AND SUCCINATE-COENZYME Q REDUCTASE IN THE MITOCHONDRIAL ELECTRON TRANSPORT CHAIN

Granger and Lehninger have identified the sites of inhibition of mitochondrial respiration in cytotoxic activated macrophage injured L1210 cells permeabilized with digitonin (Granger and Lehninger, 1982). They found that cytotoxic activated macrophages directly affected the mitochondrial respiratory chain. NADH-coenzyme Q reductase and succinate-coenzyme Q reductase, the proximal reductases in the electron transport system, were markedly inhibited. This results in closure of the two major sites for entry of electrons into the mitochondrial electron transport system. Therefore, oxidation of the major mitochondrial substrates generated by the Krebs cycle reactions (NAD-linked substrates and succinate) is blocked. Furthermore, cytotoxic activated macrophage inhibition of mitochondrial respiration is selective since electron flow in more distal portions of the electron transport system remains intact. It was observed that the respiratory chain between coenzyme Q and O_2 via cytochrome a-a_3 is functional in L1210 cells following cytotoxic activated macrophage induced injury.

ACONITASE, A KREBS CYCLE ENZYME CONTAINING AN IRON-SULFUR CLUSTER, IS INHIBITED IN TUMOR CELLS COCULTIVATED WITH CYTOTOXIC ACTIVATED MACROPHAGES

It is of interest that NADH-coenzyme Q reductase and succinate-coenzyme Q reductase, which Granger and Lehninger showed are selectively inhibited in L1210 cells cocultivated with cytotoxic activated macrophages, contain most of the iron-sulfur clusters in the mitochondrial electron system. Iron-sulfur centers could be a site of iron loss and could explain cytotoxic activated macrophage induced inhibition of these enzymes. To test this possibility, we examined aconitase activity in digitonin permeabilized L10 guinea pig hepatoma cells and L1210 cells. Aconitase, although not catalyzing a redox reaction, is a Krebs cycle enzyme containing a (4Fe-4S) cluster (Kent et al., 1985). Results show that inhibition of aconitase is an early event in the development of activated macrophage mediated cytotoxicity in L10 and L1210 target cells (J. C. Drapier and J. B. Hibbs, Jr., unpublished data).

ACONITASE ACTIVITY CAN BE RESTORED IN L10 CELLS BY REMOVING THEM FROM ACTIVATED MACROPHAGE MONOLAYERS AND INCUBATING THEM WITH FERROUS IRON OR FERROUS IRON PLUS THIOSULFATE

It has been known for many years that aconitase is reversibly inactivated by mild oxidative conditions. Recent studies utilizing Mössbauer spectroscopy showed that oxidative stress results in conversion of the [4Fe-4S] cluster of the active enzyme to an [3Fe-4S] cluster of the inactive enzyme by loss of an iron atom (Kent et al., 1982; Beinert et al., 1983; Kent et al., 1985). Upon incubation of the inactive enzyme in the presence of ferrous iron, or ferrous iron plus a reducing agent, the [3Fe-4S] cluster is converted to the active [4Fe-4S] cluster. It is of interest that we were able to restore aconitase activity in L10 cells that had been cocultivated with cytotoxic activated macrophages for six hours by removing the L10 cells from the macrophage monolayers and incubating them for one hour in culture medium supplemented with ferrous iron or ferrous iron plus thiosulfate (J.C. Drapier and J.B. Hibbs, Jr, unpublished observations). This is strong evidence that activated macrophage mediated inhibition of aconitase in L10 target cells is submolecular and mediated by iron removal from that enzyme's iron-sulfur center. Furthermore, the [4Fe-4S] $\rightleftharpoons$ [3Fe-4S] interconversion of the cluster could represent a regulatory function for the iron-sulfur center of aconitase that is modulated by an activated macrophage mediated mechanism.

SUMMARY

The experiments reviewed here suggest the reproducible pattern of metabolic inhibition induced in target cells by cytotoxic activated macrophages may be caused by iron loss from the target cells. This results in inhibition of certain enzymes that require iron for catalytic activity (aconitase, NADH-coenzyme Q reductase, and succinate-coenzyme Q reductase are examples). Enzymes with iron-sulfur centers appear to be particularly vulnerable to inhibition by the activated macrophage mediated mechanism of iron removal. It is possible activated macrophage induced metabolic changes in target cells are an exaggeration of normal biochemical mechanisms involved in the control of cellular proliferation.

REFERENCES

Beinert H, Emptage MH, Dreyer J-L, Scott RA, Hahn JE, Hodgson KO, Thomson AJ (1983). Iron-sulfur stoichiometry and structure of iron-sulfur clusters in three iron proteins: Evidence for [3Fe-4S] clusters. Proc Natl Acad Sci USA 80:393-396.

Cook JL, Hibbs JB Jr, Lewis Am Jr (1980). Resistance of simian virus 40-transformed hamster cells to the cytolytic effect of activated macrophages. A possible factor in species-specific viral oncogenicity. Pro Natl Acad Sci USA 77:6773-6777.

Cook JL, Hibbs JB Jr, Lewis AM Jr (1982). DNA virus-transformed hamster cell - host effector cell interactions: Level of resistance to cytolysis correlated with tumorigenicity. Int J Cancer 30:795-803.

Granger DL, Lehninger L (1982). Sites of inhibition of mitochondrial electron transport in macrophage-injured neoplastic cells. J Cell Biol 95:527-535.

Granger DL, Taintor RR, Cook JL, Hibbs JB Jr (1980). Injury of neoplastic cells by murine macrophages leads to inhibition of mitochondrial respiration. J Clin Invest 65:357-370.

Hibbs JB Jr, Granger DL (1982). Activated macrophage-induced cytostasis and inhibition of aerobic energy metabolism in transformed cells: Evaluation of lytic and nonlytic target cell responses. In Mizuno D, Cohn ZA, Takeya K, Ishida N (eds): "Self-Defense Mechanisms: Role of Macrophages," Tokyo: University of Tokyo Press, pp 319-333.

Hibbs JB Jr, Taintor RR, Vavrin Z (1984). Iron depletion: Possible cause of tumor cell cytotoxicity induced by activated macrophages. Biochem Biophys Res Commun 123(2):716-723.

Kent TA, Dreyer J-L, Kennedy MC, Huyhn BH, Emptage MH, Beinert H, Münch E (1982). Mössbauer studies of beef heart aconitase: Evidence for facile interconversions of iron-sulfur clusters. Proc Natl Acad Sci USA 79:1096-1100.

Kent TA, Emptage MH, Merkle H, Kennedy MC, Beinert H, Münck E (1985). Mössbauer studies of aconitase: Substrate and inhibitor binding, reaction intermediates, and hyperfine interactions of reduced 3Fe and 4Fe clusters. J Biol Chem 260(11):6871-6881

Weinberg JB, Hibbs JB Jr (1977). Endocytosis of red blood cells or haemoglobin by activated macrophages inhibits their tumoricidal effect. Nature 269(5625):245-247.

ACONITASE, A KREBS CYCLE ENZYME WITH AN IRON-SULFUR CENTER, IS INHIBITED IN TUMOR TARGET CELLS AFTER COCULTIVATION WITH CYTOTOXIC ACTIVATED MACROPHAGES[1]

Jean-Claude Drapier and John B. Hibbs, Jr.

VA Medical Center and Department of Medicine
Division of Infectious Diseases
University of Utah School of Medicine
Salt Lake City, Utah 84148

INTRODUCTION

The ways macrophages exert antitumor activity are not well defined. Much attention has been focused on the search for effector molecules but so far, little has been concluded about basic mechanisms leading to target cell alteration. A complementary approach is to analyze at a biochemical level, the metabolic changes that occur in tumor target cells as a result of macrophage-mediated injury.

From previous studies, it is known that cytotoxic activated macrophage-injured tumor cells develop cytostasis as well as inhibition of mitochondrial respiration (Granger et al., 1980). Also, it was observed that two non heme iron-containing enzymes of the respiratory chain, namely NADH-coenzyme Q reductase (Complex I) and succinate-coenzyme Q reductase (Complex II) were strongly inhibited in mouse L1210 leukemia cells cocultivated with cytotoxic activated macrophages (Granger and Lehninger, 1982) and in mouse EMT-6 adenocarcinoma cells cultivated in the presence of cytotoxic activated macrophage conditioned medium (Kilbourn et al., 1984). Recent experiments show that L1210 cells and L10 guinea pig hepatoma cells cocultivated with cytotoxic activated macrophages lose a portion of their iron-59 label (Hibbs et al, 1984). This observation suggested that removal of iron from enzymes that require iron for catalytic activity could be responsible for the pattern of metabolic inhibition caused in target cells by cytotoxic activated

[1]Supported by the Veterans Administration, Washington, D.C. and the Fogarty International Center, Bethesda, MD.

macrophages. The present studies were undertaken to address this question by measuring activity of aconitase in digitonin-permeabilized L10 and L1210 cells. Aconitase, although not catalyzing a redox reaction, is a Krebs cycle enzyme containing an iron-sulfur center essential for its catalytic activity (Kent et al., 1982).

METHODS

Aconitase, Complex I and Complex II were assayed polarigraphically in target cells after cocultivation and removal from the macrophage monolayers. Cells were then treated with 0.007% digitonin (Fiskum et al., 1980). After washing, endogenous substrates are depleted and oxygen consumption becomes dependent on exogenous-added substrates. Figure 1 illustrates the Krebs cycle and the

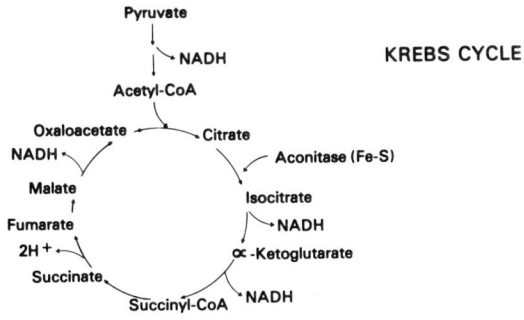

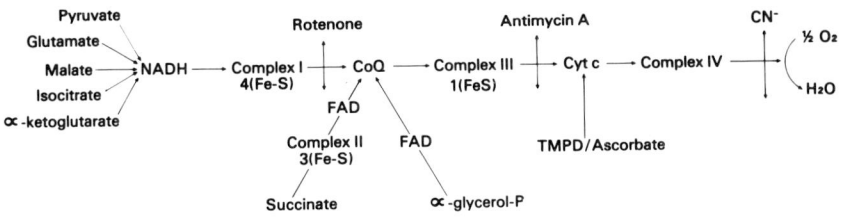

Figure 1.

electron transfer chain. Aconitase catalyses the interconversion of citrate and isocitrate with cis-aconitate as an intermediate. Isocitrate, the product of aconitase, is oxidized to α-ketoglutarate in the subsequent Krebs cycle reaction yielding NADH which reduces Complex I of the respiratory chain. The rate of consumption of O_2 (the final electron acceptor of the electron transport system) is directly related to the rate of electron transport and, if citrate is the only respiratory substrate, to aconitase activity. Therefore, sequential measurements of citrate and isocitrate-dependent O_2 consumption allow determination of aconitase and Complex I activities. Rotenone, by blocking Complex I, inhibits O_2 uptake. Addition of succinate which bypasses the rotenone block, permits measurement of respiration through Complex II.

RESULTS AND DISCUSSION

Table 1 shows that respiration on citrate is less efficient than respiration on other NAD-linked substrates, e.g. malate or isocitrate. Therefore, citrate isomerization to isocitrate is a limiting step and citrate-dependent O_2 uptake is directly proportional to aconitase activity. As shown in Figure 2, measurement of aconitase activity as well as different segments of the electron transport system can be made in the same sample by using specific inhibitors.

Target cells were cocultivated with thioglycolate or proteose peptone-elicited macrophages (stimulated macrophages) and Bacillus Calmette Guerin-activated macrophages (cytotoxic activated macrophages). No modification in aconitase activity was observed in target cells during a 20 h coculture with stimulated macrophage as compared to control cells (target cells cultivated alone). However, activity sharply plummeted between 2 and 6 hours when cytotoxic activated macrophages were used as effector cells. Aconitase activity in both L10 and L1210 cells was undetectable after 7 h of coculture. Target cells, at this time, no longer multiply but are not severely damaged since they exclude trypan blue and, after removal from the cytotoxic activated macrophage monolayer, they recover in fresh medium. Thus, aconitase inhibition is not a consequence of a target cell death. Isocitrate (or malate) dependent respiration (Complex I) and succinate-dependent respiration (Complex II) were reduced in L10 target cells 80% and 60% respectively after 22 h coculture with cytotoxic

TABLE 1. Substrate oxidation rate of L10 and L1210 cells (ng atoms O/min/10⁶ cells). Five x 10⁶ L10 cells or 12x10⁶ L1210 were permeabilized with 0.007% digitonin and state 3 of respiration (presence of ADP and Pi) was measured with various respiratory substrates. TMPD = tetramethylphenylenediamine.

Substrate	L10 Cells	L1210 Cells
Glutamate	7.5	ND*
Pyruvate	3.5	ND
α-Ketoglutarate	14.5	ND
Isocitrate	12.5	4.0
Citrate	11.5	3.0
Malate	13.0	4.0
Succinate	14.5	6.5
α-Glycerol-Phosphate	3.5	ND
TMPD + Ascorbate	30.0	9.0

* ND = not done.

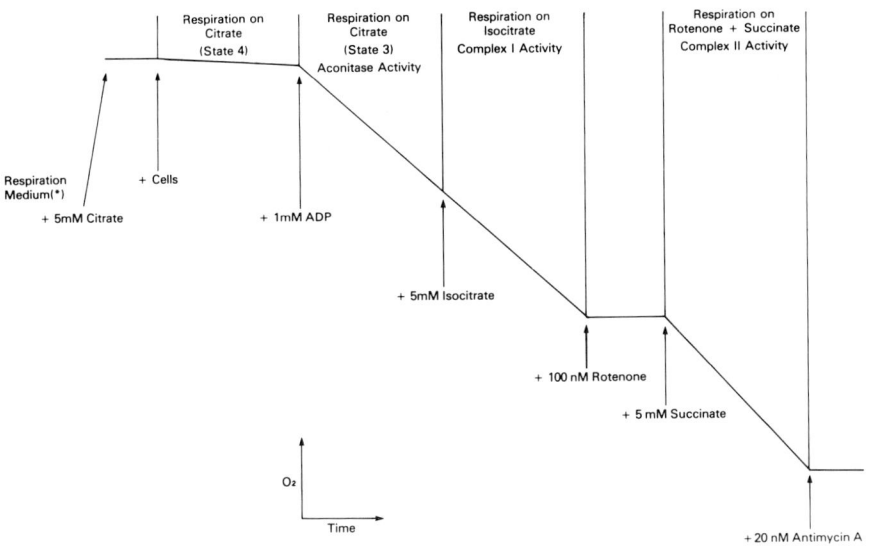

Figure 2. Typical trace of L10 cell O_2 consumption. In the presence of ADP, state 3 respiration was measured with citrate, isocitrate and succinate as respiratory substrates. *Respiration medium: 0.25 M sucrose, 20 mM HEPES, pH 7.2, 10 mM $MgCl_2$, 2 mMPi, 1 mM EGTA and 5 mM tartronate and 0.07% bovine serum albumin.

activated macrophages (J. C. Drapier and J. B. Hibbs, Jr., unpublished observations).

Aconitase in L10 cells was 100% and 50% active respectively after 10 h and 20 h coculture in the presence of 10 µg/ml cycloheximide. This shows that the rapid decrease of activity observed when cells are cocultivated with cytotoxic activated macrophages was not due to inhibition of protein synthesis and suggests alteration at the catalytic site could explain the observed inhibition of aconitase activity.

When isolated under aerobic conditions, aconitase is usually inactive but activity can be restored by addition of ferrous iron (Villafranca and Mildvan, 1971). Upon activation under reducing conditions, the [3Fe-4S] cluster is converted back to a cluster of [4Fe-4S] type (Kent et al, 1982). It is interesting that in our system, reincubation of cytotoxic activated macrophage-injured L10 cells in the presence of ferrous ions, led to restoration of aconitase activity (J. C. Drapier and J. B. Hibbs, Jr., unpublished observation). This strongly suggests that cytotoxic activated macrophages induce removal of a labile iron from the aconitase iron-sulfur cluster.

It should be pointed out that despite inhibition of aconitase, we observed that endogenous mitochondrial respiratory activity continues as long as Complex I and Complex II are still functional. Bypass of the aconitase reaction (and acetyl CoA and citrate as respiratory substrates) could occur if glutamate, after transamination to α-ketoglutarate, is utilized as an alternative respiratory substrate. Thus, metabolic consequences of aconitase inhibition should be investigated in the accumulation of citrate and/or diversion of its carbon atoms. Citrate can be transported out of mitochondria and used as a carbon source for the energy-requiring fatty acid and sterol synthesis through the ATP-citrate lyase reaction. In line with this, citrate can also activate acetyl CoA carboxylase, the rate-limiting enzyme in fatty acid synthesis. Besides, citrate allosterically inhibits phosphofructokinase, a regulatory enzyme of the energy-yielding glycolytic pathway. Finally, citrate could act as a chelator and carry iron through cell membranes with or without lipid peroxidation as a consequence.

SUMMARY

The present study was designated to determine if cytotoxic activated macrophages cause inhibition of aconitase, an iron-sulfur controlled Krebs cycle enzyme. After 4 h of coculture, aconitase activity declined dramatically in L10 and L1210 tumor target cells. This is an early event which occurs simultaneously with arrest of DNA synthesis. This inhibition is not the consequence of decreased protein synthesis but suggest the [4Fe-4S] cluster which is essential for the catalytic activity of aconitase, is altered by a cytotoxic activated macrophage-dependent mechanism. Release of iron by a chelator induced by the activated macrophage mediated cytotoxic mechanism or from an oxidized iron-sulfur cluster of aconitase (or both) is a possible explanation for the inhibition of enzymatic activity observed.

REFERENCES

Fiskum G, Craig SW, Decker DL, Lehninger AL (1980). The cytoskeleton of digitonin-treated rat hepatocytes. Proc Natl Acad Sci USA 77:3430-3434.

Granger DL, Lehninger L (1982). Sites of inhibition of mitochondrial electron transport in macrophage-injured neoplastic cells. J Cell Biol 95:527-535.

Granger DL, Taintor RR, Cook JL, Hibbs JB Jr (1980). Injury of neoplastic cells by murine macrophages leads to inhibition of mitochondrial respiration. J Clin Invest 65:357-370.

Hibbs JB Jr, Taintor RR, Vavrin Z (1984). Iron depletion: Possible cause of tumor cell cytotoxicity induced by activated macrophages. Biochem Biophys Res Commun 123:716-723.

Kent TA, Dreyer J-L, Kennedy MC, Huyhn BH, Emptage MH, Beinert H, Münch E (1982). Mössbauer studies of beef heart aconitase: Evidence for facile interconversions of iron-sulfur clusters. Proc Natl Acad Sci USA 79:1096-1100.

Kilbourn RG, Klostergaard J, Lopez-Berestein G (1984). Activated macrophages secrete a soluble factor that inhibits mitochondrial respiration of tumor cells. J Immunol 133:2577-2581.

Villafranca JJ, Mildvan AS (1971). The mechanism of aconitase action. J Biol Chem 246:772-779.

ESTABLISHMENT OF MACROPHAGE CELL LINES BY IN VITRO INFECTION OF MOUSE BONE MARROW (BM) CELLS WITH A RETROVIRUS CONTAINING v-RAF PLUS v-MYC ONCOGENES.

Elisabetta Blasi[1], Ulf Rapp[2], and Luigi Varesio[1]

[1]Laboratory of Molecular Immunoregulation, BRMP, DCT, NCI-FCRF, and [2]Laboratory of Viral Carcinogenesis, NCI-FCRF, Frederick, MD 21701

INTRODUCTION

Mature tissue macrophages (Mϕ) have little or no proliferative capacity and are continuously replenished by differentiating bone marrow precursors which derive from a pool of multipotent stem cells (Neumann and Sorg, 1980). Myeloid precursors can be grown in vitro in the presence of specific growth factors (GF); however, their expansion is limited by a competing process of terminal differentiation (Tushinski et al., 1982). Difficulties in isolating sufficient numbers of homogeneous normal Mϕ precursors have represented a limitation for studies on the molecular events controlling myelopoieis. Recently, it has been shown that murine myeloid precursors, grown in vitro with GF, respond with augmented self-renewal upon infection with recombinant retroviruses carrying v-myc or v-src (Spooncer et al., 1984; Adkins et al., 1984; Veenstrom et al., 1984) suggesting a cooperation between some viral oncogenes (v-onc) and certain GF. We show here that introduction of two v-onc (v-raf and v-myc) into fresh BM cells induces cell growth in the absence of a specific GF supplement. The expression of both v-onc induces the selective proliferation of a population of cells expressing phenotype and biological functions of the monocytic lineage. Depending on the culture conditions, these cells can either differentiate and cease to proliferate or grow continuously, thus mimicking the alternative pathways that can be followed by committed BM stem cells in vivo.

MATERIALS AND METHODS

Infection with Retroviruses:

BM cells from femurs of C3H/HeJ mice were separated on a Ficoll gradient and infected overnight (o.n.) with the following retroviruses: 3611 (containing v-raf), J2 (which contains a complete raf/mil hybrid oncogene and a complete myc gene consisting of the 5' half of the MH2 v-myc and the 3' half of MC29 v-myc) or J3 (derived from J2 by a 200 b.p. deletion which takes the raf/mil gene out of reading frame, v-myc remaining functional) (Rapp et al., 1985). Infections were carried out in the presence of helper virus (Moloney murine leukemic virus). Following infection, the cultures were washed and incubated in Dulbecco's Modified Essential Medium (4.5 g/l of glucose), supplemented with 10% fetal bovine serum, 4mM glutamine, 100 U/ml of penicillin and 100 ug/ml of streptomycin (all the reagents obtained from GIBCO, Grand Island, NY). The cultures were weekly counted and the ^{3}H-thymidine (^{3}H-Thy) uptake was measured after o.n. pulse of 10^5 cells with 10 µCi/ml of ^{3}H-Thy (New England Nuclear, Boston, MA).

Cytotoxicity Assay:

Mø-mediated cytotoxicity was measured in a 24 hr ^{111}Indium (^{111}In)-release assay (Blasi et al., 1984). BM cells or peritoneal Mø, obtained from C3H/HeJ mice injected with 1 ml of 3% proteose peptone 3 days before, were used as effector cells. Two x 10^5 cells/well were plated in 96-well plates (Dynatech, Alexandria, VA) and incubated o.n. in medium or with various dilutions of IFN-γ (kindly provided by Genentech, Inc., So. San Francisco, CA) and heat killed Listeria monocytogenes (HKLM) (2 x 10^6 particles/well) kindly provided by Dr. A. Celada. The effector cells were then washed, and tested for cytotoxicity against ^{111}In labelled L5178Y target cells, and the results were expressed as % specific ^{111}In release.

RESULTS

Fresh BM cells were infected o.n. with J2 (v-raf and v-myc) J3 (v-myc) or 3611(v-raf) viruses and cultured in regular medium in the absence of exogenous GF. As expected, uninfected control cells, incubated with no GF, did not grow and died in culture (Table 1). Similar results were observed when BM cells had been infected with helper virus or with viruses carrying only one oncogene. In contrast, BM cells infected with J2 virus proliferated in vitro with a peak in cell number and ^{3}H-Thy uptake 2 weeks after infection.

TABLE 1. Effects of in vitro infection of BM cells with viruses on cellularity and proliferation.

Virus	Weeks in culture		
	1	2	5
None	2×10^5* (2312)**	$<10^4$ —	— —
Helper	1.8×10^5 (1870)	$<10^4$ —	— —
3611	2×10^5 (981)	$<10^4$ —	— —
J3	2×10^5 (1020)	$<10^4$ —	— —
J2	1.5×10^5 (20781)	3×10^7 (150812)	2×10^7 (4033)

* Five$\times 10^6$ BM cells were infected o.n. and incubated in the absence of GF. The values represent the number of viable cells/culture 1, 2 or 5 weeks after infection.

**In parenthesis are shown the cpm of ^{3}H-Thy uptake/10^5 cells in an o.n. pulse.

Thus, by infection with J2 virus, transducing v-raf and v-myc oncogenes, we could show growth of BM cells (J2 cells) in vitro in the absence of GF.

By flow cytometry analysis, we classified J2 cells as belonging to the monocytic lineage, since they were more than 95% positive for MAC-1, MAC-2 and Fc receptor antigens, whereas they were negative for the markers typical of T, (Ly 1.1, Lyt 2.1 and Thy 1.2), B or pre-B (surface and cytoplasmic Ig) lymphocytes.

Furthermore, J2 cells expressed constitutively biological functions characteristic of normal mature Mø: they were highly phagocytic, positive for α-naphtylacetate esterase staining and spontaneous producers of lysozyme (data not shown).

Tumoricidal activity is a biological function exerted by Mø, upon activation with appropriate stimuli. We investigated whether J2 cells became cytotoxic after o.n. treatment with IFN-γ and HKLM, stimuli that can induce tumoricidal activity in pMø from C3H/HeJ mice (Schreiber et al., 1984).

TABLE 2. Induction of Tumoricidal Activity by IFN-γ and HKLM in J2 cells and in pMø.

Treatment		% Cytotoxicity	
IFN-γ (U/ml)	HKLM	J2 Cells	pMø
–	–	2.7	0.9
4	–	3.2	1.2
20	–	2.8	1.3
100	–	3.0	2.5
–	+	2.8	2.1
4	+	33.5	47.5
20	+	61.4	58.7
100	+	67.5	62.4

As shown in Table 2, J2 cells were not spontaneously cytotoxic against L5178Y target cells, nor did they become tumoricidal upon o.n. preincubation with IFN-γ alone. However, incubation of J2 cells with IFN-γ in the presence of HKLM resulted in the induction of tumoricidal activity. Identical results were obtained using pMø as effector cells in the cytotoxicity assay (Table 2). These findings demonstrate that J2 cells, proliferating by in vitro infection of BM with v-raf and v-myc carrying virus, are not only morphologically and phenotypically, but also functionally Mø-like cells.

Following the initial burst of growth characterized by non-adherent cells with maximal rate of proliferation 14 days after infection (Table 1), J2 cell cultures progressively lost their proliferative ability and 4 to 6 weeks after infection, the cells formed an adherent layer of resting cells. After several attempts, we found that the J2 quiescent cells could be reverted to actively proliferating cells, upon coculture with dextran-based beads (Cytodex, Pharmacia, Uppsala, Sweden). Under these culture

conditions (Figure 1), J2 cells have been kept growing for
more than 8 months. Analysis of their phenotype and
functional activities, showed that J2 cells growing in
beads are indistiguishable from J2 cells proliferating in
suspension 14 days after infection (data not shown).
Therefore, addition of beads to the quiescent cells causes
reactivation of their proliferative ability and provides
establishment of immortalized cell lines.

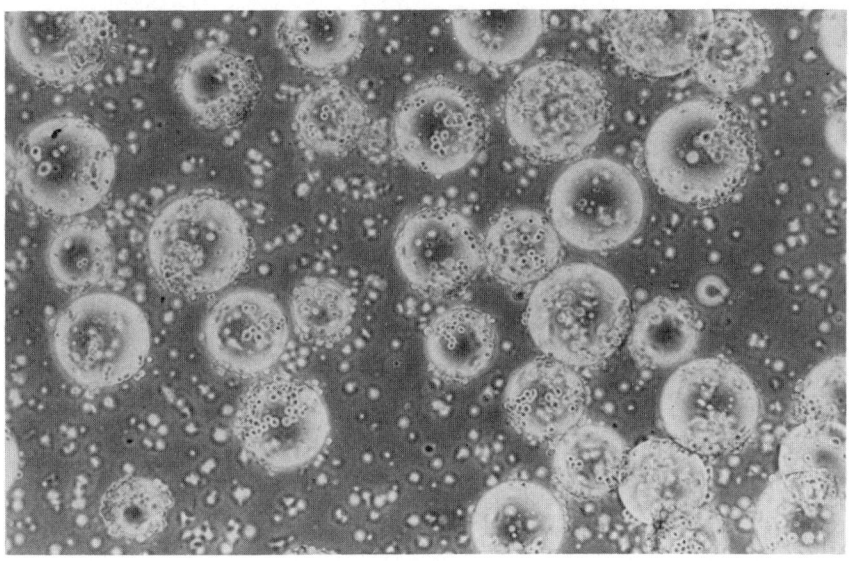

Figure 1. Morphology of the J2 cells proliferating upon
coculture with dextran-based beads.

DISCUSSION

We have demonstrated that infection of fresh BM cells
with J2 virus, carrying v-raf and v-myc oncogenes, induces
proliferation of BM cells (J2 cells), in the absence of
exogeneous GF. In contrast, viruses carrying either oncogene alone did not promote BM cell growth. These findings
indicate that a cooperation between v-raf and v-myc is
needed to induce BM proliferation in vitro. Moreover, the
fact that exogeneous GF were not required for proliferation
of J2 cells suggests that the expression of the two oncogenes might have overridden the requirement for specific
GF.

The monocytic nature of J2 cells was shown by the surface markers and by the constitutive expression of phagocytosis, lysozyme production and non-specific esterase.

Moreover, J2 cells like Mø, could be induced to become tumoricidal upon o.n. stimulation with IFN-γ and HKLM. Thus, introduction of v-raf and v-myc oncogenes in BM cells induces proliferation of a subpopulation of cells endowed with at least some biological properties similar to that of mature peritoneal Mø.

Depending upon the culture conditions, J2 cells grew continuously in suspension or formed a monolayer of resting plastic-adherent Mø. The quiescent adherent cells were indistinguishable from normal BM derived Mø. Thus, we speculate that the proliferative stimulus provided by the two oncogenes, causing the initial expansion of J2 cells, is then limited by a dominant differentiation process, which drives J2 cells to adhere and cease to proliferate.

Only J2 cells, but not normal Mø (data not shown), could be rescued from the resting differentiated stage and reverted to proliferating cells by coculture with beads, suggesting that the response to the growth promoting activity of v-raf and v-myc, down-regulated by differentiation, could be reactivated.

In conclusion, defining immortalization as continuous in vitro growth, three signals seem to be required to immortalize Mø from fresh BM cells: two oncogenes v-raf/v-myc and the beads. Because of the unique pattern of growth shown by J2 cells, our system can provide a unique experimental model to investigate the molecular events controlling proliferation and differentiation of monocytic cells.

REFERENCES

Neumann C, Sorg C (1980). Sequential expression of functions during macrophage differentiation in murine bone marrow lipid cultures. Eur. J. Immunol. 10: 834-840.

Tushinski RJ, Oliver IT, Guilbert LJ, Tynan PW, Warner JR, Stanley ER (1982). Survival of mononuclear phagocytes depends on a lineage specific growth factor that the differentiated cells selectively destroy. Cell 28: 71-81.

Spooncer E, Boettinger D, Dexter TM (1984). Continuous *in vitro* generation of multipotent stem cell clones from *src* infected cultures. Nature 310: 228-230.

Adkins B, Leutz A, Graf T (1984). Autocrine growth induced by *src*-related oncogenes in transformed chicken myeloid cells. Cell 39: 439-445.

Vennstrom B, Kahn P, Adkins B, Enrietto P, Hayman MJ, Graf T, Luciw P (1984). Transformation of mammalian fibroblasts and macrophages *in vitro* by a murine retrovirus encoding an avian v-*myc* oncogene.

Rapp UR, Bonner TI, Moelling K, Jansen HW, Bister K, Ihle J (1985). Genes and gene products involved in growth regulation of tumor cells. In Havemann K, Sorenson G, Gropp C (eds): "Recent Results in Cancer Research," Spring-Verlag, New York, Heidelberg, pp 221-236.

Blasi E, Herberman RB, Varesio L (1984). Requirement for protein synthesis for induction of macrophage tumoricidal activity by IFN-α and IFN-β but not by IFN-γ. J. Immunol. 132: 3226-3228.

Schreiber RD, Altman A, Katz DH (1982). Identification of a T cell hybridoma that produces large quantities of macrophage activating factor. J. Exp. Med. 156: 677-689.

DIFFERENCES IN FUNCTIONAL, PHENOTYPICAL AND PHYSICAL PROPERTIES OF HUMAN PERIPHERAL BLOOD MONOCYTES (Mo) REFLECT THEIR VARIOUS MATURATION STAGES

Carl G. Figdor, Anje A. te Velde, Jack Leemans and Willy S. Bont

Division of Immunology, The Netherlands Cancer Institute, Plesmanlaan 121, 1066 CX Amsterdam, The Netherlands

INTRODUCTION

Monocytes play a central role in a variety of cellular processes. There is increasing evidence that the monocyte pool consists of various functionally different subsets. However, it is not clear whether these subsets represent different states of activation, different stages of maturation, or distinct stable subpopulations. In addition, interpretation of the results is hampered since various methods (adherence, density gradient centrifugation, centrifugal elutriation) have been employed to isolate the monocyte subsets. Therefore it cannot be excluded that part of the reported monocyte heterogeneity may be attributed to activation of the cells by the isolation procedure. To prevent activation by adherence or by phagocytosis of gradient material (Wakefield et al., 1982), we developed a blood component separator (BCS) to isolate mononuclear cells without exposing the cells to body-foreign substances (Figdor et al., 1982a). Subsequently centrifugal elutriation (CE) was used to isolate and fractionate monocytes (Figdor et al., 1982b).

The aim of the present study is to investigate monocyte heterogeneity and to define the nature of this phenomenon. The differences in physical, functional and phenotypical properties described in this study strongly suggest that monocyte heterogeneity must be attributed to maturation, and not to differences in activation stages, or to the presence of stable subpopulations.

RESULTS

Human monocytes isolated as described above, were >95% pure (non-specific esterase). The data in Figure 1 demonstrate that these monocytes express only low numbers of MHC class II molecules (HLA-DR and HLA-DQ) in comparison with monocytes which were allowed to adhere for 30 min at 37°C. Furthermore the results show that adhesion results in an increased expression of MHC class II molecules and in an impaired burst of oxidative metabolites (leucigenin dependent chemiluminescence) in response to opsonized zymosan (not shown). These data indicate that adhesion leads to a non-specific activation of monocytes.

Fig. 1.

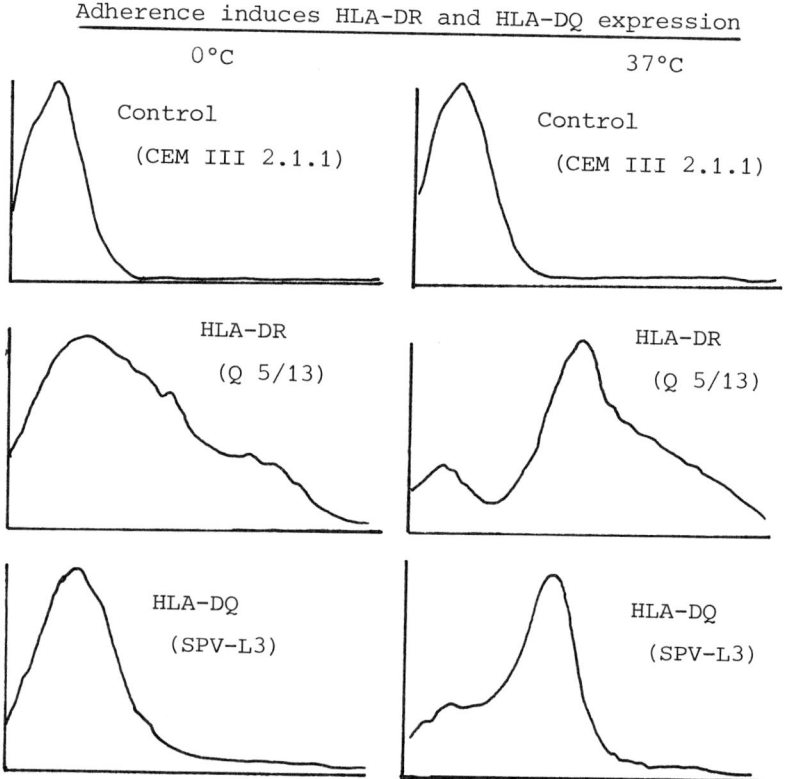

FACS analysis of CE-purified monocytes after incubation for 60 min at 37°C (adherence) or 0°C.

TABLE 1. Expression of HLA-DR and HLA-DQ on the Various Monocyte Subsets Before and After Culture

antigen	relative fluorescence intensity					
	before culture			7 days culture		
	M1	M2	M3	M1	M2	M3
HLA-DR	4.4	5.3	6.6	65.1	71.8	67.5
HLA-DQ	1.4	1.4	1.5	6.8	6.3	5.3
KLH (control)	0.3	0.3	0.5	0.4	0.1	0.1

The results in Figure 2 show that three subsets (M1, M2 and M3) of human monocytes fractionated by CE (Figdor et al., 1984) are all equally sized but differ in cell density, since they vary in protein content (Figdor et al., 1983). The monocyte subsets differ in their capacity to produce interleukin-1 (M1>M2>M3) and in their CL response to serum opsonized zymosan (M3>M2>M1) as shown in Figure 3. Furthermore, they are heterogeneous with respect to the expression of HLA-DR but not HLA-DQ (Table 1). All monocyte subsets produce equal amounts of granulocyte-macrophage colony stimulating activity and of the prostaglandins PGF_2, $F_{2\alpha}$, TXB_2, $6-K-PGF_{1\alpha}$ (not shown). The observed heterogeneity cannot be ascribed to the existence of stable subpopulations of the monocyte pool, since after 7 days of culture of the various monocyte fractions, the differences in the expression of HLA-DR (Table 1) and the CL response (not shown) are abolished. To investigate whether the heterogeneity must be attributed to differences in maturation or activation stage, we cultured the monocytes for 24 hours in the presence of IFN-γ (300 U/ml), high concentrations of LPS (1 µg/ml), low concentrations of LPS (20 ng/ml), low concentrations of LPS + IFN-γ, or in medium alone. After culture we measured the expression of both HLA-DR, HLA-DQ (Figure 4), and the CL response to opsonized zymosan (Figure 5). The data in Figures 4 and 5 illustrate that the differences between the various subsets are still present after 24 hrs of culture. In addition we observed two types of activation, first, non-specific activation caused by adherence to plastic which affected all monocyte subsets and which increased both the expression of HLA-DR (Figure 4) and HLA-DQ (not shown). Secondly, monocytes could be activated specifically by IFN-γ and/or LPS (Figures 4,5) which affected only the subsets with the higher densities.

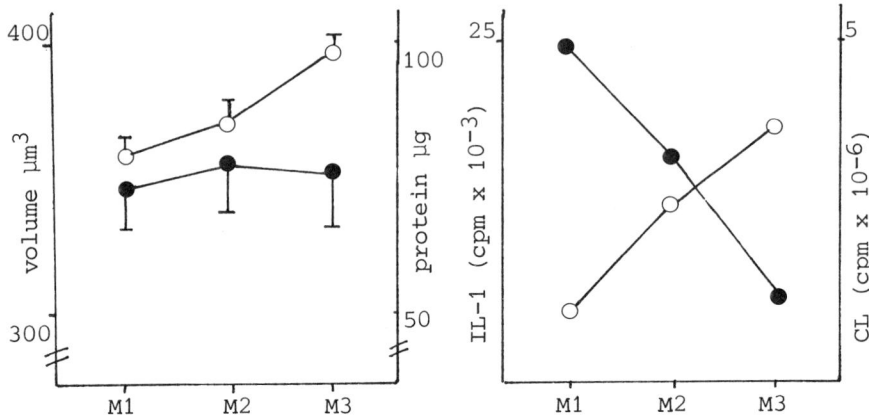

Fig. 2. Volume (●) and protein content (○) of the various monocyte fractions.

Fig. 3. IL-1 (●) production (mouse thymocyte assay) and the respiratory burst (○) (CL response to zymosan) of the monocyte subsets.

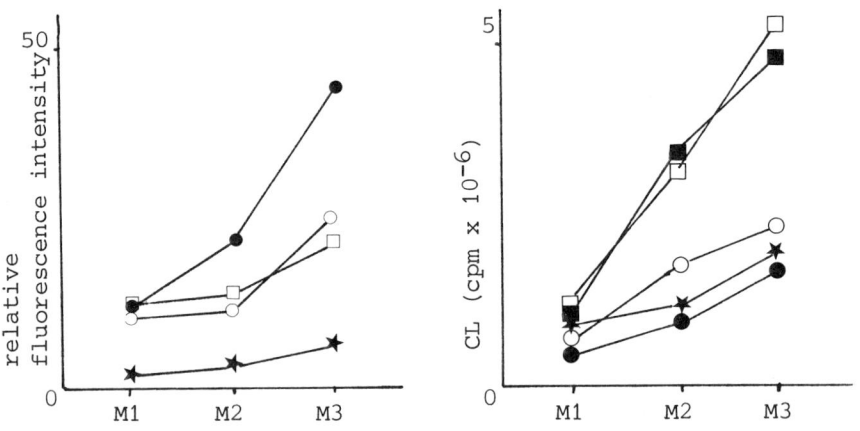

Fig. 4. The induction of HLA-DR expression by IFN-γ and LPS.
Fig. 5. Enhancement of the respiratory burst (CL response) by IFN-γ and LPS.

(★) freshly isolated monocytes; (○) 24 h culture; (□) 24 h culture + 1 µg LPS/ml; (●) 24 h culture + IFN-γ (300 U/ml) + 20 ng LPS/ml; (■) 24 h culture + IFN-γ (300 U/ml).

IFN-γ resulted in an increased expression of HLA-DR (Fig. 4) but not of HLA-DQ (not shown). IFN-γ had no effect on the burst of oxidative metabolites in response to opsonized zymosan (Fig. 5). LPS had exact opposite effects, it did not affect the expression of HLA-DR (Fig. 4) but increased the oxidative burst (Fig. 5). Whereas low concentrations of LPS were insufficient to enhance the CL response (not shown), culture of the monocytes in the presence of LPS (20 ng/ml) + IFN-γ leads to an enhanced CL response (Fig. 5), which supports the concept that IFN-γ is able to prime the monocytes, but that endotoxin is required to specifically activate the cells (Meltzer et al., 1982). Surprisingly, the monocytes with the lowest density, which represented approximately 20% of the monocyte population did not respond to LPS and/or IFN-γ. Since our isolation procedures exclude monocyte activation, these findings indicate that the monocyte subsets represent different maturation stages and that the density of the monocytes increases in parallel with maturation. The notion that monocyte heterogeneity is reflecting different maturation stages but not activation stages is supported by the observation that the differences between the monocyte subsets are still present after 24 hours of incubation (Figs. 4,5), but are abolished after 7 days of culture. Apparently, circulating peripheral blood monocytes have to reach a certain stage of maturation before they become susceptible to activation signals provided by LPS and IFN-γ.

Finally, our results indicate that controversies concerning phenotypical, functional and also physical heterogeneity of human monocytes and differences of these cells in response to activation signals may be attributed to isolation and purification procedures that result already in activation of (part of) the cells. In addition, the present data stress the importance of subtle isolation procedures to study the activation of biological functions of peripheral blood monocytes optimally.

REFERENCES

Figdor CG, Bont WS, Touw I, De Roos J, Roosnek EE, De Vries JE (1982a). Isolation of functionally different human monocytes by counterflow centrifugation elutriation. Blood 60:46-53.

Figdor CG, Bont WS, De Vries JE (1982b). Rapid isolation of mononuclear cells from buffy coats prepared by a new blood cell separator. J Immunol Methods 55:221-229.

Figdor CG, Leemans JMM, Bont WS, De Vries JE (1983). Theory and practice of centrifugal elutriation (CE). Factors influencing the separation of human blood cells. Cell Biophys 5:105-118.

Figdor CG, Van Es WL, Leemans JMM, Bont WS (1984). A centrifugal elutriation system of separating small numbers of cells. J Immunol Methods 68:73-87.

Meltzer MS, Occhionero M, Ruco LP (1982). Macrophage activation for tumor cytotoxicity: regulatory mechanisms for induction and control of cytotoxic activity. Federation Proceed 41:2198-2205.

Wakefield JStJ, Gale JS, Berridge MV, Jordan TW, Ford HC (1982). Is Percoll innocuous to cells? Biochem J 202: 795-800.

MONOCLONAL ANTIBODIES REACTIVE WITH DIFFERENT STAGES IN MURINE MACROPHAGE DIFFERENTIATION

P.J.M. Leenen[a], U. Willmer[b], F.W. Falkenberg[b], A.M.A.C. Jansen[a] and W. van Ewijk[a].
(a) Dept. Cell Biology and Genetics, Erasmus University, P.O.Box 1738, 3000 DR Rotterdam, The Netherlands. (b) Dept. Medical Microbiology and Immunology, P.O.Box 102 148, 4630 Bochum 1, FRG.

INTRODUCTION

Mononuclear phagocytes originate from the hemopoietic stem cell in the bone marrow (van Furth and Cohn, 1968). The differentiation of macrophages (MØ) is accompanied by major changes in the cellular phenotype (Walker et al., 1985). The study of these phenotypic changes is of importance as a primary step in understanding the course of MØ differentiation and the factors governing this process. Therefore, we have produced a panel of monoclonal antibodies using murine MØ as immunogen (Willmer et al., 1984). This paper describes the reactivity of these antibodies in three models of MØ differentiation:
1. bone marrow culture with CSF-1 containing conditioned medium (van der Meer et al., 1983);
2. differentiation induction of the immature M1 cell line (Ichikawa, 1969);
3. a panel of MØ cell lines aligned in a linear differentiation sequence (Leenen et al., 1985b).

Furthermore, we characterized the reactivity of these antibodies on isolated MØ and control cell populations. The results indicate that this panel of monoclonal antibodies is very useful for 1. monitoring the course of MØ differentiation in isolated models and 2. comparative studies on the differentiation of other hemopoietic lineages.

MATERIALS AND METHODS

Monoclonal antibodies

Xenogeneic monoclonal antibody producing hybridoma cell lines were established according to standard protocols. X63-Ag8.653 myeloma cells were used as fusion partner with immune DA rat spleen cells. BALB/c splenic MØ were used as immunogen. Cells were cultured in DMEM + 5% foetal bovine serum and undiluted culture supernatants were used in the various immunoassays as the source of antibodies. The antibodies were grouped in 3 clusters according to similar reactivity patterns: cluster 1: MIV 51, MIV 52, MIV 113, MIV 116; cluster 2: MIV 25, MIV 33; cluster 3: MIV 38, MIV 55. Culture supernatant of the M1/70 cell line was used as a source of anti-Mac-1 antibodies (Springer et al., 1979).

Cells

Bone marrow-derived mononuclear phagocytes were obtained by culturing bone marrow cells for 7 days in Teflon bags in the presence of CSF-1 containing conditioned medium according to Van der Meer et al. (1983). Cells were then harvested, washed and spun down on 8-well microscopic slides. The preparations were fixed in acetone and stored at $-20^{\circ}C$. Differentiation of the immature myeloid M1 cell line was induced in the following ways: selection of spontaneously adherent cells, culture in the presence of ascitic fluid, L cell conditioned medium or WEHI-3 conditioned medium (Ichikawa, 1969). Other MØ-, control populations and cell lines were obtained and prepared for the various immunoassays as described elsewhere (Leenen et al., 1985a).

Immunoassays

Indirect immunofluorescence was used for the detection of antibody binding to isolated populations and to differentiated and control M1 cells. A semi-quantitative micro-ELISA using a sheep-anti-rat-Ig-β-galactosidase conjugate was employed for the detection of antibody binding to MØ cell lines (Leenen et al. 1985a). An immunocytochemical staining using the same β-galactosidase conjugate was used for the demonstration of antibody binding to bone marrow-derived mononuclear phagocytes (Bondi et al., 1982).

RESULTS AND DISCUSSION

Antibody reactivity with isolated populations

The investigated antibodies show a clear binding to all MØ populations tested (Table 1). The degree of antibody binding, however, varies between the different MØ populations. Cluster 1 antibodies recognize a common antigen also expressed by granulocytes, thymocytes and erythrocytes. Cluster 2 antibodies bind strongly to granulocytes, whereas cluster 3 antibodies show crossreactivity with erythrocytes.

TABLE 1. Antibody reactivity with isolated populations

	Mac-1	Cluster 1	Cluster 2	Cluster 3
res.PMØ	+++	+	+	++
alv.MØ	+	+++	$\pm$	+
TG-PEMØ	++	++	+	++
PMN	++	++	+++	+
thy	−	++	+	−
ery	−	++	−	+

res.PMØ=resident peritoneal MØ; alv.MØ=resident alveolar MØ; TG-PEMØ=thioglycollate elicited peritoneal MØ; PMN= polymorphonuclear granulocytes; thy=thymocytes; ery= erythrocytes.

Antibody reactivity in MØ differentiation models

<u>Bone marrow culture with CSF-1</u>. Table 2 shows the staining patterns of the investigated antibodies on immature and mature MØ obtained from bone marrow culture in the presence of CSF-1 containing conditioned medium. Cluster 1 and 2 antibodies bind strongly to immature MØ and hardly to mature MØ. The reverse holds true for anti-Mac-1 and cluster 3 antibodies, which strongly stain mature MØ.

TABLE 2. Antibody reactivity with bone marrow-derived mononuclear phagocytes

	Mac-1	cluster 1	cluster 2	cluster 3
immature MØ	+	++	++	+
mature MØ	++	−	+	++

Immature MØ were identified as small cells with a nucleus/ cytoplasm ratio >1. Mature MØ were identified as relatively large cells with a nucleus/cytoplasm ratio <1.

Induction of MØ differentiation of M1 cells. Fig. 1 shows the antibody binding to control M1 cells and to M1 cells after induction of MØ differentiation. Mac-1 is strongly expressed on differentiated M1 cells, independent of the inducing agent. Concomitant with an increased expression of Mac-1 is the loss of cluster 1 antibody binding. The level of expression of the markers recognized by cluster 2 antibodies on differentiated M1 cells varies, depending on the inducing agent. The markers recognized by cluster 3 antibodies are induced after spontaneous differentiation or after culture with L929 conditioned medium.

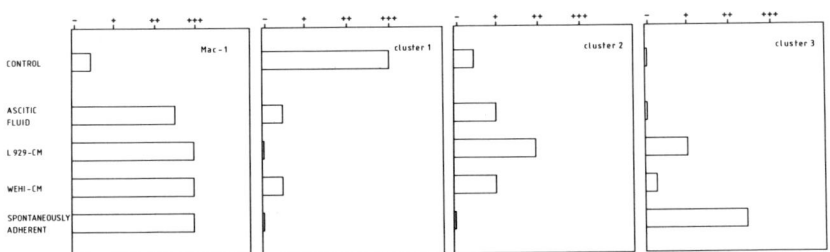

Figure 1. Antibody binding to control and differentiated M1 cells.

MØ cell lines in differentiation sequence. The binding of antibodies to a panel of MØ cell lines ordered in a linear differentiation sequence is represented in Fig. 2. The reactivity of a representative antibody from each cluster is given.

The increasing expression of Mac-1 antigen in the course of MØ differentiation was part of the characterization used to align the MØ cell lines in a differentiation sequence. MIV 51 (cluster 1) binds only to the precursor cell lines M1, RMB-1

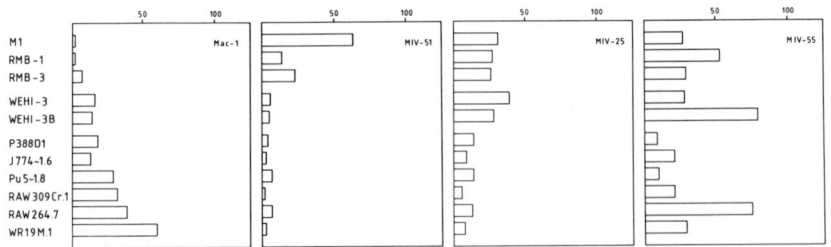

Figure 2. Antibody binding to a panel of MØ cell lines aligned in differentiation sequence. Antibody binding is expressed as a percentage of standardized positive control value (Leenen et al., 1985b).

and RMB-3. No binding of cluster 1 antibodies was detected with the immature (WEHI) cell lines nor with any of the mature MØ cell lines. The marker recognized by MIV 25 (cluster 2) antibodies is most clearly expressed by both the precursor and immature MØ cell lines and less by the mature MØ cell lines. MIV 55 (cluster 3) antibodies bind in varying degrees to precursor, immature and mature MØ cell lines.

In conclusion, cluster 1 antibodies (MIV 51, MIV 52, MIV 113, MIV 116) recognize MØ precursors in all three models of MØ differentiation. Cluster 2 antibodies (MIV 25, MIV 33) recognize MØ precursors and immature MØ in both bone marrow cultures and the cell line panel. Antibodies of the third cluster (MIV 38, MIV 55) recognize mature MØ in both bone marrow cultures and M1 differentiation. These monoclonal antibodies provide interesting tools for monitoring the course of MØ differentiation in isolated models. Furthermore, these antibodies can be used for comparative studies of MØ differentiation versus the differentiation of other hemopoietic cells.

ACKNOWLEDGMENTS

We wish to thank Mrs. Cary Meijerink-Clerkx for fast secretarial processing of this manuscript and Mr. Tar van Os and Mr. Joop Fengler for excellent photography. This work was supported by research grant 80-25 from the Netherlands Astma Foundation and grant Fa 71/11-1 from the Deutsche Forschungsgemeinschaft.

REFERENCES

Bondi A, Chieregatti G, Eusebi V, Fulcheri E, Bussolati G (1982). The use of β-galactosidase as a tracer in immunocytochemistry. Histochem 76:153-158.
Ichikawa Y (1969). Differentiation of a cell line of myeloid leukemia. J Cell Physiol 74:223-234.
Leenen PJM, Jansen AMAC, van Ewijk W (1985a). Fixation parameters for immunocytochemistry: the effect of glutaraldehyde or paraformaldehyde fixation on the preservation of mononuclear phagocyte differentiation antigens. In Bullock GR, Petrusz P (eds): 'Techniques in Immunocytochemistry, Vol. 3', London: Academic Press. In press.

Leenen PJM, Jansen AMAC, van Ewijk W (1985b). Murine macrophage cell lines can be ordered in a linear differentiation sequence. Submitted for publication.

Springer T, Galfre G, Secher DS, Milstein C (1979). Mac-1: a macrophage differentiation antigen identified by monoclonal antibody. Eur J Immunol 9:301-306.

Van der Meer JWM, Van de Gevel JS, Van Furth R (1983). Characteristics of longterm cultures of proliferating mononuclear phagocytes from bone marrow. J Reticuloendothel Soc 21:203-225.

Van Furth R, Cohn ZA (1968). The origin and kinetics of mononuclear phagocytes. J Exp Med 128:415-433.

Walker EB, Akporiaye ET, Warner NL, Stewart CC (1985). Characterization of subsets of bone marrow-derived macrophages by flow cytometry analysis. J Leukoc Biol 37:121-136.

Willmer U, Boenke B, Falkenberg FW (1984). Identification of differentiation antigens on the murine myeloid/macrophage cell line M1 by monoclonal antibodies (MABS). Immunobiol 167:163-164.

SURFACE ANTIGEN ANALYSIS OF HUMAN MACROPHAGE MATURATION AND HETEROGENEITY

Reinhard Andreesen, Klaus J. Bross and Frank Emmrich

Medizinische Klinik I, Hugstetter Str. 55, (R.A., K.J.B.), and Max-Planck-Institut für Immunbiologie, Stübeweg, (F.E.), D-7800 Freiburg, FRG

INTRODUCTION

Cell differentiation of bone marrow cells to circulating blood monocytes (mo) along the monocyte-macrophage pathway provides a common precursor pool for further maturation if these cells have left the peripheral blood and migrated to various tissue sites (van Furth, 1982). Mature macrophages (MØ) show a considerable heterogeneity of both morphology and function. It is still an open question whether predestined mo subsets exist who are attracted to the anatomic site they are designated to (Bursuker and Goldman, 1983) or whether environmental signals induce the site-specific phenotypes.

We have investigated the expression of surface antigens on MØ at maturational stages beyond the blood mo level. For this purpose an in vitro culture system was employed which allows to harvest undamaged mature MØ at sequential stages of differentiation. By using the monoclonal antibody (mAb) technique differentiation antigens of these in vitro matured MØ were defined. Interestingly, a considerable diversity was found in the expression of these differentiation antigens also among in vivo matured MØ obtained from various body fluids.

MATERIAL AND METHODS

Generation of MAX mAbs

Two months old Balb/c mice were injected 5 times at weekly intervals with 5×10^6 mo-derived MØ's cultured on teflon foils for at least 10 days. Immune spleen cells were fused with the HAT-sensitive line X63Ag8.653. Hybridoma supernatants were tested for binding to autologous B-cells, T-cells, mo and mo-derived MØ by cell-ELISA (Emmrich and Andreesen, 1985) and by the immunoperoxidase slide technique (Bross et al., 1978). Finally, 5 hybridomas were selected and subjected to re-cloning and further expansion.

OKT9 was purchased from Ortho Pharmaceutical Corp. Raritan, NJ, and a polyclonal rabbit anti-transferrin (TF) antibody from Behringwerke AG, Marburg, FRG.

Cells

Mo were isolated from the peripheral blood of healthy volunteers, separated from other mononuclear cells by adherence and cultured on hydrophobic teflon foils (Biofolie 25, Heraeus, Hanau, FRG) in RPMI 1640 plus 10% human AB-group serum essentially as described (Andreesen et al., 1983). Leukemic monocytes were obtained from the blood of patients with monocytic leukemia by density centrifugation. Pulmonary MØ were collected from the broncho-alveolar lavage fluids of healthy volunteers and patients undergoing diagnostic bronchoscopy. Pleural and peritoneal MØ were isolated from effusion fluids secondary to heart failure, portal hypertension or malignancies. Milk MØ were obtained from breast milk samples taken at day 3 to 9 post delivery.

RESULTS

A series of mAbs against MØ surface antigens was developed using mo-derived MØ for immunisation. In this report we describe 5 mAbs of the MAX.series which discriminate between MØ and mo. The reactivity pattern of these antibodies is described in Table 1. MAX. 1 and MAX. 2 detect lineage-restricted molecules of 64kD and 200 kD, respectively (unpublished own observation). MAX.3 (directed to a 68 kD molecule) behaves similar but is expressed also on cells of the megakaryocyte lineage. MAX.11 and MAX.26 are found on a minor portion of blood mo with a rapid increase in expression upon in vitro maturation. Whereas Max.11 is lineage-restricted the structure detected by MAX. 26 is also found on lymphocyte subsets, mesothelial cells, melanoma cells and some histiocytic and lymphocytic lymphomas. During MØ maturation in vitro the antigens defined by MAX.1, 2, and 3 were

Table 1: Cellular distribution of surface antigens reactive with MAX monoclonal antibodies[1]

cells[2]	Monoclonal antibody designation				
	MAX.1 (IgG1/k)	MAX.2 (IgM/k)	MAX.3 (IgG1/k)	MAX.11 (IgG1/k)	MAX.26 (IgG1/k)
monocyte-derived MØ	++[3]	+	++	++	++
adherent monocytes (day 1)	-	-	-	var	var
granulocytes	-	-	-	-	-
platelets/megakaryocytes	-	-	+	-	-
B-cells	-	-	-	-	var
T-cells	-	-	-	-	+
activated T-cells	-	-	-	-	++
permanent cell lines					
L-428 (Hodgkin cells)	-	-	-	-	-
U-937 (histiocytic lymphoma)[4]	-	-	-	+	+
DHL-1 (histiocytic lymphoma)	-	-	-	-	++
HL-60 (promyelocytic leukemia)	-	-	-	-	-
B-lymphoblastoid cells[5]	-	-	-	-	++
melanoma cells[6]	-	-	-	-	+

[1] as evaluated by immunoperoxidase staining; hybridoma supernatants were diluted 1:10

[2] all cell lines were tested at least three times; activated T cells, platelets and granulocytes were obtained from three different donors whereas MO, MO-derived MØ, B cells and T cells were obtained from ten different donors

[3] ++: more than 90% of cells reactive, +: varying reactivity ranging from 15-90%, var: reactivity varied among experiments from negative to up to 20% positive cells, -: no reactivity

[4] varying portions of positive cells on repeated tests with the same line (15-80%)

[5] LBL 6078 and LBL 3283

[6] xenotransplanted tumorgrafts Mel-1 and Mel-2 and permanent cell line Colo 38

expressed consecutively as shown in figure 1. Among several other mAbs which do not react with mo those against the TF-receptor and against surface TF could also bind to mo-derived MØ (data not shown). MAX antigens were also expressed on human MØ isolated from various body cavities (Table 2). These MØ obviously have acquired these antigens during in vivo maturation. Although heterogenous, some generalisations regarding the MAX antigen pattern can be made: MAX.3 was absent from pulmonary and breast milk MØ but present on most pleural and some peritoneal MØ. MAX.1 could be detected only on minor portions of pulmonary and peritoneal MØ but never on pleural and breast milk MØ. However, if pulmonary and peritoneal MØ were cultured in vitro the cells readily expressed these MAX antigens which were missing in situ (data not shown).

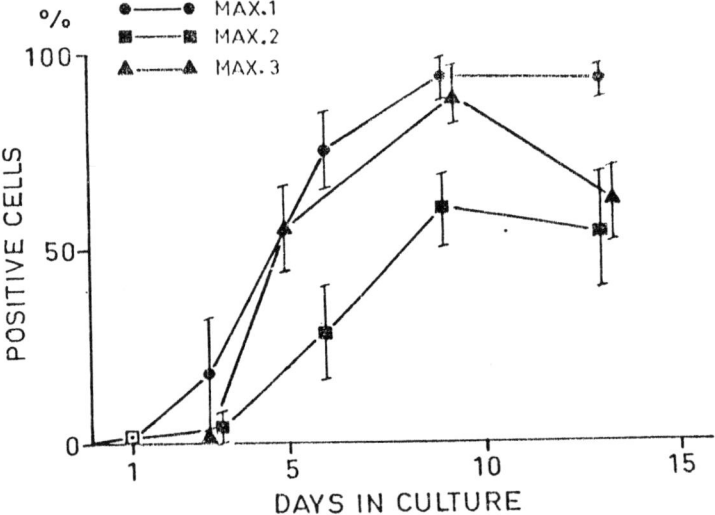

Figure 1. Sequential expression of MAX differentiation antigens during maturation on hydrophobic Teflon foils in vitro.

Table 2: Heterogeneity of human macrophages as defined by surface antigen analysis

source of macrophages	monoclonal antibody reactivity					
	MAX.1 %	MAX.2 %	MAX.3 %	MAX.11 %	OKT9 %
normal blood (n = 6)	none	none	none	21 ± 17 (0-48)	none
monocytic leukemia (n = 5)	none	none	none	57 ± 28 (2-85)	< 1
monocyte-derived (Teflon bag, n = 6)	> 90	61 ± 10	> 90	> 90	> 90
pleural effusion (n = 8)	< 1	23 ± 21 (2-61)	51 ± 28 (15-80)	41 ± 27 (10-80)	3 ± 2 (0-10)
ascites fluid (n = 12)	17 ± 18 (0-50)	16 ± 18 (0-50)	60 ± 24 (18-95)	46 ± 28 (10-90)	22 ± 16 (0-45)
alveolar lavage fluid (n = 14)	7 ± 6 (0-16)	84 ± 8	< 1	62 ± 30 (10-94)	> 90
breast milk (n = 4)	< 1	7 ± 7 (0-20)	< 1	39 ± 13	78 ± 10

DISCUSSION

The differential expression of MAX antigens which is related to various anatomic sites might indicate a functional correlation of certain membrane structures to the properties of cells residing in a given tissue. However, these site-specific MØ can be induced to express the missing antigens upon in vitro culture. This supports the hypothesis that local factors control the observed phenotypes and argues against the existence of mo subsets with commitment to differentiation into pulmonary, pleural or peritoneal MØ, respectively.

The MAX antigens seem to be unique and differ from the differentiation antigens described so far: the PAM1 (Biondi et al., 1984) is not expressed on mo-derived MØ; the 27F9 antigen (Zwadlo et al., 1985) is present on melanoma cells and differs in the molecular weight. Whether or not the MAX. antigens have any functional significance is subject to future investigations. MAX mAbs may also be useful as tools for staging of the terminal differentiation of MØ in vitro and in vivo.

REFERENCES

Andreesen R, Picht J, Löhr GW (1983). Primary cultures of human blood-born monocytes grown on hydrophobic teflon membranes. J Immunol Meth 56: 295-304.

Biondi A, Rossing TH, Bennet J, Todd RE (1984). Surface membrane heterogeneity among human mononuclear phagocytes. J Immunol 132: 1237-1243.

Bross KJ, Pangalis GA, Staatz CG, Blume KG (1978). Demonstration of cell surface antigens and their antibodies by the peroxidase-antiperoxidase method. Transplantation 25: 331-334.

Bursuker I, Goldmann R (1983). On the origin of macrophage heterogeneity: a hypothesis. RES 33: 207-220.

Emmrich F, Andreesen R (1985). Monoclonal antibodies against differentiation antigens on human macrophages. Immunol Letters 9: 321-324.

Van Furth R (1982). Current view on the mononuclear phagocyte system. Immunobiol 161: 178-185.

Zwadlo G, Bröcker TH, v Bassewitz DB, Feige U, Sorg C (1985). J Immunol 134: 1487-1492.

ANTIBODIES TO LFA-1 AND RELATED MOLECULES INHIBIT CONJUGATE FORMATION BETWEEN HUMAN PERIPHERAL BLOOD MONOCYTES AND MELANOMA CELLS

Anje A. te Velde, Gerrit D. Keizer, Jan E. de Vries and Carl G. Figdor

Division of Immunology, The Netherlands Cancer Institute, Plesmanlaan 121, 1066 CX Amsterdam The Netherlands

INTRODUCTION

Mononuclear phagocytes are thought to have appreciable levels of cytotoxicity against susceptible target cells (Mantovani et al., 1980; Fischer et al., 1983; Fidler and Kleinerman, 1984). The mechanism of target cell lysis is generally accepted to be composed of two steps (Adams et al., 1982). The first step is the formation of conjugates between the effector cell and the target cell, followed by subsequent killing of the target cell.

Recently Keizer et al. (1985b) showed that monoclonal antibodies (moabs) recognizing monocyte-associated cellular adhesion molecules (MO-CAM) are associated with monocyte functions like adhesion, migration/chemotaxis and phagocytosis. The available moabs against MO-CAMs are the anti-leukocyte function associated (LFA)-1 α and β chain and anti-Mo-1. Immunoprecipitation has demonstrated that LFA-1 is a non-covalently linked dimer of two polypeptide chains of 170 kD (α chain) and 95 kD (β chain) and that Mo-1 is a similar dimer with an α chain of 165 kD and an identical β chain (Keizer et al., 1985a). The latter antigen is associated with the function of the C3bi receptor (Beller et al., 1982).

The aim of the present study was to investigate if these MO-CAMs were involved in conjugate formation between human peripheral blood monocytes and human allogeneic melanoma target cells. To investigate this we used a single cell conjugate assay (Bonavida et al., 1983). The results demonstrate that MO-CAMs play an important role in the conjugate formation between human monocytes and melanoma target cells, and that these antigens are involved in human monocyte antibody-dependent cellular cytotoxicity (ADCC) against anti-D coated human erythrocytes.

RESULTS

FACS analyses were carried out to determine the specificity of the monoclonal antibodies recognizing MO-CAM (Table 1). These results indicate that MO-CAMs are only expressed by the effector cells and not by the target cells. Furthermore it was demonstrated that a melanoma-associated cellular adhesion molecule (MLN-CAM) is only expressed by melanoma cells.

TABLE 1. Expression of Surface Membrane Determinants[a]

antigen recognized[b]	expression on human		
	monocytes	melanoma cells	erythrocytes
keyhole limped haemocyanin (CEM)	1.2 (0%)	1 (0%)	1.5 (0%)
LFA-1 (α chain)	13.2 (95%)	1 (2%)	1.5 (3%)
LFA-1, Mo-1, p150,95 (β chain)	24.1 (97%)	0.9 (1%)	1.6 (2%)
Mo-1 (α chain)	21.4 (94%)	1.1 (4%)	1.7 (4%)
MLN-CAM-1 120/95 kD	1.2 (1%)	8 (93%)	1.5 (3%)

[a] Freshly isolated human monocytes and erythrocytes, and cultured melanoma cells (BK-mel) were labeled with moab. Data are expressed as mean relative fluorescenced index and mean percentage positive cells (between brackets).

[b] Moabs used: control : CEM; anti-LFA α chain : SPV-L7; anti common β chain : CLB54; anti-Mo-1 α chain : Bear-1; and anti-MLN-CAM-1 : AMF-7.

TABLE 2. Conjugate Formation of Activated and Non-Activated Monocytes with Melanoma Cells

monocyte activation	temperature of conjugate formation	% conjugates exp. 1	exp. 2	exp. 3
IFN-γ + LPS	30°C	34	41	49
-	30°C	21	24	30
IFN-γ + LPS	0°C	3	4	n.t.
-	0°C	5	3	n.t.

Freshly isolated monocytes were cultured for 24 h with and without 200 U IFN-γ and 20 ng LPS per ml. Effector and target cells were incubated for 30 min at 30°C and 0°C. The data shown are the percentage fluorescent monocytes conjugated to the target cells (BK-mel).

Monocytes activated by incubation in the presence of interferon-γ (IFN-γ, 200 U/ml) and LPS (20 ng/ml) for 24 h show an increased conjugate formation with human melanoma cells when compared to non-activated 24 h cultured monocytes (Table 2) and this is directly correlated with the expression of MO-CAM (results not shown). In addition, it is shown that monocyte metabolism is required to establish conjugate formation, since conjugates were only formed at 30°C and practically no conjugates were formed at 0°C.

To determined whether MO-CAMs were involved in conjugate formation, effector and target cells were incubated with anti-MO-CAM and anti-MLN-CAM antibodies. The results indicate that moab recognizing the α chain of LFA-1 and Mo-1 interferes with conjugate formation between monocytes and human melanoma cells and that conjugate formation is almost completely blocked by moab recognizing the common β chain of LFA-1 and Mo-1 (Table 3).

Furthermore it is shown that moab recognizing adhesion molecules on the melanoma target cells did not interfere with conjugate formation between monocytes and melanoma cells. Interestingly, we observed that the number of conjugates formed between monocytes and melanoma cells was much higher compared to that found between monocytes and human fibroblasts (Table 4). In addition, conjugate

TABLE 3. Inhibition of Conjugate Formation by Monoclonal Antibodies[a]

moab added[b]	exp. 1		exp. 2		exp. 3	
	% conj.	% inh.	% conj.	% inh.	% conj.	% inh.
none	32	0	41	0	30	0
anti-KLH	30	7	n.t.	–	23	23
anti-LFA-1 (α chain)	15	53	3	93	3	90
anti-LFA-1, Mo-1, p150,95 (β chain)	5	84	5	88	1	97
anti-Mo-1 (α chain)	18	44	5	88	13	57
anti-MLN-CAM-1	31	3	38	7	n.t.	–

[a] The data shown are the percentage fluorescent effector cells conjugated to the target cells (BK-mel) and the percentage inhibition of conjugate formation compared to the incubation with medium alone. E/T ratio was 1 : 1.

[b] The same moabs were used as in Table 1.

TABLE 4. Conjugate Formation of Monocytes with Melanoma Cells and Fibroblasts

target cell	% conjugate formation	
	experiment 1	experiment 2
melanoma (BK-mel)	33	41
fibroblast (human)	8	17

formation between fibroblasts and monocytes can be inhibited by anti-MO-CAM antibodies (results not shown). Finally, it was demonstrated that moab directed to the common β chain of LFA-1 and to Mo-1 α chain interfere with the ADCC of human monocytes against anti-D coated human erythrocytes (Table 5).

TABLE 5. Inhibition of ADCC of Monocytes to Anti-D Coated Human Erythrocytes with Monoclonal Antibodies

monoclonal antibody added (dilution)			$LU/10^7$ monocytes	% inhibition
medium			250	–
control CEM	(1 :	500)	210	16
	(1 :	1000)	267	–7
SPV-L7	(1 :	500)	222	11
	(1 :	1000)	250	0
CLB-54	(1 :	500)	0.1	99
	(1 :	1000)	65	74
Bear-1	(1 :	500)	143	43
	(1 :	1000)	167	33

Monocytes were incubated with ^{51}Cr-labeled, anti-D coated human erythrocytes. E/T ratio's were 0.4 and 0.2. Data shown are the number of lytic units/10^7 monocytes and the % inhibition with monoclonal antibodies compared to incubation with medium alone. One lytic unit equals the number of monocytes necessary to give 25% lysis of the target cells.

CONCLUSION

Monocyte-associated cellular adhesion molecules play an important role in the binding step of both direct cell mediated cytotoxicity and ADCC of human monocytes.

REFERENCES

Adams DO, Johnson WJ, Marino PA (1982). Mechanisms of target recognition and destruction in macrophage-mediated tumor cytotoxicity. Federation Proceed 41:2212-2221.
Beller DL, Springer TA, Schreiber RD (1982). Anti-Mac-1 selectively inhibits the mouse and human type three complement receptor. J Exp Med 156:1000-1009.
Bonavida B, Bradley TP, Grimm EA (1983). Frequency determination of killer cells by a single-cell cytotoxic assay. In: Methods in Enzymology, Vol. 93, pp. 270-280, Academic Press, Inc.

Fidler IJ, Kleinerman, ES (1984). Lymphokine-activated human blood monocytes destroy tumor cells but not normal cells under cocultivation conditions. J Clin Oncol 2: 937-943.

Fisher DG, Golightly MG, Koren HS (1983). Potentiation of the cytolytic activity of peripheral blood monocytes by lymphokines and interferon. J Immunol 130:1220-1225.

Keizer GD, Borst J, Figdor CG, Spits H, Miedema F, Terhorst C, De Vries JE (1985a). Biochemical and functional characteristics of the human leukocyte membrane antigen family LFA-1, Mo-1 and p150,95. Eur J Immunol, in press.

Keizer GD, Te Velde AA, Schwarting R, Figdor CG, De Vries JE (1985b). Myeloid cellular adhesion molecules: association with adhesion, migration, chemotaxis and phagocytosis of human monocytes. J Immunol, submitted.

Mantovani A, Polentarutti N, Peri G, BarShavit Z, Vecchi A, Bolis G, Mangioni C (1980). Cytotoxicity on tumor cells of peripheral blood monocytes and tumor-associated macrophages in patients with ascites ovarian tumors. J Natl Cancer Inst 64:1307-1315.

THE CYTOKINETIC BEHAVIOR OF RESIDENT PULMONARY ALVEOLAR MACROPHAGE IN SPLENECTOMIZED-STRONTIUM 89 MONOCYTOPENIC MICE.

Richard T. Sawyer

Division of Basic Medical Science
Mercer University School of Medicine
Macon, Georgia   31207

INTRODUCTION

While it is a widely held belief that resident macrophages (RM) are the lineal descendants of marrow-derived blood monocytes (van Furth et al., 1983), accumulating data suggests that RM are marrow-independent (Volkman et al., 1983) and self-renewing (Sawyer et al., 1982). If monocytes are necessary to sustain RM, their removal should result in a change in both RM population size and cytokinetic behavior. Failure to demonstrate changes in these parameters would support the hypothesis that RM are, in fact, marrow-independent. One experimental approach to this question has been to induce monocytopenia by selective irradiation of bone marrow by the intravenous injection of the bone-seeking isotope strontium-89 (89Sr) (Sawyer et al., 1982).

89Sr treatment renders mice monocytopenic for up to one month (Sawyer, 1985a; Volkman et al., 1983). During this period, in the virtual absence of monocytes, there are no changes in the total number/mouse of either resident peritoneal macrophages (Volkman et al., 1983) or resident pulmonary alveolar macrophages (PAM) (Sawyer, 1985a). Recent studies (Coggle and Tarling, 1984; Sawyer, 1985a) demonstrate that local proliferation of PAM, in both intact and monocytopenic mice, accounts for PAM population renewal. Further, 89Sr administration does not alter PAM cytokinetic behavior (Sawyer, 1985b). From these studies it has been concluded that monocytes are not required, in adult mice, to sustain RM populations.

It has been established that compensatory extramedullary splenic hemopoiesis occurs in 89Sr treated mice (Adler et al., 1977). Volkman et al. (1983) found that, in 89Sr treated mice, a 90% decrease in bone marrow macrophage colony forming cells was accompanied by a ten fold increase in splenic M-CFC. However, splenectomy had no effect on the total number/mouse of resident peritoneal macrophages, even at intervals beyond the population half-time. Nevertheless, the possibility remains that compensatory splenic hemopoiesis might supply input necessary to sustain PAM populations in 89Sr treated mice. This study, therefore, evaluates the effects of combined splenectomy and 89Sr induced monocytopenia on PAM population size and 3HTdR labeling kinetics.

MATERIALS AND METHODS

Female CD-1 (ICR) mice (20-25g, Charles River Breeding Laboratories) were used throughout this study and maintained under standard conditions. 89Sr, specific activity 7-8 Ci/mM, was purchased from Oak Ridge National Laboratories and injected IV at 2 uCi/g body weight on day zero. Control groups were injected IV with 200 ug nonradioactive 88Sr. Ten days after strontium treatment, when monocyte levels were undetectable, mice were injected IV with 1 uCi/g body weight 3HTdR, specific activity 2 Ci/mM (Amersham), and mononuclear phagocytes harvested by standard methods beginning one day after labeling. Each time interval represents a minimum of at least five separate experimental determinations.

Splenectomy (SPLX) was performed by standard methods on ether anesthetized mice and one month was allowed to elapse before SPLX mice were used. The experimental groups consisted of 88Sr-intact, 89Sr-intact, 88Sr-SPLX, and 89Sr-SPLX mice. There were no statistically significant differences among PAM labeling data from 88Sr-intact and 89Sr-intact mice. Thus, only data from the 88Sr-intact control group will be presented for the sake of brevity.

Methods for harvesting, identification of, enumeration of autoradiographically labeled monocytes and PAM, determination of labeling indices (LI%) and mean grain count have been described (Sawyer, 1985b). Statistical analysis was performed using an IBM-PC/AT and NWA

Multi-Functional Statistic library (Northwest Analytical Inc., Portland, OR) with Wilcoxon Signed-Ranks, and Single-variable regression analysis with multiple, linear and logarithmic curve fit programs.

RESULTS

The data presented in Table 1 show changes in the total number/mouse of white blood cells, monocytes and PAM from 88Sr-SPLX and 89Sr-SPLX mice. There were no significant changes in the total number/mouse of white blood cells, blood monocytes or PAM at the various intervals within the 88Sr-intact group; thus, the control (CTRL) represents pooled data from 88Sr-intact mice. In comparison to CTRL values there were significant ($P = 0.01$) changes in monocyte numbers as a result of SPLX alone. Values tended to return to control levels by the second week of the experiment. During the period of study monocytes were undetectable in 89Sr-SPLX, and in 89Sr-intact, mice. By contrast, there were no changes in the total number/mouse of PAM in either 88Sr/89Sr-intact or 88Sr/89Sr-SPLX mice during the one month of observation.

Table 1. Total number/mouse of WBCs, monocytes and PAM from 88Sr-SPLX and 89Sr-SPLX mice.

Day after strontium	Total WBCs $\times 10^{-6}$		Monocytes $\times 10^{-5}$		PAM $\times 10^{-5}$	
	88Sr	89Sr	88Sr	89Sr	88Sr	89Sr
1	2.4(0.4)	1.4(0.2)*	1.7*	0*	3.5	7.2
2	1.3(0.3)*	1.7(0.2)*	0.7*	0	7.9	5.0
3	3.2(1.0)	0.9(0.2)*	2.2	0	7.9	3.8
4	2.2(0.4)	2.0(0.4)	1.2*	0	9.6	4.8
5	2.1(0.4)	2.0(0.4)	1.3*	0	6.9	7.8
8	4.0(0.7)	1.3(0.4)*	2.4	0	6.8	5.6
10	3.4(1.2)	3.6(0.8)	2.0	0	8.9	7.4
12	4.2(1.3)	3.2(0.5)	2.5	0	5.2	7.6
15	5.1(1.0)	3.4(0.6)	3.1	0	8.1	8.6
20	3.3(1.0)	1.8(0.3)*	2.0	0	5.7	7.9
25	2.5(0.5)	2.3(0.4)	1.5*	0	7.0	6.5
30	3.1(0.7)	2.1(0.5)	2.0	0	5.6	6.9
CTRL	4.0(0.2)		3.0		2.5	5.0

Each interval represents the mean (SEM) of at least five separate experimental determinations.
*P = 0.01 (Wilcoxon Signed Ranks)

In this model it is important to demonstrate that monocyte kinetics were unchanged as a result of SPLX. Regression analysis of the decline in the LI for monocytes from 88Sr-intact and 88Sr-SPLX mice shows no change in halving time (about 3.5 days) resulting from SPLX alone (Table 2). In both instances the monocyte mean grain count halving time was unchanged, which suggests a generation time (TG) of about 4.3 days. Taken together these data suggest that monocyte numbers and cytokinetic behavior were essentially at control levels at the time of cytokinetic studies in 89Sr treated mice.

Table 2. Cytokinetic parameters of blood monocytes from 88Sr-INTACT and 88Sr-SPLX mice.

CYTOKINETIC PARAMETER	88Sr-INTACT	89Sr-SPLX
HALF-TIME	3.8 da	3.4 da
	(Y = -6X + 85)	(Y = -3.6X + 47)
	(R = -.96)	(R = -.93)
GENERATION TIME	4.1 da	4.5 da
	(Y = -4.9LNX+13.9)	(Y = -.28LNX+11.3)
	(R = -.99)	(R = -.97)

R = the correlation coefficient

Regression analysis of the decline in the PAM LI suggests that the PAM population half-time was unchanged as a result of either 89Sr treatment alone, SPLX alone or in 89Sr-SPLX mice (T½ ca. 8 da). Estimated population turnover times were 35 days for PAM from intact mice and 88Sr-SPLX mice and 34 days for PAM from 89Sr-SPLX mice. Regression analysis of the decline in the PAM mean grain count suggests TG increased from 4.9 days in 88Sr-intact mice to 8.2 days in 88Sr-SPLX mice while TG increased from 4.9 to 14 days in 89Sr-SPLX mice (Table 3).

Table 3. Cytokinetic parameters of PAM in the presence and absence of a spleen.

CYTOKINETIC PARAMETER	88Sr INTACT	88Sr SPLX	89Sr INTACT	89Sr SPLX
HALF-TIME	8.9 da ($R = -.99$)	8.8 da ($R = -.85$)	7.5 da ($R = -.95$)	8.0 da ($R = -.92$)
TURNOVER TIME	35 da ($R = -.71$)	35 da ($R = -.73$)	29 da ($R = -.79$)	34 da ($R = -.78$)
GENERATION TIME	4.9 da ($R = -.87$)	4.9 da ($R = -.95$)	8.2 da* ($R = -.94$)	14 da* ($R = -.92$)

* $P = 0.01$ (Wilcoxon Signed Ranks)

DISCUSSION

It can be reasonably concluded from this study that despite the combined absence of a spleen and peripheral blood monocytes there were no changes in the total number/mouse of PAM. Such treatment did not alter monocyte cytokinetic behavior in control mice. In comparison to controls, in 89Sr-SPLX mice there was no change in either the PAM population half-time or estimated turnover time. There were, however, significant increases in the generation time. In 88Sr treated mice TG increased from 4.9 da to 8.2 da as a result of SPLX, whereas in 89Sr treated mice TG increased from 4.9 da to 14 da in the SPLX group. This is highly suggestive that PAM cell cycle parameters were altered in the 89Sr-SPLX group as a result of 89Sr treatment. Alternatively, since there were no demonstrable alterations in the decline of the PAM population LI in this group, such changes might also reflect inaccuracy in measuring cell cycle times using 3HTdR labeling techniques. This question could be resolved by flow cytometry analysis of PAM cell cycle parameters in 89Sr treated mice.

Collectively the data show that PAM populations are not sustained by the obligatory daily influx of peripheral blood monocytes. It is also clear that in 89Sr-monocytopenic mice PAM population renewal is not the result of compensatory extramedullary splenic hemopoiesis since PAM population size was unaltered at intervals well in excess of the population half-time. These findings refute those of Blusse et al. (1979) who claimed that 16% of the peripheral blood monocyte pool enters the alveoli giving rise to the PAM population. They fully support previous studies (Sawyer et al., 1982; Sawyer, 1985a, 1985b; Volkman et al., 1983) showing that in adult mice PAM are sustained independent of bone marrow input. As originally suggested by Volkman (1976) PAM, and other RM populations, are more probably autochthonous in adult mice. (Supported by HL30619).

REFERENCES

van Furth, R. and W. Sluter (1983) Current views on the ontogeny of macrophages and humoral regulation of monocytopoiesis. Trans. Roy. Soc. Trop. Med. Hyg. 77:614.

Volkman, A., N.C. Chang, P.H. Strausbach and P.S. Morahan (1983) Differential effects of chronic monocyte depletion on macrophage proliferation. Lab. Invest. 49:291.

Sawyer, R.T, P.H. Strausbach and A. Volkman (1982) Resident macrophage proliferation in mice depleted of blood monocytes by strontium-89. Lab. Invest. 49:165.

Sawyer, R.T. (1985a) The significance of local resident pulmonary alveolar macrophage proliferation to population renewal. J. Leuko. Biol. (in press).

Coggle, J.E. and J.D. Tarling (1984) The proliferation kinetics of pulmonary alveolar macrophages. J. Leuko. Biol. 35:317.

Sawyer, R.T. (1985b) The cytokinetic behavior of pulmonary alveolar macrophages in monocytopenic mice. J. Leuko. Biol. (in press).

Adler, S.S., F.E. Trobaugh and W.H. Knospe (1977) Hemopoietic stem cell dynamics in 89Sr marrow ablated mice. J. Lab. Clin. Med. 89:592.

Blusse, A.B., R. van Furth (1979) Origin, kinetics and characteristics of pulmonary macrophage in the normal steady state. J. Exp. Med. 149:1504.

Volkman A. (1976) Disparity in the origin of mononuclear phagocyte populations. J. Reticuloendothel. Soc. 19:249.

Section VI. Microbial-Host Interactions

MACROPHAGES AND HOST DEFENSE: INDUCTION OF ANTIMICROBIAL EFFECTOR REACTIONS OF ACTIVATED MACROPHAGES

Carol A. Nacy, Monte S. Meltzer, Anne H. Fortier Micheal G. Gilbreath, David L. Hoover

Department of Immunology, Walter Reed Army Institute of Research, Washington, District of Columbia 20307-5100

INTRODUCTION

The immune system functions both as a migratory sensory organ to detect alterations in tissue integrity, and as an amplification system to efficiently mobilize cells that can reassert homeostatic balance for protection of tissues against invasion by outside agents (microorganisms) or destruction from within (unregulated cell division). The complex interactions that occur between cells and humoral factors during immune reactions precludes the isolation of any of these individual participants for a discussion of host defense. Nonetheless, the ubiquitous presence of macrophages in tissues, their participation in both the afferent and efferent phases of immunity, strongly suggests that macrophages play a pivotal role in these protective responses.

Under steady-state conditions, resident tissue macrophages preserve the integrity of their environment through various phagocytic and secretory activities. The actual products secreted by a given macrophage vary with its differentiative pathway and microenvironment in specific tissue (Table 1). Some secretory products are constituitively produced by both resident tissue macrophages and inflammatory cells (lysozyme and components of complement); secretion of other products is particularly enhanced in inflammatory and activated macrophages as a result of endocytosis, interaction with membrane active reagents (LPS), or factors from activated lymphocytes.

Table 1. Partial list of macrophage secretory products.

Acid hydrolases	Monokines
Proteinases	Interleukin 1
Lipases	CSF
Arginase	Interferon
Bioactive lipids	Neutral proteases
Prostaglandins	Nucleotide metabolites
Leukotrienes	Plasma proteins
Thromboxane	Coagulation proteins
Chemotactic factors	Complement components
Enzyme inhibitors	Fibronectin
Lipoprotein lipase	alpha-2-microglobulin
Lysozyme	Reactive oxygen metabolites

In acute inflammatory reactions, both the influx of circulating monocytes and the local proliferation of tissue macrophages increases dramatically. Secretion still remains a major function of these cells: macrophage secretory products influence both the degree and chronicity of inflammation, as well as facilitate induction of antigen-specific immune responses (Table-1). During inflammation, however, the repertoire of mononuclear phagocytes expands to include other specialized activities. Among these reactive changes are the nonspecific effector activities that macrophages acquire after interaction with soluble lymphocyte products (lymphokines, LK) eary in immune responses: destruction of antigenically unrelated microorganisms and neoplastic cells. The signals and sequence of events that lead to the activation of macrophages for these nonspecific effector activities has been of particular interest to our laboratory over the last several years. To analyze the changes that occur in macrophages exposed to LK, we use an obligate intracellular pathogen which multiplies in phagolysosomes of macrophages, Leishmania major (formerly L. tropica major). This microorganism has several attributes that facilitate our analyses:

(1) L. major preferentially replicates in phagolysosomes, and is intrinsically resistant to the natural degradative armamentarium of the macrophage,
(2) the obligatory intracellular existence of L. major suggests that the parasite is sequestered in nature from

most humoral host defense mechanisms and developing immune reactions, and
(3) the central effector cell for both humoral and cellular immunity, the macrophage, is the only host cell that Leishmanias infect in vivo.

The macrophage must undergo extraordinary intracellular changes in order to effect parasite elimination, or be itself eliminated, for successful resolution of disease. That changes can be induced in the macrophage that affect macrophage-parasite interactions has been demonstrated in vivo with immunomodulating agents, and in vitro with antigen or mitogen-stimulated LK (Pappas and Nacy, 1983; Nacy, et.al., 1981b). We document two distinct alterations in macrophage function that affect this obligate intracellular parasite: macrophage resistance to infection and intracellular destruction of the parasite.

RESISTANCE TO INFECTION

Macrophage resistance to infection is induced by pretreatment of macrophages with LK prior to exposure to L. major, and is observed as a decrease in the percentage of cells that phagocytose parasites in LK-treated cultures compared to medium-treated controls. Resistance to infection has these characteristics:
(1) rapid in onset: occurs with as little as 4 hr LK treatment before infection, and is maximal (60-70% decrease in infected cells) with 20 hr of LK pretreatment (Oster and Nacy, 1984);
(2) long-lived: can be demonstrated for up to 72 hr after LK treatment (Oster and Nacy, 1984);
(3) induced in vivo with immunomodulating agents, such as BCG (Pappas and Nacy, 1984);
(4) not parasite specific: has been demonstrated with other species of Leishmania, rickettsiae, Trypanosoma cruzi, and Legionella pneumophila (all obligate or facultative intracellular parasites) (Miller and Twohy, 1969; Hoff, 1975; Nacy and Meltzer, 1979, Horwitz and Silverstein, 1981; Nacy and Meltzer, 1982);
(5) induced by a factor(s) in LK of molecular weight approximately 55 kd (Nacy, et al 1981a).

The recent availability of purified recombinant gamma interferon (gammaIFN) enabled us to ask whether this LK was responsible for induction of activated macrophage resistance to infection. Figure 1 is a dose response of spleen cell-derived LK and murine gammaIFN (obtained from Genentech, S. San Francisco, CA) for induction of this effector activity. Although the LK for resistance to infection elutes from sizing gels in approximately the same molecular weight region as naturally glycosylated gammaIFN, the recombinant gammaIFN did not induce this effector reaction, nor did monoclonal antibodies prepared against recombinant gammaIFN (H21) interfere with the LK dose response:

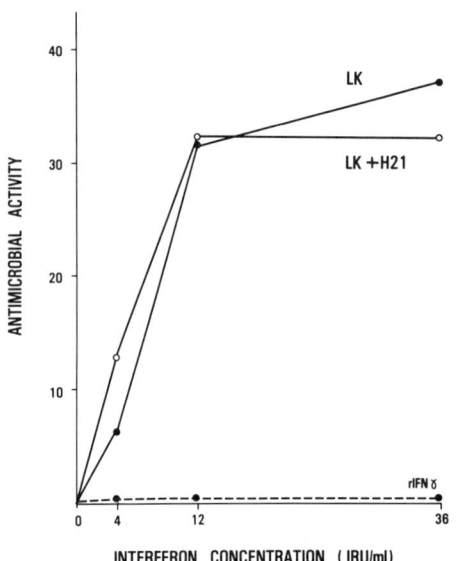

Figure 1. Induction of macrophage resistance to infection. Macrophages were treated with activating agents for 6 hr, washed, and then infected with parasites for 1 hr. H21 monoclonal antibody was added to certain cultures at a concentration that neutralized antiviral activity of 1000 IRU/ml gammaIFN.

Whether macrophage resistance to infection reflects extracellular killing of parasites, or an alteration of the macrophage membrane that influences capacity of parasites to enter the intracellular environment of the cell, remains a mystery. The mechanism responsible for this change in macrophage-parasite interaction may be elucidated when the reaction can be induced by a relatively pure LK preparation. Our recent observation that the murine T cell line EL-4 (Meltzer subline) produces a factor that induces macrophage resistance to infection in the absence of detectable gammaIFN suggests that this immunoregulatory factor can now be produced in quantity for purification and physicochemical analysis, as well as characterization of its biological activities.

INTRACELLULAR KILLING

The second major alteration that LK induces in macrophage-L. major interactions is intracellular destruction of the parasite. This effector activity can be dissociated from resistance to infection by exposing macrophages to L. major first, and then treating the cells with LK after infection (Nacy et.al., 1981b). In this case, we can effect the elimination of 90-100% of intracellular parasites without affecting viability of the macrophage. The LK that regulate this effector reaction elute from sizing gels at 10-15,000, 50,000, and 130,000 kd (Nacy et.al., 1981a). One of these activating factors is clearly gammaIFN, and dose responses of the recombinant murine gammaIFN demonstrate that as little as 3-5 IRU/ml is sufficient to induce maximal intracellular killing (Nacy et.al., 1985). GammaIFN is not the only activating factor in LK capable of inducing intracellular destruction of L. major: removal of gammaIFN from LK by affinity chromatography with monoclonal anti-gammaIFN antibodies (H21) leaves residual (50-60% of total) LK activity for induction of intracellular killing (Nacy et.al., 1985; Hoover et.al., 1985).

LK-induced intracellular destruction of L. major is a complex process that requires the interaction of cells and signals in a multi-stage reaction sequence (Nacy et.al, 1984). Infected macrophages exposed to certain signals found exclusively in LK (priming signals) are not microbicidal, but are exceptionally responsive to second (trigger) signals supplied by factors in LK, secreted products from certain neoplastic cells, or LPS that induce expression of the effector reaction. Priming and triggering for intracellular destruction of L. major occurs in the activation of macrophages by both gammaIFN and IFN-depleted LK. Treatment of macrophages with 12 IRU/ml gammaIFN or 1/6 LK for as little as 5 hr induces microbicidal activities; treatment of macrophages with 12-fold less activating agent is not sufficient to induce intracellular killing (Figure 2). Microbicidal activity of these primed, but not activated macrophages could be restored, however, by supplying trigger signals (homologous activation factor or LPS) in high concentration for a single 1 hr pulse. That priming with low concentrations of activating factor actually induces changes in the macrophage is demonstrated with medium-treated cells: these cells did not become activated for intracellular killing with the 1 hr high concentration pulse (Figure 2):

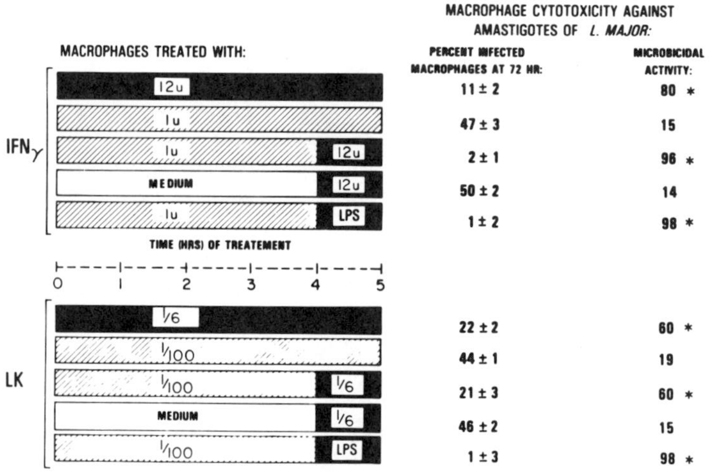

Macrophages treated with:	Percent infected macrophages at 72 hr:	Microbicidal activity:
IFNγ: 12u	11 ± 2	80 *
IFNγ: 1u	47 ± 3	15
IFNγ: 1u / 12u	2 ± 1	96 *
IFNγ: MEDIUM / 12u	50 ± 2	14
IFNγ: 1u / LPS	1 ± 2	98 *
LK: 1/6	22 ± 2	60 *
LK: 1/100	44 ± 1	19
LK: 1/100 / 1/6	21 ± 3	60 *
LK: MEDIUM / 1/6	46 ± 2	15
LK: 1/100 / LPS	1 ± 3	98 *

Figure 2. Treatment sequence for activation of macrophage intracellular killing by gammaIFN and nonIFN LK.

In an homologous system, then, priming and triggering can be demonstrated with both gammaIFN and nonIFN LK, and LPS (50 ng/ml) serves as a triggering factor for both of these activation agents. The pathways for activation of macrophages for intracellular destruction of L. major by gammaIFN and the nonIFN LK must, however, be distinct. In the presence of polymixin B (PMB), 12 IRU/ml gammaIFN will trigger gammaIFN primed cells, but not LK primed cells; 1/6 LK will trigger LK primed macrophages, but not gammaIFN primed cells (Figure 3):

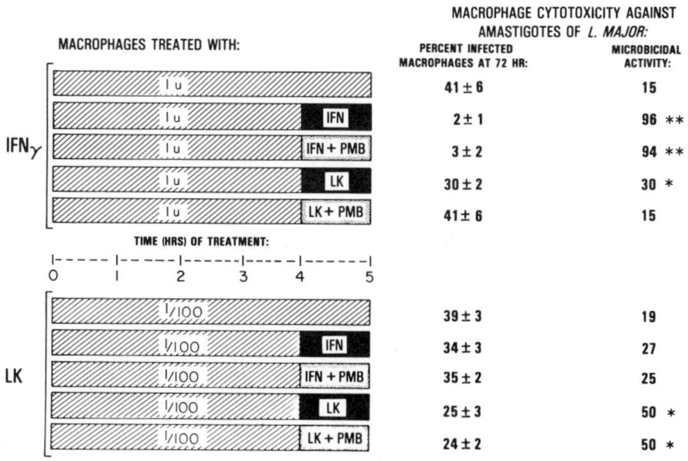

MACROPHAGES TREATED WITH:	MACROPHAGE CYTOTOXICITY AGAINST AMASTIGOTES OF L. MAJOR:	
	PERCENT INFECTED MACROPHAGES AT 72 HR:	MICROBICIDAL ACTIVITY:
IFNγ: 1u	41 ± 6	15
1u / IFN	2 ± 1	96 **
1u / IFN + PMB	3 ± 2	94 **
1u / LK	30 ± 2	30 *
1u / LK + PMB	41 ± 6	15
LK: 1/100	39 ± 3	19
1/100 / IFN	34 ± 3	27
1/100 / IFN + PMB	35 ± 2	25
1/100 / LK	25 ± 3	50 *
1/100 / LK + PMB	24 ± 2	50 *

Figure 3. Treatment sequence for activation of macrophage intracellular killing by IFNgamma and nonIFN LK.

Although reciprocol priming and triggering does not occur with IFNgamma and nonIFN LK, there must be at least one step in common in the sequential activation of macrophages for intracellular killing induced by these two activation stimuli. Suppressor factors obtained from phorbol myristate acetate-treated EL-4 thymoma cells (Meltzer subline) will completely abrogate both LK and gammaIFN-induced intracellular killing by macrophages in the first hr of the priming step (Nacy, 1984). The activation cascade for both gammaIFN and nonIFN LK has at least one initial step in common, but the metabolic pathways diverge at 1-2 hr into priming, and remain distinct for each activation stimuli. Our current concept of the activation of macrophages for intracellular destruction of L. major is depicted in Figure 4.

It is not yet clear whether the multiple pathways for activation of macrophages reflect differential induction of distinct killing mechanisms, or whether each

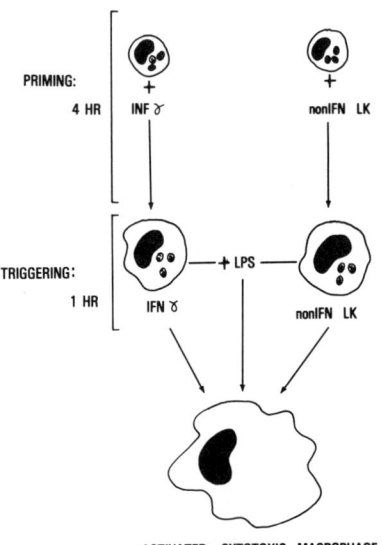

Figure 4. Sequential steps in the activation of macrophages for intracellular killing of L. major.

lead, through different metabolic pathways, to the generation of a single killing mechanism for destruction of obligate intracellular parasites.

REFERENCES

Hoover DL, Finbloom DS, Crawford RM, Nacy CA, Gilbreath MG and Meltzer MS (1985). A lymphokine distinct from gamma interferon that activates human monocytes to kill Leishmania donovani in vitro. J Immunol 136: (in press, December).

Horwitz MA and Silverstein SC (1981). Activated human monocytes inhibit the intracellular multiplication of Legionaire's disease bacteria. J Exp Med 154: 1618-1628.

Miller HC and Twohy DW (1969). Cellular immunity to Leishmania donovani in macrophages in culture. J

Parisitol 55:200-207.
Nacy CA (1984). Macrophage activation to kill Leishmania tropica: identification of a soluble T cell factor that suppresses lymphokine-induced intracellular killing of amastigotes. J Immunol 133:448-453.
Nacy CA and Meltzer MS (1979). Macrophages in resistance to rickettsial infections: macrophage activation in vitro for killing of Rickettsia tsutsugamushi. J Immunol 123: 2544-2599.
Nacy CA and Meltzer MS (1982). Macrophages in resistance to rickettsial infections: strains of mice susceptible to the lethal effects of Rickettsia akari show defective macrophage rickettsiacidal activity in vitro. Infect Immun 36:1096-1101.
Nacy CA, Leonard EJ and Meltzer MS (1981a). Macrophages in resistance to rickettsial infections: characterization of lymphokines that induce rickettsiacidal activity in macrophages. J Immunol 126:204-207.
Nacy CA, Meltzer MS, Leonard EJ and Wyler DJ (1981b). Intracellular replication and lymphokine-induced destruction of Leishmania tropica in C3H/HeN mouse macrophages. J Immunol 127:2381-2386.
Nacy CA, Oster CN, Meltzer MS and James SL (1984). Activation of macrophages for intracellular and extracellular destruction of parasites In Adams DO and Hanna MG (eds): "Contemporary Topics in Immunobiology" vol 14, New York: Academic Press, pp 147-170.
Nacy CA, Fortier AH, Schreiber RD, Buchmeier N and Meltzer MS (1985). Macrophage activation to kill Leishmania tropica: macrophages can be activated to kill amastigotes by both gamma interferon and noninterferon lymphokines. J Immunol 135 (in press, November)
Oster CN and Nacy CA (1984). Macrophage activation to kill Leishmania tropica: kinetics of macrophage response to lymphokines that induce antimicrobial activities against amastigotes. J Immunol 132:1494-1500.
Pappas MG and Nacy CA (1983). Antileishmanial activities of macrophages from C3H/HeN and C3H/HeJ mice treated with Mycobacterium bovis strain BCG. Cell Immunol 80:217-222.

BIOLOGICAL FUNCTIONS IN VITRO AND IN VIVO OF CLONED AUTOREACTIVE T CELLS FROM MYCOBACTERIUM BOVIS BCG-INFECTED MICE

I. Müller, A. Rolink, N. Freudenberg and S.H.E. Kaufmann

Max-Planck-Institut für Immunbiologie (I.M., S.H.E.K.), Freiburg, FRG, Basel Institute for Immunology (A.R.), Basel, Switzerland, and Institut für Pathologie (N.F.), Universität Freiburg, FRG

INTRODUCTION

It has been proposed that chronic infections can provide adequate stimuli for the induction of autoreactive T cells in vivo and that self-Ia reactive T cells are important in the regulation of the immune response against the infectious agent (e.g., Janeway et al., 1984). Pathogenic mycobacteria are intracellular microorganisms which cause chronic infectious diseases and lead to an enhanced expression of Ia antigens in vivo. In the present study we describe autoreactive T-cell hybridomas and T-cell clones derived from mice infected with the intracellular microorganism Mycobacterium bovis BCG which displayed multiple biological activities in vitro and induced autoimmune phenomena in vivo.

MATERIALS AND METHODS

C57BL/6 mice were infected subcutaneously (s.c.) with live BCG and 2 weeks later draining lymph nodes were collected. T cells were cultured in the presence of syngeneic irradiated spleen cells and 2×10^6/ml killed BCG. Cultures were restimulated weekly with irradiated syngeneic accessory cells (AC) and antigen and cloned at limiting diluting conditions after 4 weeks of culture. Cloned T cells were maintained by weekly restimulation with irradiated syngeneic AC and interleukin 2 (IL-2) containing supernatants. For functional assays cells were purified over a ficoll-urovision-gradient. T-cell hybrids were generated and tested as previously described (Müller and Kaufmann, 1985).

RESULTS

Several T-cell clones derived from long-term cultured LNC of BCG immune mice were tested for antigen reactivity. These clones were stimulated by syngeneic AC alone (Table 1). They also grew in medium containing 0.25% normal mouse serum and could be stimulated by syngeneic AC pretreated with chloroquine which blocks processing of soluble antigens (data not shown). One of these clones, designated 10H12, was chosen for further analysis. For determination of the biological activities of clone 10H12 in vitro, purified T cells were stimulated with irradiated syngeneic AC and supernatants tested for IL-2, interferon (IFN), and interleukin 1 (IL-1) activities. Table 2 shows that the cultures contained IL-2, IFN, and IL-1. Furthermore, the biological activities could be blocked by anti-IA^b or anti-L3T4, but not by anti-IA^K or anti-Lyt 2.2 monoclonal antibodies. Addition of monoclonal anti-IA^b or anti-L3T4 antibodies to IL-2 activated T cells had no influence indicating, that the antibodies were not toxic and inhibited only the antigen- but not the lymphokine-induced activation of 10H12 T cells. The response of the autoreactive T cell clone was H-2 restricted. For adequate stimulation, T cells and AC had to share the H-2I-A^b locus (Table 3).

TABLE 1   Reactivity pattern of T-cell clones[*]

T cell clone	BCG	AC	Proliferative response (cpm)
1A8	+	+	61,229
	−	+	74,653
	−	−	973
10E7	+	+	8,790
	−	+	7,070
	−	−	398
10B1	+	+	23,569
	−	+	23,468
	−	−	181
10H12	+	+	8,471
	−	+	11,440
	−	−	252
No T cells	+	+	65
	−	+	67

[*] 1×10^4 cloned T cells were stimulated with 2×10^5 irradiated syngeneic AC in the presence or absence of 2×10^6 heat-killed BCG as antigen. After 4 d of culture the proliferative response was determined.

Furthermore the cells had the penotype Thy 1^+, $L3T4^+$ $Lyt2^-$. We conclude that the T-cell clone was of the helper/inducer type and self-Ia reactive.

TABLE 2. Biological activities of cloned autoreactive T cells*

Stimulation with:	Monoclonal Antibody	Biological activities		
		Il-1 (cpm)	IL-2 (cpm)	IFN
AC	-	5,799	14,685	+
AC	α-L3T4	788	42	-
AC	α-IA^b	n.t.	1,223	n.t.
IL-2	-	19,248	76,101	+
IL-2	α-L3T4	18,497	63,162	+
IL-2	α-IA^b	n.t.	57,926	n.t.
-	-	954	32	-

*$3x10^3$ cloned T cells were stimulated with $5x10^5$ irradiated syngeneic AC or 10% IL-2 in the presence or absence of 10% monoclonal α-L3T4 or α-IA^b antibodies. 24 h later cell free supernatants were collected and tested for IL-2 and IFN activity. Supernatants for the determination of IL-1 induction were removed after 72 h. n.t. = not tested.

TABLE 3 Genetic restriction of cloned autoreactive T cells*

Mouse Strain	H-2-Complex				Proliferation (cpm)
	K	I-A	I-E	D	
C57BL/6	b	b	b	b	6,795
B10A.(4R)	k	k	b	b	108
B10A.(5R)	b	b	k	d	4,905
B10. MBR	b	k	k	q	106
B10. BR	k	k	k	k	122
DBA/2	d	d	d	d	96
B6.C-H2^{bm1}	.	b	b	b	11,597
B6.C-H2^{bm12}	b	.	b	b	76
BALB/B	b	b	b	b	1,424

*$3x10^3$ 10H12 T cells were incubated with $5x10^5$ irradiated AC from different donor strains. Proliferation was measured after 4 d of culture.

To evaluate whether these autoreactive T cells were also active in vivo, they were injected intraveneously (i.v.) into syngeneic sublethally irradiated or untreated recipient mice. T-cell recipients developed autoantibodies within 2 weeks and became moribund after 5 weeks (Table 4). Histological examination revealed prominent lymphoproliferative foci in spleens, livers, lungs and kidneys of T-cell recipients (Fig.1). Spleen cells from these mice proliferated in the absence of feeder cells or IL-2. The mutated cells were Thy 1.2^+, $L3T4^+$, $Lyt\ 2^-$ (data not shown). Currently we investigate whether the transformed mutants are host, or T-cell graft, derived. It is notable that another autoreactive T-cell clone, 10B1, caused a scleroderma-like disease in syngeneic recipient mice (data not shown).

To study the possibility that the emergence of autoreactive T cells was related to the mycobacterial infection and not due to long-term culture conditions we established T-cell hybridomas from short-term cultured LNC of mice infected with BCG. Most of the T-cell hybridomas showed exclusive responsiveness to BCG or purified protein derivate (PPD) of mycobacteria at one concentration of antigen. Only a small percentage of cells could be stimulated by both antigens. Interestingly, approximately 1/3 of the T-cell hybridomas were autoreactive (Table 5). Since the T cells were immortalized after 7d of in vitro cultivation the antigen recognition pattern closely reflected the in vivo situation.

TABLE 4 In vivo effects of cloned autoreactive T cells[*]

Treament of C57BL/6 mice		Serum-antibodies		
350 R	Injection	ANA	α-Thymocytes	Enhanced IgG
+	T cells	2/3	3/3	3/3
+	-	0/2	0/2	0/2
-	T cells	0/3	2/3	1/3
-	-	0/3	0/3	0/3

[*]Cloned T cells were injected 4 days after restimulation. Mice were injected in weekly intervals. 1st Injection: 2×10^6 T cells/mouse; 2nd: 1×10^6 T cells/mouse; 3rd: 3×10^5 T cells/mouse. Serum was removed 2 weeks after the first injection and tested as described (Van der Veen et al., 1981).

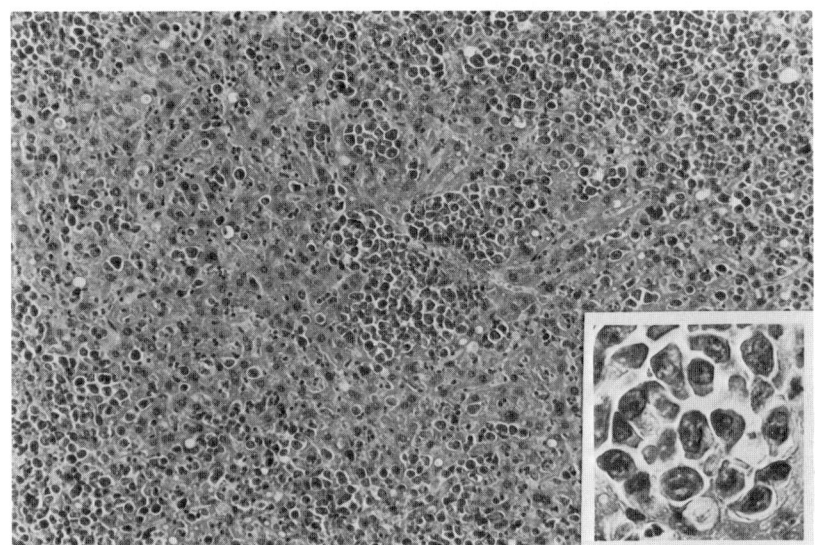

Figure 1. Lymphoproliferative focus of the mouse liver following transfer of autoreactive 10H12 T cells. Primary magnification: 100 X. Hematoxylin Eosin staining. Inset: higher magnification of a lymphoproliferative focus. Primary magnification: 630 X.

TABLE 5 Reactivity pattern of T-cell hybridomas derived from BCG-immune LNC*

Reactive to:			Percent of reactive hybridomas
AC	AC+PPD	AC+BCG	
+	−	−	24.6
−	+	−	23.1
−	−	+	33.8
+	+	−	6.2
+	−	+	4.6
−	+	+	4.6
+	+	+	3.1

*Lymph node cells from BCG immunized mice were fused with BW 5147 and hybridomas selected in HAT medium. Of 981 wells 36.7% showed cell growth. Of these, 18% released IL-2 in response to AC, AC+ PPD, and/or AC + BCG. The percent distribution of IL-2 secreting hybridomas is indicated in the table.

DISCUSSION

It is known that BCG stimulates Il-1 secretion (Meltzer and Oppenheim, 1977) and expression of Ia antigens (Beller et al., 1980) and that mycobacteria can inhibit phagolysosome fusion in macrophages thereby preventing adequate processing of mycobacterial antigens (Goren et al., 1976). We therefore suggest that mycobacteria are particularly apt to activate self-reactive T cells in vivo. It is unclear whether autoreactive T cells were stimulated because they had some affinity for self plus mycobacterial antigens or whether they represented distinct T-cell populations. Autoreactive T cells of the sort described may play a role in the immune response generated in mycobacterial infections and could be both beneficial (activation of mycobacteriocidal macrophages) and detrimental (induction of autoimmune responses) for the host.

ACKNOWLEDGEMENTS

This work received financial support from the World Health Organization as part of its Programme for Vaccine Development.

REFERENCES

Beller DI, Kiely JM, Unanue ER (1980). Regualtion of macrophage populations. I. Preferential induction of Ia-rich peritoneal exudates by immunologic stimuli. J Immunol 124: 1426-1432.
Goren MB, D'Arcy Hart P, Young MR, Armstrong JA (1976). Prevention of phagosome-lysosome fusion in cultured macrophages by sulfatides of Mycobacterium tuberculosis. Proc Nat Acad Sci USA 73:2510-2514.
Janeway CA Jr, Bottomly K, Babich J, Conrad P, Conzen S, Jones B, Kaye J, Katz M, McVay L, Murphy DB, Tite J (1984). Quantitative variation in Ia antigen expression plays a central role in immune regulation. Immunol Today 5: 99-104.
Meltzer MS, Oppenheim JJ (1977) Bidirectional amplification of macrophage-lymphocyte interactions: enhanced lymphocyte activation factor production by adherent mouse peritoneal cells. J Immunol 118: 77-82.
Müller I, Kaufmann SHE (1985). Antigen-reactivity pattern of T-cell hybridomas from Mycobacterium bovis BCG-infected mice. Infect Immun 49 in press.
Van der Veen F, Rolink AG, Gleichmann E (1981). Diseases caused by reactions of T lymphocytes to incompatible structures of the major histocompatibility complex IV. Autoantibodies to nuclear antigens. Clin Exp Immunol 46: 589-596.

PROTECTION AGAINST LISTERIA MONOCYTOGENES WITH A CLONOTYPIC ANTISERUM

Stefan H.E. Kaufmann, Klaus Eichmann, Ingrid Müller and Laura J. Wrazel

Max-Planck-Institut für Immunbiologie, 7800 Freiburg, FRG

INTRODUCTION

Protection against intracellular bacterial pathogens depends on cell-mediated immunity and effective vaccination is best achieved with live organisms (Hahn and Kaufmann, 1981). However, the use of live vaccines causes several unresolved problems and novel vaccination strategies should be considered (Kaufmann, 1984). Recently, several groups have generated clonotypic antibodies which can specifically block and/or stimulate the homologous T-cell clone (e.g., Haskins et al., Meuer et al., 1983, Ertl et al., 1984). It is conceivable that clonotypic antibodies directed against T cells which confer protection against intracellular pathogens can induce protection. We have established T-cell clones with specificity for the intracellular bacterium Listeria monocytogenes with protective activity and raised clonotypic antisera against these T-cell clones. Using these clontypic antisera we have analysed whether clonotypic antibodies can provide an alternative for vaccination against intracellular pathogens and thereby allow one to circumvent the dependence on live vaccines.

MATERIALS AND METHODS

Mice (C57Bl/6) were immunized with 2×10^5 live organisms of L. monocytogenes EGD subcutaneously (s.c.) and 8 days later draining lymphnodes were collected. T cells were cultured in the presence of heat-killed L. monocytogenes (HKL) and syngeneic irradiated spleen cells and afterward cloned and recloned under limiting dilution conditions (Kaufmann, 1984). L. monocytogenes specific T-cell clones were propagated in the presence of HKL, syngeneic spleen cells and interleukin 2 (IL-2) containing supernatants. To determine the capacity of these T-cell clones to adoptively mediate protection, 3×10^5 T cell, together with 2×10^5 live L. monocytogenes, were injected s.c. into one hind footpad and 2 days later bacterial numbers in footpads were determined (Kaufmann, 1984). Some of the T cell clones were immortalized by fusion to the AKR thymoma line BW5147.G.1.4 Oua^r.1 using polyethyleneglycol 1500 (Kaufmann et al., 1985). Hybridomas were selected in medium containing hypoxanthine, aminopterin, thymidine, and ouabain. T-cell hybridomas were stimulated with syngeneic spleen cells and HKL and after 24h cell-free supernatants were transferred to an IL-2 addicted cell line (CTLL-2). Antigen-specific hybridoma cells were irradiated and then injected intraveneously (i.v.) into (C57Bl/6 x AKR) F_1 mice at weekly intervals. After the fifth immunization, mice were bled once a week and sera were tested for blocking of antigen specific IL-2 secretion by hybridomas. Antisera with clonotypic activity were injected s.c. either alone or emulsified in complete Freund's adjuvant (CFA). Afterward, mice were challenge infected i.v. with live L. monocytogenes and 2 days later bacterial numbers in spleens were determined (Kaufmann et al, 1985).

RESULTS

Adoptive protection conferred by 3 L. monocytogenes-specific T-cell clones is shown in Table 1. Clones 26.1.1 and 26.1.2

TABLE 1. Local transfer of protection by L. monocytogenes-specific T-cell clones*

T cell clone	Log protection against EGD	Log protection against ATCC19114
26.1.1	1.6	0.2
26.1.2	1.3	0.4
26.1.3	1.8	1.9

*Cloned T cells (3×10^5) together with 2×10^5 live L. monocytogenes EGD or ATCC 19114, respectively, were injected s.c. into one hind footpad. Bacterial numbers in footpads were determined 2 days later. From Kaufmann, 1984.

conferred protection against L. monocytogenes EGD but not against L.monocytogenes ATCC 19114 while clone 26.1.3 could protect against both strains. Thus, clones 26.1.1 and 26.1.2 were specific for an epitope present on EGD but not on ATCC 19114 and clone 26.1.3 recognized an epitope shared by both bacterial strains. Clones 26.1.1 and 26.1.3 were fused with BW 5147 and the resulting T cell hybridomas,TLm1 and TLm2, respectively used for further studies. Both T cell hybridomas maintained the antigen-specificty and genetic restriction of the parental clones (Table 2). Mice were immunized with TLm1 cells and sera tested for their capacity to block antigen-induced IL-2 secretion by TLm1 and TLm2 cells (Table 3). Two out of 8 antisera were identified which blocked antigen-stimulation of TLm1 but not of TLm2 cells. We conclude from these findings that these two antisera were clonotypic for TLm1 cells.

Mice were injected s.c. with anti-TLm1 antiserum either alone or in CFA and afterward infected i.v. with live L. monocytogenes EGD. Control mice received antiserum without blocking activity.

TABLE 2. Antigen specificity and H-2-restriction of TLm1 and TLm2*

Accessory cells	L.monocytogenes-strain	IL-2 activity (cpm)	
		TLm1	TLm2
(C57Bl/6xAKR)F_1	EGD	19,400	13,400
C57Bl/6	EGD	21,400	12,400
AKR	EGD	600	300
B10.A(4R)	EGD	700	400
B10.A(5R)	EGD	16,800	7,600
B10.MBR	EGD	700	500
(C57Bl/6xAKR)F_1	ATCC 19114	900	10,200
(C57B/6xAKR)F_1	None	900	700
None	EGD	500	400
None	None	200	300

* Hybridoma cells (1 x 10^5), HKL (10^7) and accessory cells (2 x 10^5) were cultured in a total volume of 0.2 ml for 24 h and afterward supernatants tested for IL-2 activity. From Kaufmann et al., 1985.

TABLE 3. Specific blocking of IL-2 production by antisera raised against TLm1 cells

Preincubation	IL-2 activity (cpm)	
	TLm1	TLm2
Antiserum I	1,300	12,600
Antiserum VII	1,900	13,700
Normal mouse serum	9,800	14,600
No antiserum	12,400	14,000

*Hybridoma cells (1×10^5) were preincubated with antiserum I or VII (final dilution 1:50) for 2 h. Afterward, 10^7 HKL and 2×10^5 accessory cells from (C57Bl/6xAKR)F_1 mice were added. After 24 h 100 µl supernatants were removed and tested for IL-2 activity. From Kaufmann et al., 1985.

As shown in Table 4, mice pretreated with anti-TLm1 antiserum in CFA were significantly protected against listeriosis. Some mice injected with anti-TLm1 antiserum alone were also protected, although protection in this group was not statistically significant. Mice were vaccinated with anti-TLm1 antiserum and afterward infected with L. monocytogenes EGD or ATCC 19114, respectively (Table 5). Vaccination was only effective against strain EGD and

TABLE 4.* Vaccination against L. monocytogenes with anti-TLm1 antiserum

Group	Vaccination regime	Log protection
A	Anti-TLm1 antiserum alone	1.02
B	Control antiserum alone	0.14
C	Anti-TLm1 antiserum in CFA	1.57
D	Control antiserum in CFA	0.27

*Mice ((C57Bl/6xAKR)F1) were vaccinated (s.c.) with 50 µl 1/10 diluted antiserum alone or in CFA. After 5 or 8 days, respectively, mice were infected with 3×10^5 live L. monocytogenes EGD. Protection in spleens was determined 2 days later. Significant differences ($p < 0.05$): C vs D (Wilcoxon test). From Kaufmann et al., 1985.

TABLE 5. Vaccination with anti-TLm1 antiserum is antigen-specific*

Group	Vaccination regime	Challenge	Log protection
A	Anti-TLm1 antiserum	EGD	1.12
B	Control antiserum	EGD	0.16
C	Anti-TLm1 antiserum	ATCC19114	0.24
D	Control antiserum	ATCC19114	0.29

*Mice (C57Bl/6) were vaccinated (s.c.) with 50µl 1/10 diluted antiserum in CFA. After 8 days, mice were infected with 3×10^5 live L. monocytogenes EGD or ATCC19114, respectively. Protection in spleens was determined 2 days later. Significant differences ($p < 0.05$): A vs B (Wilcoxon test). From Kaufmann et al., 1985.

not against strain ATCC 19114. Thus, the clonotypic vaccine was antigen-specific. Anti-TLm1 antiserum was used for vaccination of C57Bl/6 or BALB/C mice. As shown in Table 6, both mouse strains could be protected against subsequent L. monocytogenes infection. Thus, vaccination with clonotypic antiserum was genetically nonrestricted.

Table 6. Vaccination with anti-TLm1 antiserum is genetically nonrestricted*

Group	Vaccination regime	Recipient	Log protection
A	Anti-TLm1 antiserum	C57Bl/6	1.28
B	Control antiserum	C57Bl/6	0.20
C	Anti-TLm1 antiserum	BALB/C	1.47
D	Control antiserum	BALB/C	0.14

*C57Bl/6 or BALB/C mice, respectively, were vaccinated (s.c.) with anti-TLm1 antiserum in CFA. After 8 days, mice were infected with 3×10^5 live L. monocytogenes EGD, and protection in spleens was determined 2 days later. Significant differences ($p < 0.05$): A vs B and C vs D (Wilcoxon test). From Kaufmann et al., 1985.

DISCUSSION

We have used clonotypic antibodies directed against L. monocytogenes-specific T cells with protective activity for active vaccination against listeriosis. This vaccination was antigen-specific and genetically non-restricted. The T-cell clone 26.1.1 was capable of adoptively protecting mice against L. monocytogenes EGD but not against ATCC 19114 and the clonotypic vaccine was of comparable antigen-specificity. On the other hand, the clonotypic vaccine could induce protection in an allogeneic enviroment while antigen-recognition by the T-cell clone 26.1.1 and its hybridoma TLm1 was H-2I-A restricted. Thus, the T cells used for raising the clonotypic antiserum determined the antigen-specificity, but not the genetic restriction, of the protective reaction induced by the clonotypic vaccine. Clonotypic antibodies may therefore allow vaccination of different individuals in the absence of the etiological agent. Such a strategy may be of particular interest for vaccination against pathogens, from which sufficient amounts of pure antigen preparations are not readily available, as is the case with Mycobacterium leprae.

REFERENCES

Ertl HCJ, Homans S, Tournas S, Finberg RW (1984). Sendai virus specific T cell clones. V. Induction of virus-specific response by antiidiotypic antibodies directed against a T-helper cell clone. J Exp Med 159: 1778-1783.

Hahn H, Kaufmann SHE (1981). The role of cell-mediated immunity in bacterial infections. Rev Infect Dis 3: 1221-1250.

Haskins K, Kubo R, White J, Pigeon M, Kappler J, Marrack P (1983). The major histocompatibility-restricted antigen receptor on T cells. I. Isolation with a monoclonal antibody. J Exp Med 157: 1149-1169.

Kaufmann, SHE (1984). T cell clones and their products: Experimental clues for the immunoprophylaxis and immunotherapy of intracellular bacterial infections? Infection 12: 124-130.

Kaufmann SHE (1984). Acquired resistance to facultative intracellular bacteria: relationship between persistence, cross-reactivity at the T-cell level, and capacity to stimulate cellular immunity of different Listeria strains, Infect Immun 45: 234-241.

Kaufmann SHE, Eichmann K, Müller I, Wrazel LJ (1985). Vaccination against the intracellular bacterium Listeria monocytogenes with a clonotypic antiserum. J Immunol 134: 4123-4127.

Meuer SC, Fitzgerald UA, Hussey RE, Hodgedon JC, Schlossman SF Reinherz EL (1983). Clonotypic structures involved in antigen-specific human T cell function. J Exp Med 157: 705-719.

THE SYNTHETIC ANALOGA OF BACTERIAL LIPOPROTEIN ARE POTENT IMMUNOADJUVANTS IN COMBINATION WITH OR COVALENTLY LINKED TO ANTIGEN

W. G. Bessler, A. Lex, B. Suhr, A. Ortmann, S. Schlecht, H. Bühring, C. Muller, J. Metzger, K.H. Wiesmüller, G. Jung

Arbeitsbereich Mikrobiologie und Immunologie, Institut für Organische Chemie, and Medizinische Klinik der Universität, Tübingen, and Max-Planck-Institut für Immunbiologie, Freiburg, FRG.

INTRODUCTION

The lipoprotein from the outer cell wall of <u>Escherichia coli</u> has been shown to stimulate murine B-lymphocytes into both proliferation and immunoglobulin secretion (Bessler and Braun 1975, Melchers et al.1975) The part of lipoprotein responsible for the biological activity resides in the N-terminal lipopeptide region (Bessler et al.1977, Resch et al.1981). A synthetic lipopentapeptide prepared by us contained the same amino acid sequence as the native lipopeptide, but differed in its fatty acid composition in containing solely palmitic acid residues (Wiesmüller et al. 1983).This compound, S-(2,3-bis(palmitoyloxy)-(2RS)-propyl)-N-palmitoyl-(R)-cysteinyl-(S)-seryl-(S)-seryl-(S)-aspara-

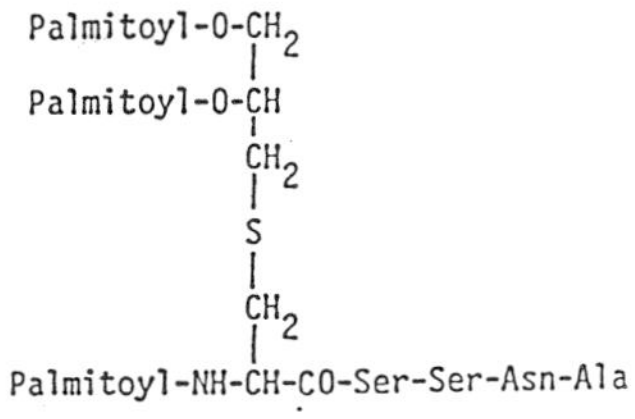

```
        Palmitoyl-O-CH₂
               |
        Palmitoyl-O-CH
               |
              CH₂
               |
               S
               |
              CH₂
               |
        Palmitoyl-NH-CH-CO-Ser-Ser-Asn-Ala
```

Figure 1. Molecular structure of tripalmitoyl pentapeptide.

ginyl-(S)-alanine (tripalmitoyl-pentapeptide, fig.1), is an active mitogen and polyclonal mouse B-lymphocyte activator in vitro and in vivo (Bessler,Cox et al. 1985, Johnson et al.1983). As shown here, tripalmitoyl pentapeptide constitutes a potent adjuvant of the humoral response, if given in combination with antigen (trinitrophenylated sheep red blood cells). It was also able to enhance the protective capacity of bacterial vaccines. Lastly it was possible to enhance the antigen-specific in vivo and in vitro immune response against weakly immunogenic peptides by coupling them covalently to the lipopeptide adjuvants.

MATERIALS AND METHODS

Lymphocytes: Balb/c mice (5-14 weeks of age), were obtained from Ivanovas, Kisslegg, FRG. Lymphocytes were prepared as previously described (Bessler,Suhr, Bühring et al.1985).
Reagents: Lipopeptides were prepared by chemical synthesis (Wiesmüller et al.1983). Before addition to the cultures the adjuvants were suspended in 20 mM Hepes-buffered Eagles Minimal Essential Medium (MEM; Flow Laboratories, Meckenheim/Bonn, FRG) with 2.5 µg/ml Triton X 100 by the aid of sonification (6 x 10 sec, 100 W; Braun Labsonic 1510 sonifier, Melsungen, FRG). Coupling of lipopeptide adjuvant to antigen was performed as described (Bessler,Suhr,Bühring et al 1985).
Hemolytic plaque assay: The development of immunoglobulin-secreting cells was measured using a plaque assay against highly trinitrophenylated sheep red blood cells (Rittenberg and Pratt 1969).
Protection Experiments: Mice were injected intraperitoneally with 0.2 ml of the respective bacterial suspension with or without adjuvant or with adjuvant alone, on days 0 and 14. On day 24 the immunized as well as nonimmunized mice were intraperitoneally infected with S. typhimurium C5.
ELISA: The amount and class of immunoglobulin secreted during splenocyte cultures was determined by ELISA (McKearn 1980).

RESULTS

To determine whether tripalmitoyl pentapeptide had the capacity to act as an in vitro adjuvant, its effect on the primary antibody response to TNP-SRBC and SRBC was evaluated. As shown in fig. 2, tripalmitoyl pentapeptide alone in concentrations ranging from 0.1 - 3 µg/ml exhibited only a weak stimulatory effect, as measured by the determination of plaque-forming cells (PFC) against TNP-SRBC. Optimal polyclonal activation of B-lymphocytes was seen at mitogen concentrations around 10 - 33 µg/ml. The addition of TNP-SRBC (1×10^2 to 1×10^7/ml) to adjuvant free cultures induced only a minimal increase in plaque-forming cells against TNP-SRBC. In contrast, supplementation of splenocyte cultures with both tripalmitoyl pentapeptide and TNP-SRBC resulted in a marked enhancement of PFC in vitro immune response (fig.2, open circles). A maximal number of plaque-forming cells was found at a tripalmitoyl pentapeptide-concentration of 33.3 µg/ml (closed squares) and 1×10^7 TNP-SRBC/ml. Thus, the addition of tripalmitoyl pentapeptide increased the specific humoral response to TNP-SRBC 10 - 100fold, depending on antigen- and adjuvant concentration.

Tripalmitoyl pentapeptide was also able to enhance the protective capacity of a S.typhimurium S-form vaccine. Table 1 shows that a vaccine dosage reduced to 1/10 (10^7) evoked a clearly inferior protection as compared with the full dose (10^8). Both groups differed significantly from one another as regards the mortality rates (p = 0.001). A supplementa-

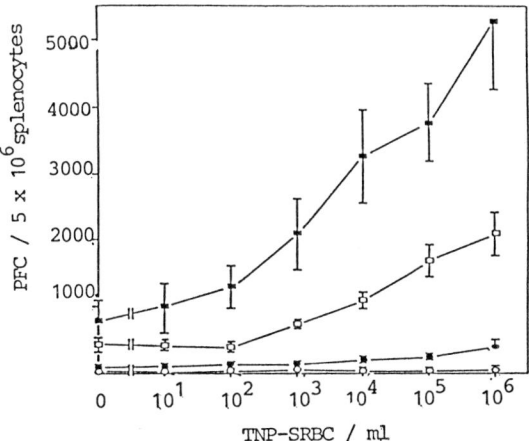

Figure 2. Enhancement of the primary antibody response by tripalmitoyl pentapeptide. 5×10^6 viable Balb/c splenocytes were cultured for 4 days in the presence of different TNP-SRBC-concentrations and either 0 µg (O), 0.33 µg (●), 3.33 µg (□), or 33.3 µg (■) tripalmitoyl pentapeptide/ml. Direct PFC, triplicate experiments ± standard deviations.

tion of the reduced vaccine dose using 175 µg of adjuvant led to an effectiveness as high as the full vaccine dose (10^8).

The synthetic lipopeptides turned also out to be potent adjuvants of the antibody response towards antigens with low immunogenicity, after coupling them covalently to the compounds. The resulting conjugates were highly active immunogens, and they induced antigen-specific immunoglobulin production (IgG and IgM) in vivo and in vitro. Using the in vivo approach (Fig.3) we obtained, via a single i.p. administration, specific antibodies against e.g. the non-immunogenic tetradecapeptide EGF-R 516-529 of the extracytoplasmatic region of the epidermal growth factor receptor, as measured by ELISA. Figure 3 shows the elicitation of specific anti-Pep 14 antibodies after a single in vivo immunization with the adjuvant-antigen conjugate. 2 weeks after i.p. immunization with 0.2 micromole of conjugate-solution, a drastic increase in serum antibody titer was detected. The application of antigen, or of the antigen adjuvant mixture, had no effect at any concentration, and the adjuvant alone exhibited only a weak stimulatory effect at the highest concentration applied.

Table 1. Protection of NMRI mice against infection with S. typhimurium C5 by immunization[a] with acetone killed homologous S. typhimurium S-form bacteria, and mixtures of homologous bacteria and tripalmitoyl pentapeptide.

Vaccine[a]	Single dose[b] bacteria	Addition of adjuvant[c]	LD_{50}[e]
None (infection control)			8.5×10^1
S.typhimurium	10^8	–	2.0×10^7
	10^7	–	3.2×10^5
	10^7	TPP (175µg)	2.0×10^7

[a] The immunization were effected by two injections
[b] Acetone killed bacteria
[c] µg/mouse/immunization
[d] Infection doses of 2.0×10^0 etc. bacteria. The infection was performed 14 days after the second immunization
[e] LD_{50} values represent the final mortality after 15 days
[f] Increase of LD_{50} in comparison to infection control.

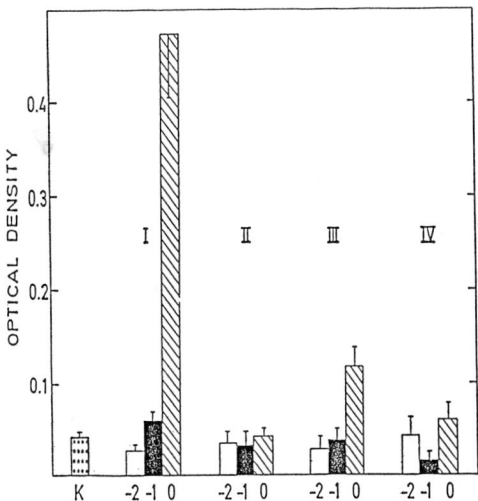

Figure 3. Elicitation of specific antibodies against Pep 14 after in vivo immunization (groups of 3-5 mice) with conjugate (I), Pep 14 (II), Tripam-Cys-Ser (III), a mixture of Tripam-Cys-Ser and Pep 14 (IV), and medium control (K). Mice were injected with 0.2 ml of 10^{0} mM, 10^{-1} mM, and 10^{-2} mM solutions of the corresponding substances. Antibody titer was determined by ELISA assay (4). Pep 14 specific antibody titer was calculated by substracting BSA-specific antibody titer from BSA-Pep 14 antibody titer. Ordinate: optical density at 405 nm, abscissa: mM concentrations of injected solutions (negative decadic logarithm) (comp. Bessler, Suhr, Bühring et al.1985).

A further series of experiments was performed to examine whether the conjugates were able to induce specific antibody formation in vitro. Thus, conjugate and controls were applied to in vitro cell cultures of Balb/c mouse splenocytes. The table shows that 5 to 7 days after in vitro administration of the conjugate, a marked specific anti-Pep 14 response could be monitored by the ELISA test. Application of antigen alone or of adjuvant alone had a minor effect. Interestingly, in contrast to the in vivo results described above, the adjuvant antigen mixture was also active, though to a lesser extent and only at higher doses, where also the adjuvant alone exhibited an effect.

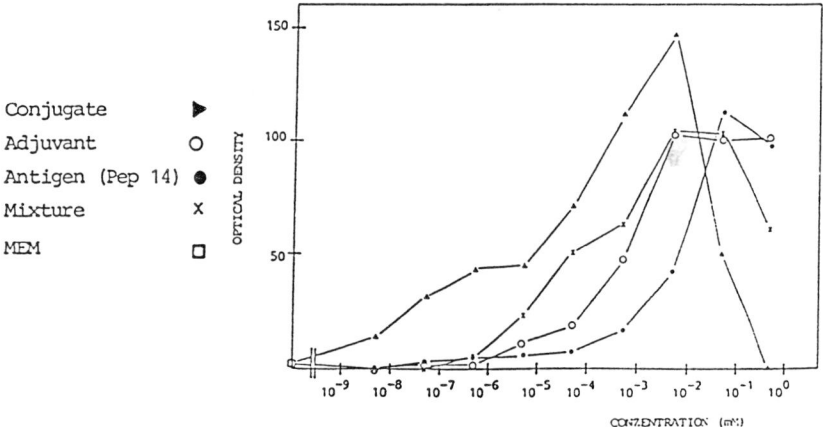

Figure 4. Production of specific antibodies against Pep 14 in vitro as measured by ELISA (optical density at 405 nm). Results of one representative experiment out of four experiments. Cultures were performed in triplicate as described in Material and Methods. Pep 14 specific antibody titers were determined as described in the legend to fig. 2. Titers of BSA-specific antibodies ranged from 0,000 to 0,034 for all determinations. Means of at least 3 determinations $\pm$ SD. (comp. Bessler,Suhr,Bühring et al.1985)

DISCUSSION

In this communication the adjuvant capacity of tripalmitoyl pentapeptide towards trinitrophenylated sheep red blood cells is shown. Augmentation of the antibody response by tripalmitoyl pentapeptide was highly dose-dependent, with optimal stimulation occurring at 10-30 µg/ml. The adjuvant effect could only be obtained when tripalmitoyl pentapeptide and antigen were administered at the same time. In the primary antibody response against TNP-SRBC in the presence of tripalmitoyl pentapeptide IgM- as well as IgG-antibodies were produced (data not shown).

In the protection experiments with tripalmitoyl pentapeptide in vivo we could show that mice could be immunized against Salmonella typhimurium with only 10% of the amount of bacteria needed without adjuvant. Thus, the new synthetic adjuvant will be a valuable tool for the application with a variety of vaccines, reducing the amount of vaccine and minimizing side effects (Schlecht et al., in preparation).

Using lipopeptides as adjuvants covalently linked to antigen we could show, that a single injection of the Tripam-Cys-Ser-Pep 14 conjugate elicited a high level of specific antibodies.The method of covalently coupling adjuvants to antigen has been described before for muramyldipeptide-antigen conjugates, which were used to amplify the immune response against viral peptide sequences (Arnon et al.1980). In fact, as early as 1974 Coutinho et. al. coupled bacterial LPS to hapten and thus obtained a specific immune response at a very low hapten dose. Synthetic vaccines have since been described by several groups (Chedid 1984,Delbende 1983,Sela 1983). The experimental procedure of covalently coupling weakly immunogenic antigens to lipopeptides may have a wide range of applications. Advantages of these low molecular weight, chemically well-defined carrier-antigen-adjuvant conjugates are: relatively easy prepa-ration, routine incorporation in Merrifield syntheses, production of specific antibodies within 1 - 2 weeks after single administration, no severe skin reactions since no Freund's adjuvant is required, high efficiency also in vitro providing elegant screening possibilities in gentechnology. It is obvious that our approach is not restricted to peptides as antigens.

REFERENCES

Arnon, R., Sela M., Parant L. and L.Chedid. 1980. Antiviral response elicited by a completely synthetic antigen with built-in adjuvanticity. Proc. Natl. Acad. Sci. 77: 6769.

Bessler, W.G., and V. Braun. 1975. Mitogenität von Lipoprotein aus der äußeren Membran von Escherichia coli gegenüber Lymphozyten verschiedener Spezies. Z. Immun. Forsch. 150: 193.

Bessler, W.G., M. Cox, A. Lex, B. Suhr, K.H. Wiesmüller, and G. Jung. 1985. Synthetic lipopeptide analogues of bacterial lipoprotein are potent polyclonal activators for murine B-lymphocytes. J. Immunol. (in press)

Bessler, W., K. Resch, E. Hancock, and K.Handtke. 1977. Induction of lymphocyte proliferation and membrane changes by lipopeptide derivatives of the lipoprotein from the outer membrane of Echerichia coli. Z. Immun.- Forsch. 153:11.

Bessler, W., B. Suhr, H.-J. Bühring, C. P. Muller, K.-H. Wiesmüller, G. Becker, and G. Jung. 1985. Specific antibodies elicited by antigen covalently linked to a synthetic adjuvant. Immunobiology, in the press (1985).
Coutinho, A., E. Gronowicz, W.W. Bullock and G. Möller, 1974. Mechanism of thymus-independent immunocyte triggering. J. Exp. Med. 139: 74.
Chedid,L. 1984. The present status of synthetic vaccines, respective roles of adjuvant, carrier and antigen. In: Proc. Forum Peptides, Cap d'Adge.
Delbende C. 1983. Approach to a synthetic vaccination against cholera. In: Peptides, Pierce, Rockford: 877.
Johnson, R.B.,S. Köhl, K.-H. Wiesmüller, G. Jung, and W.G. Bessler. 1983. Synthetic analogues of the N-terminal lipid part of bacterial lipoprotein are B-lymphocyte mitogens in vitro and in vivo. Immunobiol. 165 :27.
McKearn, T.J. 1980. Binding hybridoma antibodies to polyvinyl chloride microtiter dishes. In: Monoclonal Antibodies. Eds.: R.H. Kennett, T.J. McKearn, and K.B. Bechtol. Plenum Press, New York, p. 388.
Melchers, F., V. Braun, and C. Galanos. 1975. The lipoprotein of the outer membrane of Escherichia coli: A B-lymphocyte mitogen. J. Exp. Med. 142: 473.
Resch, K., and W. Bessler. 1981. Activation of lymphocyte populations whith Concanavalin A or with lipoprotein and lipopeptide from the outer cell wall of Escherichia coli: Correlation of early membrane changes with induction of macromolecular synthesis. Eur. J. Biochem. 115: 247.
Rittenberg, M.B., and K.J. Pratt. 1969. Trinitrophenyl plaque-assay primary response of Balb/c mice to soluble and particulate immunogen. Proc. Soc. Exp. Biol. Med. 132: 575.
Sela M. 1983. From synthetic antigens to synthetic vaccines. Biopolymers. 22: 419.
Wiesmüller, K.H., W. Bessler, and G. Jung. 1983. Synthesis of the mitogenic S-(2,3-Bis(palmitoyloxy)propyl)-N-palmitoyl-pentapeptide from the Escherichia coli lipoprotein. Hoppe-Seyler's Z. Physiol. Chem. 364: 593.

Section VII. Role of Leukocytes in Host Defense

MAST CELLS IN HOST DEFENSE

John Bienenstock[*] and Dean Befus[**]

[*]Dept. Pathology, McMaster University, Hamilton Ontario, Canada.
[**]Dept. Microbiology and Immunology, University of Alberta, Calgary, Alberta, Canada.

The classical view of mast cells and basophils is that they are involved in allergic or immediate hypersensitivity types of reactions. This occurs as a result of their sensitization with IgE through binding to high affinity IgE receptors on their membranes. When these receptors are cross-linked immunologically by antigen or anti-IgE, secretion of preformed substances such as histamine occurs through a complex series of events involving granule association with the membrane and exocytosis. This event signals the synthesis of nonpreformed mediators such as leukotrienes and platelet-activating factor (Pinckard 1983). These substances are then subsequently secreted. It is through the secretion of mast cell contents that many of the biological effects associated with allergies appear to be mediated and the reader is referred elsewhere for reviews of these complex events (Ishizaka 1984, Befus et al. 1985).

We will briefly touch upon the fact that mast cells may be involved in a variety of reactions to injury and even in the physiological control of certain aspects of homeostasis in an as yet incompletely understood manner.

Let us turn first to the fact that mast cells may be heterogeneous in respect to tissue site of origin within a species and also with respect to the same site of origin between species. The best example of the latter may be the observations of Pearce and co-workers who have shown that peritoneal mast cells from mice, rats and hamsters may vary totally in their response to both secretagogues and to anti-allergic compounds (Leung et al. 1984, Pearce et al. 1985). In respect to the former it is now clear that in the rat the mast cells found especially in the lamina propria of the intestine may differ in many respects from those found in connective tissues and perhaps best characterized by the peritoneal mast cell (PMC) (Befus et al. 1982, Pearce et al. 1982, Bienenstock et al. 1982). The intestinal mucosal mast cell, (IMMC), differs from the PMC and other connective tissue mast cells by virtue of histochemical properties which reflect the granule content. If fixatives such as neutral formalin are used the IMMC granules are difficult to visualize by subsequent staining, whereas the use of lead-based stains such as Mota's reveals both mast cell types. This histochemical heterogeneity is seen in the mucosa of the intestine as well as that of the bronchus and has been identified in a number of species including man. However, only in the rat have these histochemical differences been shown to correlate with functional differences. The IMMC appear to be derived from bone marrow precursors which may circulate. The mature cell found in the intestine arises as a result of growth and differentiative factors which are in part T-cell derived and which in the mouse have been shown to be due to interleukin 3 (IL-3) (Ihle et al. 1983). It is possible that IMMC have a different lineage from that of the PMC although recent work from Kitamura and his group have suggested that PMC may be converted into a different histochemical type (IMMC) after injection into the gastrointestinal tissue itself (Nakano et al. 1985). This suggests that the micro environment and the soluble factors released there are the important determining factors in deciding whether the cell will become an IMMC mucosal or PMC type of cell.

As can be seen in Table 1 we have shown that there are major differences in response to a variety of secretagogues between peritoneal and IMMC. Of particular interest is the total lack of response to compound 48/80 and bee venom peptide 401 by IMMC and the similar lack of response to several neuropeptides such as VIP (Shanahan et al. 1985) and the non-responsiveness to endorphins (Shanahan et al. 1984). The response to substance P while less than that of the peritoneal counterpart is highly significant in our view and raises questions about the modulation of mast cell activity in the intestine and in inflammatory states where the levels of substance P are markedly elevated locally.

TABLE 1

MAST CELL HETEROGENEITY IN THE RAT

Secretagogue	Mast Cell Source	
	Peritoneum	Intestine
Antigen, anti-IgE	++	++
Neutrophil cationic protein C3a, C5a, Dextran, Polylysine	++	?
48/80, Bee Venom peptide 401	++	0
Ionophores	++	+/++
Substance P	++	+
VIP, Somatostatin, Bradykinin, Neurotensin	++	0
Dynorphin, B-Endorphin, Neoendorphin	++	0

From the point of view of anti-allergic compounds, disodium chromoglycate is totally without effect on the rat IMMC whereas doxantrazole (Wellcome) is almost equipotent (Pearce et al. 1982). It is interesting that quercetin, a flavonoid, as well as some other derivative compounds are equipotent against both types of cells (Pearce et al. 1984). Mast cell hyperplasia is known to occur in a variety of situations which include responses in lymphoid tissues to antigen and the extraordinary increase which was shown by Burnet to occur in the thymuses of NZB mice which led him first to the hypothesis that mast cells were derived from lymphocytes (Burnet 1965), an observation which after careful work seems no longer tenable. Mast cell increases are found in the intestine in graft versus host disease (Mowat and Ferguson 1982) and in both Crohn's disease and ulcerative colitis (Lloyd et al. 1975). In the lung increases are found associated with pulmonary hypoxia, asbestosis (Wagner et al. 1984), pulmonary fibrosis (Kawanami et al. 1979) and in the broncho-alveolar washings of patients with many different forms of interstitial lung disease (Tomioka et al. 1984). Mast cell increases are also known to occur in osteoporotic bone, callus formation and in scar tissue of many sorts including keloids (Claman 1985). Various solid tumors have been associated with mast cell hyperplasia which include especially neurofibromata.

In sectioned peripheral nerves mast cell numbers increase up to six times normal in association with the repair process (Olsoon 1968).

In many chronic inflammatory states increases of mast cells are common. One example of this might be the synovium in rheumatoid arthritis (Crisp et al. 1984). Another less obvious example would be scleroderma of the skin which resembles changes occurring in chronic graft versus host disease (Claman 1985). In one acute type of inflammation, the response of the intestine to nematode infection is massive mast cell hyperplasia (Befus et al. 1982).

How then can these disparate observations be linked together? In the case of nematode infection it is known that mast cells are involved together with eosinophils in killing schistosomula larvae (Capron et al. 1978). Mast cells may well be involved in, but not obligatory for, the expression of delayed hypersensitivity (Askenase and Van Loveren 1983) although controversy exists about this (Galli and Dvorak 1984). Mast cells have been shown to be directly cytotoxic for fibrosarcoma and other tumour cells (Farram and Nelson 1980). This may occur through a mechanism separate from the normal secretory degranulation process since prior degranulation with 48/80 does not diminish the cytotoxic potential which occurs at effector to target ratios of less than 1 (Ernst et al. 1985).

PMC contain heparin whereas IMMC contain an oversulfated proteoglycan called chondroitin sulfate diB (Stevens and Austen 1985). Heparin is associated with the inhibition of lymphocytes (Frieri and Metcalfe 1983) and smooth muscle proliferation, appears capable of stimulation of angiogenesis (Azizkhan et al. 1980) and some _in vitro_ tumour growth, as well as blocking phagocytosis (Victor et al. 1981) and the damage done by eosinophil derived major basic protein. The effect of chondroitin sulfate diB in these systems is not known. Intestinal mucosal mast cells probably synthesize and release leukotrienes (particularly LTC_4), in preference to prostaglandins such as PGD_2, whereas the reverse is true for peritoneal mast cells (Schwartz and Austen 1984). Prostaglandins such as PDE_2 have inhibitory effects on many T and B functions. Leukotrienes such as LTB_4 inhibit lymphocyte proliferation and lymphokine mediated activation through T suppressor cells.

Histamine has a very complex series of actions (Beer and Rocklin, 1984), which include inhibition of monocyte synthesis of the second component of complement, inhibition of release of histamine, and the chemotactic response by basophils, whereas it stimulates eosinophils through an H1 receptor to increase the number of C3b receptors on its surface. All of the other activities of histamine indicated above are through the H2 receptor. The inhibitory effects of histamine on T cells include migration inhibition factor and interferon synthesis, proliferation to mitogen, antigen and mixed leukocyte reactions, cytotoxic T cell activity and a decrease in expression of IgE and IgG receptors on T lymphocytes. An interesting series of effects of histamine mediated through the H2 receptor has been shown in the granulomatous reaction induced by schistosomes (Weinstock et al. 1983, Chensue et al. 1983). Cimetidine blocks the effect of histamine and enhances granuloma size through its effect on histamine activated T suppressor cells.

We have recently shown that histamine may have different effects on fibroblasts which range from stimulation of proliferation to inhibition depending on the stage of cell cycle of the fibroblast (Jordana et al. 1985). Thus mast cell products may be involved in the promotion of fibroblast synthesis of collagen and the formation of fibrous tissue. Indeed, most granules may be phagocytosed by fibroblasts and have effects upon them (Atkins et al. 1985). This suggests an extremely complex series of events which must be highly regulated in the normal situation whereas in situations where antigen persists or in other, presumably genetically defined circumstances such as keloid formation, excess fibrous tissue is formed. This is compatible with observations of 50 fold increases in mast cells and histamine content in the pulmonary fibrosis induced by bleomycin in the rat (Goto et al. 1984).

It has been shown that psychological conditioning can induce a learned release of histamine and this suggests at least some neurohumoral regulation of mast cell secretion (Russell et al. 1984). Our own observations about neuropeptide modulation of histamine secretion by mast cells (Shanahan et al. 1985) and the significant literature on mast cell/nerve interaction quoted above (Olsoon 1968, Newson et al. 1983), all suggest mechanisms whereby this may occur. This promotes the suggestion that mast cells may be amplification cells between the inflammatory response and the central nervous system, placed locally at the site of inflammation. Direct nerve mast cell interdigitation has been shown in ultrastructural studies (Newson et al. 1983) and we have observed regular such relationships in the intestine of rats undergoing mast cell hyperplasia (Tomioka et al. 1985). It is particularly interesting in this regard that in anaphylaxis induced by antigen in rat intestine, major changes in terms of ion flux in epithelial cells occurs (Perdue et al. 1984). That this change in homeostasis was due to mast cell products was suggested by the inability of disodium chromoglycate to affect this in any way whereas doxantrazole, which is effective on rat IMMC, reversed the changes. Similarly, antigen-induced changes in short circuit current of the colonic epithelium have been shown in guinea pigs sensitized with cow's milk and subsequently challenged with B-lactoglobulin. This change was shown to be reversed by the prior administration of indomethicin, an inhibitor of prostaglandin synthetase. Thus, the immune system interacts with the epithelium to alter the normal physiological state in several different models.

Conclusions

Mast cells appear to be involved in a variety of inflammatory events both in the acute and chronic stages. Their products released on stimulation differ according to the type of mast cell involved and the tissue site in which it is found, and therefore their modulatory effects, are not always the same. Mast cell responses are probably part of a homeostatic mechanism involved in repair but which in many different sets of circumstances encountered in biology and seen as "disease" are dysregulated, and in some yet unknown manner, involved in the pathogenesis of these disorders.

REFERENCES

Askenase PW, Loveren HV (1983). Delayed-type hypersensitivity: activation of mast cells by antigen-specific T-cell factors initiates the cascade of cellular interactions. Immunology Today 4:259-264.

Atkins FM, Friedman MM, Rao PVS, Metcalfe DD (1985). Interactions between mast cells, fibroblasts and connect-

ive tissue components. Int Archs Allergy appl Immunol 77:96-102.
Azizkhan RG, Azizkhan JC, Zetter BR, Folkman J (1980). Mast cell heparin stimulates migration of capillary endothelial cells in vitro. J Exp Med 152:931-944.
Beer DJ, Rocklin RE (1984). Histamine induced suppressor cell activity. J Allergy Clin Immunol 73:439-452.
Befus AD, Pearce FL, Gauldie J, Horsewood P, Bienenstock J (1982). Mucosal mast cells: 1. Isolation and functional characteristics of rat intestinal mast cells. J Immunol 128:2475-2480.
Befus D, Pearce F, Bienenstock J (1985). Intestinal mast cells in pathology and host resistance. In Brostoff J, Challacombe SJ (eds): "Food Allergy and Intolerance," London: Saunders. In Press.
Bienenstock JB, Befus AD, Pearce F, Denburg J, Goodacre R. (1982). Mast cell heterogeneity: derivation and function, with emphasis on the intestine. J Allergy Clin Immunol 70:407-412.
Burnet FM (1965). Mast cells in the thymus of NZB mice. J Pathol Bacteriol 89:271-284.
Chensue SW, Boros DL, David CS (1983). Regulation of granulomatous inflammation in murine schistosomiasis. II. T suppressor cell-derived, I-C subregion-encoded soluble suppressor factor mediates regulation of lymphokine production. J Exp Med 157:219-230.
Claman HN (1985). Mast cells, T cells and abnormal fibrosis. Immunology Today 6:192-195.
Crisp AJ, Chapman CM, Kirkham SE, Schiller AL, Krane SM (1984). Articular mastocytosis in rheumatoid arthritis. Arthritis Rheum 27:845-851.
Cuthbert AW, McLaughlan P, Coombs RRA (1983). Immediate hypersensitivity reaction to B-lactoglobulin in the epithelium lining the colon of guinea pigs fed cow's milk. Int Archs Allergy appl Immunol 72:34-40.
Ernst P, Lee T, Befus AD, Bienenstock J (1985). Unpublished observations.
Farram E, Nelson DS (1980). Mouse mast cells as anti-tumour effector cells. Cell Immunol 55:294-301.
Frieri M, Metcalfe DD (1983). Analysis of the effect of mast cell granules on lymphocyte blastogenesis in the absence and presence of mitogens: identification of heparin as a granule-associated suppressor factor. J Immunol 131:1942-1948.
Galli SJ, Dvorak AM (1984). What do mast cells have to do with delayed hypersensitivity. Lab Invest 50:365-368.

Goto T, Befus D, Low R, Bienenstock J (1984). Mast cell heterogeneity and hyperplasia in bleomycin-induced pulmonary fibrosis of rats. Am Rev Respir Dis 130:797-802.

Ihle JN, Keller J, Oroszlan S, Henderson LE, Copeland TD, Fitch F, Prystowsky MB, Goldwasser E, Schrader JW, Palaszynski E, Dy M, Lebel B (1983). Biologic properties of homogeneous interleukin 3. Demonstration of WEHI-3 growth factor activity, mast cell growth factor activity, P cell-stimulating factor activity, colony-stimulating factor activity, and histamine-producing cell-stimulating factor activity. J Immunol 131:282-287.

Ishizaka K (1984). Mast cell activation and mediator release. Progr Allergy 34:1-336

Jordana M, Gauldie J, Befus AD, Newhouse M, Bienenstock J (1985). Effect of histamine on proliferation of human adult lung fibroblasts. Submitted.

Kawanami O, Forram VJ, Fulmer JD, Crystal RG (1979). Ultrastructure of pulmonary mast cells in patients with fibrotic lung disorders. Lab Invest 40:717-734.

Leung KBP, Barrett KE, Pearce FL (1984). Differential effects of anti-allergic compounds on peritoneal mast cells of the rat, mouse and hamster. Agents Actions 14:461-467.

Lloyd G, Green FHY, Fox H, Mani V, Turnberg LA (1975). Mast cells and immunoglobulin E in inflammatory bowel disease. Gut 16:861-866.

Mowat AM, Ferguson A (1982). Intraepithelial lymphocyte count and crypt hyperplasia measure the mucosal component of the graft-versus-host reaction in the mouse small intestine. Gastroenterology 83:417-423.

Nakano T, Sonoda T, Hayashi C, Yamatodani A, Kanayama Y, Yamamura T, Asai H, Yonezawa T, Kitamura Y, Galli SJ (1985). J Exp Med. In Press.

Newson B, Dahlstrom A, Enerback L, Ahlman H (1983). Suggestive evidence for a direct innervation of mucosal mast cells. Neuroscience 10:565-570.

Olsoon Y (1968). Mast cells in the nervous system. Int Rev Cytology 24:27-70.

Pearce FL, Befus AD, Gauldie J, Bienenstock J (1982). Mucosal mast cells. II. Effects of anti-allergic compounds on histamine secretion by isolated intestinal mast cells. J Immunol 128:2481-2486.

Pearce FL, Befus AD, Bienenstock J (1984). Mucosal mast cells. III. Effect of quercetin and other flavonoids on antigen-induced histamine secretion from rat intestinal

mast cells. J Allergy Clin Immunol 73:819-823.
Pearce FL, Ali H, Barrett KE, Befus AD, Bienenstock J, Brostoff J, Ennis M, Flint KC, Hudspith B, Johnson NM, Leung KBP, Peachell PT (1985). Functional characteristics of mucosal and connective tissue mast cells of man, rat and other animals. Int Archs Allergy appl Immunol 77:274-276.
Perdue MH, Chung M, Gall DG (1984). Effect of intestinal anaphylaxis on gut function in the rat. Gastroenterology 86:391-397.
Pinckard RN (1983). Platelet-activating factor. Hosp Practice 18:67-76.
Russell M, Dark KA, Cummins RW, Ellman G, Callaway E, Peeke HVS (1984). Learned histamine release. Science 225:733-734.
Schwartz LB, Austen KF (1984). Structure and function of the chemical mediators of mast cells. Progr Allergy 34: 271-321.
Shanahan F, Lee TDG, Bienenstock J, Befus AD (1984) The influence of endorphins on peritoneal and mucosal mast cell secretion. J Allergy Clin Immunol 74:499-504.
Shanahan F, Denburg JA, Fox J, Bienenstock J, Befus AD (1985). Mast cell heterogeneity: effects of neuroenteric peptides on histamine release. J Immunol 135: In Press
Stevens RL, Katz HR, Seldin DC, Austen KF (1985). Biochemical characteristics distinguish subclasses of mammalian mast cells. In Befus AD, Bienenstock J, Denburg J (eds). "Mast Cell Heterogeneity", New York: Raven Press.
Tomioka M, Ida S, Shindoh Y, Ishihara T, Takishima T (1984). Mast cells in bronchoalveolar lumen of patients with bronchial asthma. Am Rev Resp Dis 129:1000-1005.
Tomioka M, Simon G, Bienenstock J. Mast cell-nerve interaction in rat intestine. In preparation.
Victor M, Weiss J, Elsbach E (1981). Heparin inhibits phagocytosis by polymorphonuclear leukocytes. Infect Immun 32:295-299.
Wagner MMF, Edwards RE, Moncriell CB, Wagner JC (1984). Mast cells and inhalation of asbestos in rats. Thorax 39: 539-544
Weinstock JV, Chensue SW, Boros DL (1983). Modulation of granulomatous hypersensitivity: V. Participation of histamine receptor positive and negative lymphocytes in the granulomatous response of Schistosomiasis mansoni-infected mice. J Immunol 130:423-427.

THE ROLE OF THE EOSINOPHIL IN HOST DEFENSE

D.G. Colley, S.J. Stewart, E.K. Duncan and W.E. Secor

VA Medical Center, (D.G.C., S.J.S.), Departments of Microbiology, (D.G.C., E.K.D., W.E.S.) and Medicine (S.J.S.), Vanderbilt University School of Medicine, Nashville, TN 37203

INTRODUCTION

Eosinophils are myeloid cells capable of various immune and inflammatory functions (Beeson and Bass, 1977; Butterworth, 1977; Colley and James, 1979; Weller and Goetzl, 1979; Mahmoud and Austen, 1981). Peripheral blood eosinophilia is associated with several disease states including tissue-dwelling parasitic infections, allergic reactions, some neoplasms, and the hypereosinophilic syndrome. Eosinophil production, migration and function can be influenced by T lymphocytes and their products (Colley, 1980a). In some hypersensitivity states eosinophils may modulate the degree of inflammation (Austen, 1978). A major function proposed for eosinophils is the killing of extracellular targets such as helminths (Ellner and Mahmoud, 1982; Butterworth, et al., 1982; Capron et al., 1982).

T LYMPHOCYTE CONTROL OF EOSINOPHILS

T cell control of eosinophils was first shown in regard to parasite larvae and soluble antigens by Beeson's and Speirs' groups, respectively (Colley,1980b). Recent data implicate L3T4+ T cells in the maintenance of peripheral blood eosinophilia (Figure 1). Mice with eosinophilia due to patent *Schistosoma mansoni* infection were injected with ascites fluid containing 1 mg monoclonal anti-L3T4 (from hybridoma GK1.5) and their eosinophilia was monitored. Eosinophilia was decreased by this treatment.

Presumably, this is secondary to the documented decrease in L3T4+ lymphocytes.

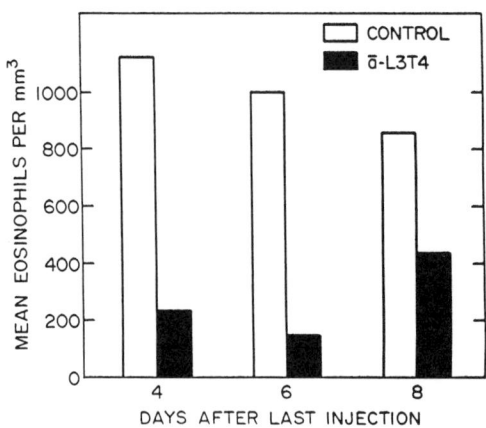

Figure 1. Peripheral blood eosinophil levels 4, 6, and 8 days after iv injection of anti-L3T4 monoclonal antibody into CBA/J mice infected for 8 weeks with S. mansoni.

Several lymphokines affect eosinophils (Colley, 1980a). Eosinophil-differentiating factor, produced by T cell clones or hybrids, stimulates the differentiation of eosinophils in liquid bone marrow cultures (Sanderson, et al., 1985). This 46 kD material is neither IL-2 nor IL-3.

Eosinophil Stimulation Promoter (ESP)

The T cell-dependent lymphokine ESP (Colley, 1980a,b; Rand and Colley, 1982) has been described in murine and human systems. Although often associated with helminth-related immune responses, ESP is generated in response to concanavalin A, phytohemagglutinin, or specific antigens. ESP is usually assayed by measuring the distance of migration of eosinophils out of an agarose droplet. Recently we have determined that a colorimetric assay of viable cells, in which mitochrondrial enzymes cleave the tetrazolium salt MTT to a dark blue formazan product (Mosmann, 1983) is also an efficient assay of ESP activity (Figure 2). Extensive physicochemical characterization of ESP has not been done.

It is hoped that this task will be assisted by the recent observation that ESP activity precipitates between 60-80% saturated ammonium sulfate (Figure 3).

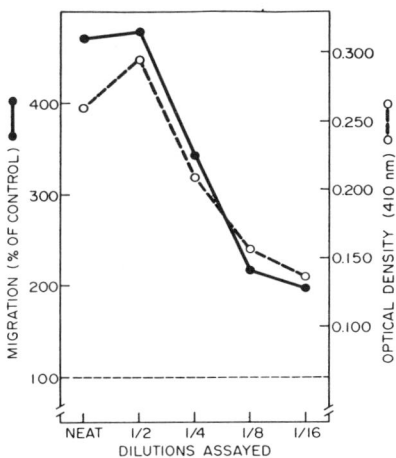

Figure 2. Eosinophil migration measured either microscopically (solid line) or as conversion of MTT (Sigma M2128; 500 ug/ml) to formazan by viable migrating cells.

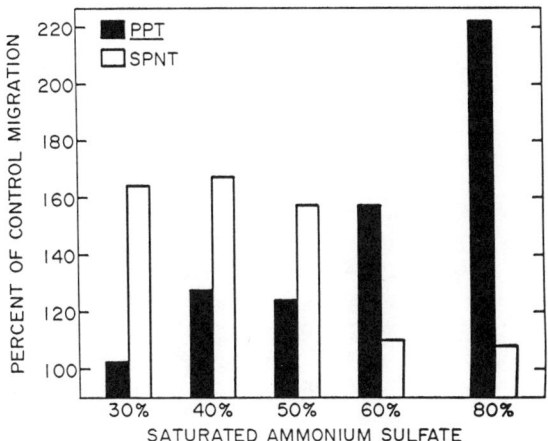

Figure 3. ESP activity in culture supernatants (SPNT, ☐) or saturated ammonium sulfate precipitates (PPT, ■).

In a series of studies (Rand and Colley, 1982), our laboratory examined arachidonic acid metabolism in murine eosinophils. Incubation of murine eosinophils with ESP led to 2-3 fold increases in production of 12-HETE. Furthermore, 12-HETE and LTB4 caused eosinophil migration, while 15-HETE inhibited migration and synthesis of 12-HETE. All these metabolites are produced by murine eosinophils. Relatively selective inhibitors of lipoxygenase pathways of arachidonate metabolism inhibited ESP-induced eosinophil migration, while only very high levels of some cyclooxygenase inhibitors had an effect. Passively transferred, Indium-111 labeled eosinophils efficiently localized to ESP intradermal injection sites. This in vivo effect of ESP was abrogated by lipoxygenase pathway inhibitors.

THE POSSIBLE ROLE OF EOSINOPHILS IN HOST DEFENSE

Destruction of Schistosome Eggs

ESP is produced by schistosome egg-induced hepatic granulomas from S. mansoni-infected mice. In vitro ESP activates normal eosinophils to destroy schistosome eggs (Phillips and Colley, 1978). There is also in vivo evidence of an egg-destroying role of activated eosinophils during schistosomiasis (Olds and Mahmoud, 1980). Injections of anti-eosinophil serum led to more schistosome eggs retained in the livers of infected mice, indicating that the antiserum interfered with egg destruction.

Cytotoxicity for Larval Helminths

Eosinophils can kill a variety of parasite larvae in vitro (Capron, et al., 1982; Ellner and Mahmoud, 1982). The list of susceptible targets ranges from protozoans to worms. The most studied system is the killing of Schistosoma mansoni schistosomula, but the cytotoxicity of eosinophils for larval forms of nematodes such as Trichinella spiralis and Onchocera volvulus also is clear. Eosinophil degranulation is required, and the events that lead to cell-to-parasite attachment and subsequent degranulation usually involve antibodies or complement as ligands. The process begins with cell-to-parasite binding, degranulation, very firm binding, and ultimately larval killing

(Butterworth, et al., 1982). Because the target is often considerably larger than the eosinophil, a unique feature of this effector cell may be its ability to bind firmly and focally deposit its granular materials on large invaders.

The mechanisms of destruction used by eosinophils appear combinatory. The eosinophil's basic granular proteins, such as Major Basic Protein, Eosinophil Cationic Protein and Eosinophil-derived Neurotoxin are directly cytotoxic to various cells and parasites. The eosinophil peroxidase-hydrogen peroxide-halide, and phospholipase systems also are active in the killing process. The former can prepare helminth targets for enhanced killing by other cell types (Jong, et al., 1984). Mast cell components, lymphokines and monokines can augment the efficacy of eosinophil-mediated cytotoxicity (Capron, et al., 1982; Pincus, et al., 1984; Veith, et al., 1984). Activation is often mediated through increased expression of receptors for various ligands, such as Fc and/or C3b receptors (Butterworth, et al., 1982).

Several other lines of evidence indicate that eosinophils participate in host defense mechanisms. In vivo use of anti-eosinophil sera, mentioned above in regard to schistosome egg destruction, has abrogated concomitant immunity against challenge schistosomes (Mahmoud, et al., 1975) and has resulted in increased larval loads in the muscles of T. spiralis-infected mice (Grove, et al.,1977). Histopathologic studies have observed eosinophils in the right place at the right time to be responsible for killing some invading parasites (von Lichtenberg, et al., 1985). While incriminating, such evidence does not yet seem convincing. Capron et al. (1984) showed that rats exposed to S. mansoni cercariae, followed by local adoptive transfer of antibody-coated eosinophils, express significant levels of protection.

PRELIMINARY DATA ON AN ANTI-EOSINOPHIL MONOCLONAL ANTIBODY

We recently have begun to develop new tools for the dissection of the roles which eosinophils play in immunobiology. We are evaluating a monoclonal antibody (6B4) produced by a hybridoma obtained from a fusion of spleen cells from a Lewis rat immunized with mouse eosinophils and the Y3 Louvain rat myeloma. Monoclonal 6B4 reacts strongly with purified eosinophils, but not neutrophils, in a cellular ELISA system. The antibody inhibits ESP-stimulated migration, and thus may react either with a cell surface receptor for ESP or some migration-related structure. Immunoprecipitation of surface-iodinated purified eosinophil lysates with 6B4 precipitates a major iodinated component of 75 kD and a minor band of 37 kD (data not shown).

We have evaluated the in vivo effect of 6B4 on schistosome egg antigen (SEA)-induced 5, 24 and 48 hr skin tests in the pinna of mice infected with S. mansoni for 8 weeks (Figure 4). Administration (ip) of 3 ml of 6B4 supernatants over a 24 hr period decreased subsequent SEA-induced 24 and 48 hr cell-mediated reactions, but not 5 hr Arthus-type reactions. Pre-absorption of 6B4 by an anti-immunoglobulin immunoabsorbant reversed this suppression. Histopathologic evaluation of the skin test sites revealed a dramatic decrease in the tissue eosinophilia normally observed (Colley, 1980a) at 48 hr in such sites.

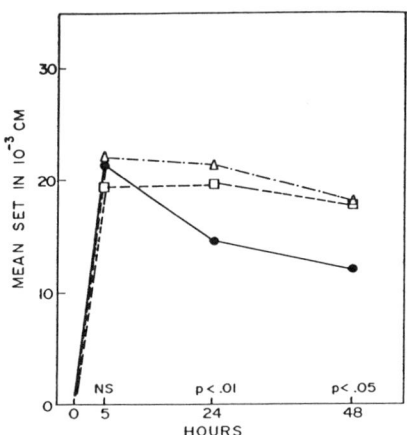

Figure 4. Specific ear thickening (SET) due to intradermal injection of 15 ug of SEA after injection of either 6B4 supernatant (●——●), 6B4 supernatant absorbed with anti-immunoglobulin (△--△) or RPMI 1640. Mice were infected with 40 cercariae of S. mansoni 8 week previously.

SUMMARY

The eosinophil remains an enigma. Despite elucidation of its cytotoxic capabilities, certain mediators of its migration and localization, and its potential as a regulatory cell, there remains a need to define the eosinophil's in vivo activities and the mediators of those activities. Monoclonal antibodies and molecular biology may provide the tools required to properly define the eosinophil's role in various areas of immunobiology.

REFERENCES

Austen KF (1978). Homeostasis of effector systems which can also be recruited for immunologic reactions. J Immunol 121:793-805.
Beeson PB, Bass DA (1977). In "Major Problems in Internal Medicine" (LH Smith, Jr., ed.), Vol. XIV. Philadelphia: Saunders.
Butterworth AE (1977). The eosinophil and its role in immunity to helminth infection. Curr Top Microbiol Immunol 77:127-168.
Butterworth AE, Taylor DW, Veith MC, Vadas MA, Dessein A, Sturrock RF, Wells E (1982). Studies on the mechanisms of immunity in human schistosomiasis. Immunological Rev 61:5-39.
Capron A, Dessaint JP, Haque A, Capron M (1982). Antibody-dependent cell-mediated cytotoxicity against parasites. Prog Allergy 31:234-267.
Capron M, Nogueira-Queiroz JA, Papin JP, Capron A (1984). Interactions between eosinophils and antibodies: In vivo protective role against rat schistosomiasis. Cell Immunol 83:60-72.
Colley DG (1980a). Lymphokine-related eosinophil responses. Lymphokine Reports 1:133-155.
Colley DG (1980b). Lymphocyte products. In Mahmoud, AAF, Austin, KF (eds): "The Eosinophil in Health and Disease," New York: Grune & Stratton, pp 293-309.
Colley DG, James SL (1979). Participation of eosinophils in immunological systems. In Gupta S, Good RA (eds): "Cellular, Molecular, and Clinical Aspects of Allergic Disorders," New York: Plenum, pp 55-86.
Ellner JJ, Mahmoud AAF (1982). Phagocytes and worms: David and Goliath revisited. Rev Inf Dis 4:698-714.

Grove DI, Mahmoud AAF, Warren KS (1977). Eosinophils and resistance to Trichinella spiralis. J Exp Med 145:755-759.

Jong EC, Chi EY, Klebanoff SJ (1984). Human neutrophil-mediated killing of schistosomula of Schistosoma mansoni: augmentation by schistosomal binding of eosinophil peroxidase. Am J Trop Med Hyg 33:104-115.

Mahmoud AAF, Warren KS, Peters PA (1975). A role for the eosinophil in acquired resistance to Schistosoma mansoni infection as determined by anti-eosinophil serum. J Exp Med 142:805-813.

Mahmoud AAF, Austen KF (1980). "The eosinophil in health and disease." New York: Grune & Stratton.

Mosmann T (1983). Rapid colorimetric assay for cellular growth and survival: Application to proliferation and cytotoxicity assays. J Immunol Meth 65:55-63.

Olds GR, Mahmoud AAF (1980). Role of host granulomatous response in murine schistosomiasis mansoni. Eosinophil-mediated destruction of eggs. J Clin Invest 66:1191-1199.

Phillips SM, Colley DG (1978). Immunologic aspects of host responses to schistosomiasis: Resistance, immunopathology, and eosinophil involvement. Prog Allergy 24:49-182.

Pincus SH, Dessein A, Lenzi H, Vadas MA, David J (1984). Eosinophil-mediated killing of schistosomula of Schistosoma mansoni: Oxidative requirement for enhancement by eosinophil colony stimulating factor (CSF-α) and supernatants with eosinophil cytotoxicity enhancing activity (E-CEA). Cell Immunol 87:424-433.

Rand TH, Colley DG (1982). Lymphokine-mediated regulation of murine eosinophils. In Yoshida T, Torisu M (eds): "Immunobiology of the Eosinophil," New York: Elsevier Biomedical, pp 13-27.

Sanderson CJ, Warren, DJ and Strath M (1985). Identification of a lymphokine that stimulates eosinophil differentiation in vitro. Its relationship to interleukin 3, and functional properties of eosinophils produced in cultures. J Exp Med 162:60-74.

Veith M, Taylor DW, Thorne K, Richardson BA, Butterworth, AE (1984). Studies on the enhancement of human eosinophil function by mononuclear cell products in vitro. Clin Exp Immunol 58:603-610.

von Lichtenberg F, Correa-Oliveira R, Sher A (1985). The fate of challenge schistosomula in the murine anti-schistosome vaccine model. Am J Trop Med Hyg 34:96-106.

Weller PF, Goetzl EJ (1979). The regulatory and effector roles of eosinophils. Adv Immunol 27:339-371.

Platelet-Neutrophil Interactions in the Eicosanoid Pathway

Aaron J. Marcus, Lenore B. Safier, Harris L. Ullman, M. Johan Broekman, Naziba Islam, Thomas D. Oglesby, Robert R. Gorman and Clemens von Schacky

Departments of Medicine, Divisions of Hematology-Oncology, New York Veterans Administration Medical Center, New York 10010; Cornell University Medical College, New York 10021; and Department of Experimental Sciences, The Upjohn Company, Kalamazoo, Michigan 49001

INTRODUCTION

Eicosanoids are defined as oxygenated derivatives of 20-carbon polyunsaturated fatty acids, predominantly arachidonate. Several eicosanoids, their intermediates (some of which are very transient), and precursors are labile substances which exert biological effects in the microenvironment of cells which participate in their formation (Marcus, 1984). In this sense, they can be regarded as autacoids (Marcus, 1978). It therefore follows that a specific biological event in vivo would involve more than one cell type which is anatomically in proximity to another. A given physiological or pathological stimulus or event is likely to involve several cell types. For example, a thrombus or inflammatory site might involve combined biological and biochemical activities of leukocytes, platelets, endothelial cells and smooth muscle cells.

Research strategy in our laboratory has recently evolved from the realization that intravascular thrombosis and inflammation represent multicellular events. Our studies have been specifically directed toward elucidation of mechanisms by which eicosanoids are formed and/or inactivated during cellular interactions.

The biochemical mechanisms in tissues for transforming arachidonic acid are ubiquitous, but usually reflect the enzymatic capacity of a given cell. Therefore, in the microenvironment, the possibility exists for an admixture and interaction between eicosanoid products and intermediates which can then generate compounds with biological effects which might not have been anticipated on the basis of theory.

CLASSIFICATION OF CELL-CELL INTERACTIONS IN THE EICOSANOID PATHWAY

We have demonstrated (Marcus, et al., 1980, Marcus, et al., 1984) and recognized the potential for in vitro conversion of eicosanoid intermediates and end products to new metabolites which could not have been synthesized by a single cell type alone, and might have heretofore unrecognized biological properties. This concept may be pertinent with regard to formation of hemostatic platelet plugs or arterial thrombi. It can be observed microscopically, that platelets, leukocytes and endothelial cells which possess active eicosanoid pathways are in positions of plasma membrane contact during these events. The early inflammatory process may also be analogous, in that circulating leukocytes closely adhere to blood vessel surfaces prior to migration between endothelial cells. At this point there is also considerable approximation of cell membranes (Lewis and Austen, 1984). Since neutrophils have been identified during formation of thrombi, our studies have been extended to evaluation of platelet-neutrophil interactions.

We have arbitrarily classified cell-cell interactions in the 20:4 6 pathway into two broad areas: (1) Two cells in close proximity can share a common precursor. One example is released arachidonate from stimulated platelets (whether aspirin treated or not) with subsequent entry into a stimulated neutrophil for synthesis of LTB_4 and 5-HETE (Marcus, et al., 1982). Secondly, endoperoxides from stimulated platelets can be metabolized by endothelial cells to prostacyclin (Marcus, et al., 1980). (2) One cell can transform the product of another into a new metabolite which neither cell can synthesize alone. An example is 5-lipoxygenation of platelet 12-HETE to 5S,12S-DiHETE, when both the platelet and neutrophil have been stimulated by ionophore in vitro. Another instance is the omega-hydroxylation of platelet 12-HETE by the neutrophil to 12S,20-DiHETE, when only the platelet has been stimulated by thrombin or collagen.

STIMULATION OF PLATELET-NEUTROPHIL SUSPENSIONS WITH IONOPHORE A23187

Most clinical and laboratory studies of arachidonic acid metabolism in platelets have involved the cyclooxygenase pathway, which produces mainly thromboxane. The platelet lipoxygenase-pathway which catalyzes formation of 12-hydroxy acids has been studied in less detail because direct effects of hydroxy acids on platelet function have not been observed to any appreciable extent. In contrast, the main pathway of arachidonate metabolism in neutrophils, involves the 5-lipoxygenase enzyme and has been studied in detail. This is because the 5-lipoxygenase catalyzes oxygenation of arachidonate to leukotriene B_4. In 1982, we devised a system for studying interactions between human platelets and neutrophils (Marcus, et al., 1982). This was carried out by incubation of combined suspensions of [^{3}H]arachidonate-labeled platelets with unlabeled neutrophils. This was followed by stimulation with ionophore A23187 after which lipid extraction, thin-layer radiochromatography and high-performance liquid chromatography (HPLC) were carried out. Several radioactive metabolites, not produced by stimulated platelets alone were detected in this incubation system. The most important metabolite identified was LTB_4. Also, present were 5S,12S-DiHETE, 5-HETE and trihydroxyeicosatetraenoic acids (THETEs).

Since platelets were the only source of radioactivity in these experiments, LTB_4, DiHETE, and 5-HETE were therefore produced from precursor(s) originating in platelets upon ionophore stimulation. These experiments represented the first direct demonstration of the platelet contribution to formation of neutrophil-derived leukotrienes and hydroxy acids.

The results were extended with utilization of platelets from donors who had ingested aspirin. Thus, only three platelet-derived precursors were available to the neutrophils: arachidonic acid, 12-HPETE, and 12-HETE. We therefore studied effects of adding arachidonate or 12-HETE to neutrophil suspensions.

INCUBATION OF NEUTROPHILS WITH IONOPHORE A23187 AND WITH EITHER [^{14}C]ARACHIDONATE OR [^{3}H]12-HETE

When we added one micromolar ionophore and 5.7 micromolar [^{14}C]arachidonate to neutrophils, LTB$_4$, 5S,12S-DiHETE and 5-HETE formed (THETE was also identified). However, in these experiments formation of 5S,12S-DiHETE was attributable to contaminating platelets in the neutrophil suspension. Importantly, neutrophils exposed to 5.7 micromolar [^{14}C]arachidonate, but not stimulated with ionophore did not produce these metabolites.

When 2 micromolar ionophore and 9.4 nM [^{3}H]12-HETE were added to neutrophils, we noted production of 5S,12S-DiHETE which was therefore synthesized from platelet 12-HETE. No LTB$_4$ was formed from radiolabeled 12-HETE.

Results of these experiments indicated that radiolabeled platelet-derived 12-HETE was the precursor of labeled 5S,12S-DiHETE synthesized by neutrophils when [^{3}H]arachidonate-labeled platelets and unlabeled neutrophils were stimulated by ionophore. In addition, the experiments demonstrated that platelet arachidonate could serve as precursor of neutrophil LTB$_4$ and 5-HETE.

The importance of LTB$_4$ in the inflammatory and allergic processes is well-known. Demonstration of a platelet contribution to LTB$_4$ formation under conditions of ionophore stimulation is presently of theoretical interest, but as stimuli for LTB$_4$ in vivo are characterized in the future, this reaction should take on further clinical significance. Thus, we developed the hypothesis that platelet-neutrophil interactions can generate new eicosanoids, capable of modulating normal or abnormal homeostasis. Platelets from patients who have ingested aspirin are still capable of releasing free arachidonate and considerable quantities of 12-HETE. In fact, 12-HETE is produced as long as free arachidonate is available in the platelet. These phenomena may eventually take on clinical importance.

EICOSANOID METABOLISM IN PLATELET-NEUTROPHIL SUSPENSIONS EXPOSED TO PLATELET AGONISTS (THROMBIN OR COLLAGEN)

In the experiments described above, combined platelet-neutrophil suspensions were stimulated by an agent which initiates arachidonate metabolism in both neutrophils and platelets (ionophore). A separate group of experiments was designed to ascertain whether eicosanoid metabolism would be initiated in a platelet-neutrophil suspension wherein only a platelet agonist for eicosanoid metabolism was added (Marcus, et al., 1984). The stimulus utilized was either thrombin (5 U/ml) or collagen (30 micrograms/ml). Upon addition of these agonists to cell suspensions containing [^{3}H]arachidonate-labeleled platelets and unlabeled neutrophils, production of a labeled compound which could not be synthesized by platelets or neutrophils alone was detected. This was a new eicosanoid, subsequently identified as 12S,20-dihydroxyeicosatetraenoic acid (12,20-DiHETE). The product was identified initially by thin-layer radiochromatography wherein its R_f value did not coincide with any previously identified eicosanoid.

Lack of production of radiolabeled 5-HETE, indicated that thrombin or collagen did not initiate arachidonic acid metabolism in neutrophils. Therefore, 12,20-DiHETE was synthesized by neutrophils from an eicosanoid produced by stimulated platelets. This conclusion was additionally supported when 5.7 micromolar [^{14}C]arachidonate (a non-stimulatory concentration for neutrophils, but capable of activating platelets) was added to an unlabeled platelet-neutrophil mixture. Under such conditions, 12,20-DiHETE was produced. In sharp contrast, when platelet-neutrophil suspensions were stimulated by ionophore A23187, formation of 12,20-DiHETE was minimal, but 5S,12S-DiHETE was produced.

Since 12,20-DiHETE was produced when platelet donors had ingested aspirin, involvement of 12-HETE from the platelet lipoxygenase pathway appeared likely. In control experiments aspirin-treated platelets produced mainly 12-HETE when stimulated by thrombin. In contrast, when a radiolabeled platelet-neutrophil suspension was exposed to thrombin, 12-HETE decreased and 12,20-DiHETE appeared.

In the next group of experiments, we attempted to ascertain whether 12-HETE was indeed the precursor of 12,20-DiHETE. [^{3}H]12-HETE (9.4 pmoles/ml) was added to an unlabeled neutrophil suspension. The radioactive product was identified as 12,20-DiHETE. Production of unlabeled 12,20-DiHETE was measured by reversed-phased HPLC under several different experimental conditions (Marcus, et al., 1984). 12,20-DiHETE was rechromatographed on thin-layer plates following its elution from a reversed-phase HPLC column. The R_f value was identical to that obtained in the earlier thin-layer radiochromatographic studies. An ultraviolet absorption spectrum of the isolated material after esterification and straight-phase HPLC showed an absorption maximum at 235 nm. This spectrum was similar to that of the parent compound, 12-HETE.

The purified, esterified product obtained by straight-phase HPLC was converted to the trimethylsilyl ether and analyzed by gas chromatography/mass spectrometry. The derivatized product eluted from an SE-30 column with an equivalent chain length value of C-24.6. Mass spectrometry studies indicated that the compound was a dihydroxy derivative of arachidonic acid. The base peak of 295 strongly suggested that the additional hydroxylation was present between C-12 and C-20. After hydrogenation, the mass spectrum suggested that the additional hydroxyl group was located at C-20. Confirmation was obtained by gas chromatography/mass spectrometry of the derivative from catalytic hydrogenation, Jones oxidation, and methylation (Marcus, et al., 1984).

Results of studies of cell-cell interactions also have implications for clinical trials, since platelets from patients who ingest aspirin can still release free arachidonate upon stimulation. This arachidonate can then interact with other cell types in production of products in the lipoxygenase pathway having biological activities yet to be described.

ACKNOWLEDGMENTS

This work was supported by grants from the Veterans Administration, National Institutes of Health HL 18828 10 (SCOR), HL 29034, RR 05396, the New York Heart Association, the Edward Gruenstein Fund, the Sallie Wichman Fund, and the Deutsche Forschungsgemeinschaft. Dr. Broekman is an Established Investigator of the American Heart Association.

REFERENCES

Lewis RA, Austen KF (1984). The biologically active leukotrienes. Biosynthesis, metabolism, receptors, functions, and pharmacology. J Clin Invest 73: 889-97.

Marcus AJ (1984). The eicosanoids in biology and medicine. J Lipid Res 25: 1511-6.

Marcus AJ, Safier LB, Ullman HL, Broekman MJ, Islam N, Oglesby TD, Gorman RR (1984). 12S,20 Dihydroxyicosatetraenoic acid: A new icosanoid synthesized by neutrophils from 12S-hydroxyicosatetraenoic acid produced by thrombin- or collagen-stimulated platelets. Proc Natl Acad Sci USA 81: 903-7.

Marcus AJ, Broekman MJ, Safier LB, Ullman HL, Islam N, Serhan CN, Rutherford LE, Korchak HM, Weissmann G (1982). Formation of leukotrienes and other hydroxy acids during platelet-neutrophil interactions in vitro. Biochem Biophys Res Commun 109: 130-7

Marcus AJ, Weksler BB, Jaffe EA, Broekman MJ (1980). Synthesis of prostacyclin from platelet-derived endoperoxides by cultured human enothelial cells. J Clin Invest 66: 979-86

Marcus AJ (1978). The role of lipids in platelet function: with particular reference to the arachidonic acid pathway. J Lipid Res 19: 793-826.

ROLE OF GTP-BINDING PROTEINS IN THE REGULATION OF THE HUMAN NEUTROPHIL

Pramod M. Lad, Charles V. Olson, Iqbal S. Grewal, Marianne Frolich, Paula A. Smiley, and Stephen J. Scott

Kaiser Regional Research Laboratory
4953 Sunset Boulevard, Los Angeles, CA 90027

INTRODUCTION

The human neutrophil plays an important role in both host defense and inflammation. Chemotaxis, superoxide generation (SOG) enzyme release (ER) and aggregation are observed in response to occupancy of the f-met-leu-phe (FMLP), C5a and platelet activating factor (PAF) receptors. The phenomenon of capping, in which crosslinked receptor sites are moved to one end of the cell prior to their removal by internalization, is observed in response to lectins (concanavalin-A) and immune complexes. Phagocytosis is promoted by receptors for Fc, C3b and mannose-6-phosphate. A question of importance is the manner in which cell surface receptors transduce extracellular signals to carry out a range of complex functions. It is known that GTP-binding proteins play an important role in the actions of peptide hormones and neurotransmitters (Lad, et al, 1977a, b). However, their role in the action of mediators of inflammation has remained largely unknown.

Bacterial toxins (cholera and pertussis) are ADP-ribosyltransferases which selectively modify the Ns and Ni components and are thus useful probes in evaluating the role of GTP binding proteins in receptor action. Recent studies suggest that the f-met-leu-phe receptor is regulated by a particular GTP-binding protein, termed Ni, which is selectively modified by pertussis toxin (PT) (Koo and Snyderman, 1983; Lad, et al 1985a). As a result of this modification, the FMLP receptor is uncoupled from its regulatory protein resulting in a loss of receptor action. The target enzymes

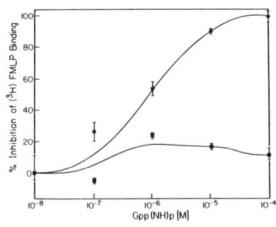

Fig. 1. Gpp(NH)p-mediated alteration of [^{3}H] fMet-Leu-Phe binding. PT treatment (15 ug/ml, incubated for 35 min at 30°C) was carried out prior to the binding study in a buffer containing NAD and arginine. Membranes were then diluted directly into the assay. Control membranes were similarly treated without PT. Control (top curve) and toxin-treated (lower-curve) membranes are shown. Total binding ranged from 125 to 150 fmol/mg. Details are given in (Lad, et al (1985a).

to which an FMLP-Ni complex might be coupled have also been explored and a role involving both cyclic AMP and calcium seems to be indicated. Evidence for distinct Ni related sequences which are involved in the regulation of chemotaxis, capping and phagocytosis is presented below.

RESULTS AND DISCUSSION

Our initial studies of the role of GTP binding proteins were directed at the role of Ns in receptor regulation and transduction in the human neutrophil. Purified plasma membranes were prepared in which receptor sensitivity of the adenylate cyclase system was retained. In these membranes we were able to establish that both the PGE_1 and beta adrenergic receptors activate adenylate cyclase through Ns and cause a shift in the affinity of beta agonists for their receptor. Under these conditions FMLP activation of adenylate was not observed suggesting that the Ns GTP-binding

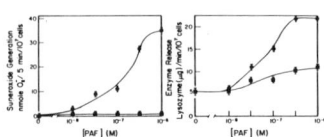

Fig. 2. Effects of pertussis toxin pretreatment on PAF mediated SOG (left panel) and ER (right panel). Human neutrophils were pretreated with (lower curves) or without (upper curves) pertussis toxin and tested for functional responses as indicated. The details of cell preparations, toxin pretreatment and function tests are given in (Lad, et al 1985a, b)

protein was not involved in the actions of FMLP. Concurrently, the FMLP receptor modulation by Gpp(NH)p was demonstrated (Koo and Snyderman, 1983). As Ns was not involved in the actions of the FMLP receptor, a logical choice was the mediation of Ni. Analysis of this protein has been facilitated by the work of Okajima and Ui; 1984, who had previously demonstrated that PT selectively modifies this protein and that modification of Ni is associated with an uncoupling of the receptor from its regulatory protein.

These observations led us to test the effect of PT on the regulation of the FMLP receptor by Gpp(NH)p. The results shown in Figure 1 indicate that (a) Gpp(NH)p causes a dissociation of FMLP from its receptor in a dose dependent manner and (b) pretreatment of the membranes with PT results in the abolition of the regulation of the receptor by Gpp-(NH)p. The role of the PT substrate in the regulation of multiple receptors and functions in the human neutrophil was then examined. For the FMLP receptor, it has been demonstrated that superoxide generation, enzyme release, aggregation, chemotaxis and shape change are inhibited as a result of PT pretreatment (Lad, et al 1985a, b; Volpi, et al 1985). Our experiments indicate that PAF as well as C5a mediated effects on neutrophil functions are similarly inhibited (Lad, et al 1985b). We conclude that protein as well as lipid mediators of inflammation act through Ni to exert their effects on the neutrophil.

Another set of receptors is involved in crosslinking of cell surface sites and hence induce exocytosis of granule constituents. Two examples of such ligands are immune

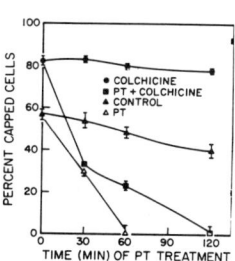

Fig. 3. Distribution of FITC-con-A in human neutrophils. Control and PT-treated neutrophils were suspended in modified HBSS at a concentration of 5×10^6 cells/ml. The cells were then treated with buffer or colchicine (10^{-5}M) and subsequently exposed to FITC-Con-A (10 ug/ml). The details of the PT treatment and the capping reaction are outlined in (Lad, et al 1985b).

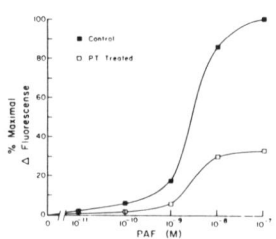

Fig. 4. Transduction mechanisms associated as the neutrophil Ni GTP-binding protein. Whole cells loaded with Quin2 were treated with pertussis toxin as described in the legends to figures 1 & 2. Change in fluorescence of Quin2 loaded cells was monitored at different PAF concentrations. Details of these assays are provided in Lad, et al 1985a, b.

complexes and lectins such as concanvalin-A (con-A). While con-A and heat aggregated IgG both cause ER and SOG, ER occurs only from secondary granules. Chemotaxis is not observed in response to these ligands and although shape change is observed, it is accompanied by cap formation in a structure referred to as a "bleb". Because of both the similarity and differences in the actions of these receptors from those for FMLP, C5a and PAF, we have examined the role of Ni in both the secretory response and capping. The form of the inhibition observed differs from that observed with FMLP and PAF. For the latter, inhibition involves a significant effect on both the Vmax as well as Kact. By contrast for con-A and heat aggregated IgG, the inhibition is predominately a K act effect. Conditions can be designed in which complete inhibition of FMLP or PAF responses is noted without an appreciable effect on con-A mediated effects where saturating concentrations of both ligands are utilized. A study of the capping reaction however reveals that PT completely abolishes this reaction at very low concentrations (Figure 3) while CT is without effect. Abolition of capping is not due to the induction of unstable caps, but is due to the abolition of an element essential to cap formation. These studies indicate that the Ni protein plays a central role in cap formation but plays only an attenuating role in the secretory responses of agents which cause cell surface crosslinking. Recent results also indicate that, under conditions in which chemotaxis and capping are completely inhibited, phagocytosis and adhesion are unaltered (Lad, et al (1985b). Thus the Ni protein plays a minor role in the regulation of these pathways.

Transduction mechanisms that may be involved in the actions of FMLP and PAF were analyzed. The first was adenlate cyclase (Lad, et al 1985a). Our initial results suggested that only a small inhibitory effect was observed when effects on basal adenylate cyclase activity were tested. However, when cyclase was primed with PGE_1 or forskolin, a significant inhibition was noted, albeit at concentrations higher than required for chemotaxis or secretory responses. Calcium is thought to be central to the actions of chemoattractant receptors. Calcium uptake, efflux, exchange of membrane bound calcium and calcium mobilization have all been observed in response to receptor occupancy. Our efforts are directed at characterizing the role of Ni in these processes. Calcium mobilization was measured by changes in the fluorescence of Quin2 loaded cells. Complete abolition of FMLP and PAF-mediated Quin2 fluorescence change was observed after PT pretreatment (Lad, et al (1985b). Only partial inhibition of calcium uptake was observed when tested under conditions of complete abolition of calcium mobilization. Both Ni dependent and independent processes of calcium uptake are involved in response to FMLP or PAF. Calcium efflux and exchange of membrane bound calcium are currently being examined. An important result from these studies is that regulation of calcium levels inside the cells is achieved by multiple mechanisms only a component of which is under Ni control.

Does Ni regulation of two distinct processes imply a single mechanism? Our results (Lad, et al (1985b) indicate that chemotaxis occurs with substantial mobilization of calcium which is inhibited by PT. By contrast, very little mobilization of calcium is noted at lectin concentrations under which substantial capping is observed. Colchicine, an agent which enhances capping, causes no enhancement of calcium mobilization. Also capping is a slow process and no sustained calcium rise is observed during the duration of capping. These results point to two possibilities: either threshold effects of internal calcium are involved or a process other than calcium mobilization (exchange of membrane-bound calcium) may be important. Experiments to distinguish between these possibilities are now being carried out.

In conclusion, our results suggest that GTP-binding proteins play an important role in the regulation of inflammation. The anologies to the action of other hormones and neurotransmitters suggest similar mechanisms may be involved in receptor action in the central nervous system as well as in endocrine and immune systems.

REFERENCES

Koo C, Lefkowitz RJ and Snyderman R (1983). Guanine nucleotides modulate the binding affinity of the oligopeptide chemoattractant receptor on human polymorphonuclear leukocytes. J. Clin Invest. 72:748-753.

Lad PM, Welton AF and Rodbell M (1977). Evidence for distinct guanine nucleotide sites in the regulation of the glucagin receptor and adenylate cyclase. J. Biol Chem 252:5280-5284.

Lad PM, Yamamura H and Rodbell M (1977). GTP stimulates and inhibits adenylate cyclase in fat cell membranes through distinct regulatory processes. J. Biol Chem 252:7964-7967.

Lad PM, Olson CV and Smiley PA (1985a). Association of the N-formyl-met-leu-phe receptor in human neutrophils with a GTP-binding protein sensitive to pertussis toxin. Proc Nat Acad Sci 82:869-873.

Lad PM, Olson CV, Grewel IS and Scott SJ (1985b). A pertussis toxin sensitive GTP-binding protein regulates multiple receptors, calcium mobilization and lectin induced capping. Proc Nat Acad Sci (USA) in press.

Okajma F and Ui M (1984). ADP-ribosylation of the specific membrane protein by IAP is associated with inhibition of chemotactic/peptide induced arachidonate release in neutrophils. J. Biol Chem 259:13863-13871.

Verghese MW, Smith CD, Snyderman R (1985). Potential role for a guanine nucleotide regulatory protein in chemoattractant receptor-mediated polyphosphoinositide metabolism, calcium mobilization and cellular responses by leukocytes. Biochem Biophy Res Commun 127:450-457.

Volpi M, Naccache PH, Molski TFP, Shefcyr J, Huang CK, Marsh ML, Munoz J, Becker EL and Sha'afi RI (1985). Pertussis toxin inhibits FMLP but not PMA stimulated changes in rabbit neutrophils. Proc Nat Acad Sci 82:2708-2712.

CHEMOTACTIC PROPERTIES OF SYNTHETIC COLLAGEN-LIKE PEPTIDES

Debra L. Laskin and Richard A. Berg

Department of Pharmacology & Toxicology, Rutgers University (D.L.L.) and Department of Biochemistry (D.L.L., R.A.B.), UMDNJ-Rutgers Medical School, Piscataway, New Jersey 08854

INTRODUCTION

Damage to interstitial collagens is associated with the rapid migration of monocytes and PMNs to the site of tissue injury (Campbell and Senior, 1981). Phagocyte accumulation is mediated by chemotactic factors released by damaged tissues. It has been reported that human types I, II and III collagens and peptide fragments of digested collagen are chemotactic for fibroblasts and monocytes, but not PMNs (Postlethwaite et al., 1976;1978). Stecher (1975) found, that while purified bacterial collagenase was a potent chemoattractant for PMNs, degradation products of collagen were inactive. In fact, these products appeared to inhibit the chemotactic activity of collagenase. In contrast to these findings, Chang and Houck (1970) observed that both native soluble collagen and collagen degradation products are chemotactic for PMNs in vivo. In support of these latter observations, we report here that small molecular weight synthetic polypeptides consisting of triplet units of proline (P), hydroxyproline (H) and glycine (G), the predominant amino acids present in collagen, as well as bovine dermal collagen digested by bacterial collagenase or cyanogen-bromide are potent chemoattractants for PMNs. Chemotactic activity is concentration dependent and related to the size and structure of the synthetic collagen-like fragments. These results suggest that PMN accumulation in tissue following injury may be mediated, in part, by release of chemotactic peptides derived from connective tissue.

MATERIALS AND METHODS

The preparation of collagenase and cyanogen bromide digests of bovine collagen and the synthesis of collagen-like polypeptides have been described previously (Berg et al., 1977; Sage & Bornstein, 1962; Sakakibara et al., 1968; 1973). Human peripheral blood PMNs were prepared from normal healthy donors by sedimentation in dextran (6%) followed by centrifugation on a Ficoll-Hypaque gradient. Chemotaxis of PMNs through millipore filters was measured using the modified Boyden chamber technique (Boyden, 1962). For our studies, we used a 48 well microchemotaxis chamber (Neuro Probe, Inc.) as previously described (Laskin & Rovera, 1985).

RESULTS

Initially, we compared the chemotactic activity of collagenase (CG) and cyanogen bromide (CB) digests of bovine collagen with the chemoattractant, f-met-leu-phe (fMLP). Both digests of collagen were potent chemoattractants for PMNs (Table 1). In fact, the activity of the CG digest was comparable to that observed with fMLP in the same concentration range. Induction of chemotaxis by the collagenous peptides was dose-related reaching a maximum with 100 nM. Tryptic peptides of bovine serum albumin (BSA) displayed no chemotactic activity for PMNs thus demonstrating the specificity of the response for digested collagen.

We next examined the chemotactic activity of two synthetic collagen-like polypeptides containing the repeating triplet amino acid sequences, P, P and G in pentameric $(PPG)_5$ and decameric $(PPG)_{10}$ forms. Both of these peptides induced chemotaxis in a dose-related fashion (Table 2). $(PPG)_5$, the shorter synthetic peptide, was found to be approximately 1.5 times more active as a chemoattractant than the longer peptide, $(PPG)_{10}$ at each concentration tested.

Table 1. Comparison of the chemotactic activity of CG- and CB-digested collagen with fMLP and trypsin digested BSA.

Conc. (nM)	Chemotaxis (cells/10 oil fields ± SE)			
	BSA	CG	CB	fMLP
0	68.2± 5.1	73.4± 6.7	69.6± 2.4	77.4± 6.6
1	71.4± 7.8	396.3±14.2	311.2± 8.1	377.4± 9.1
10	75.6± 6.7	482.3±11.2	440.1±10.9	583.1±10.3
100	69.1± 4.9	523.1± 9.9	459.2±12.6	550.3±13.4

Table 2. Induction of chemotaxis by synthetic collagen-like peptides.

Conc. (nM)	Chemotaxis (cells/10 oil fields ± SE)	
	$(PPG)_5$	$(PPG)_{10}$
0	72.4± 3.2	69.6± 5.1
1	284.4± 8.8	173.4±11.5
10	399.1±13.4	270.8±12.8
100	373.6± 9.1	286.0±10.4

We also examined a series of synthetic peptides containing the amino acids P, H, and G in repeating triplet sequences of $(PHG)_1$, $(PHG)_5$ and $(PHG)_{10}$. $(PHG)_5$ was found to be the most potent of the H containing synthetic peptides tested producing a maximal stimulation at 1 nM (Table 3). Increasing the length of the PHG fragment from 5 to 10 subunits decreased its activity as a chemoattractant. The single subunit, $(PHG)_1$ was chemotactic for PMNs, but only in the concentration range of 10-100 nM.

Table 3. Induction of chemotaxis by H containing peptides.

Conc. (nM)	Chemotaxis (cells/10 oil fields ± SE)		
	$(PHG)_1$	$(PHG)_5$	$(PHG)_{10}$
0	80.1± 5.5	78.4± 4.2	82.3± 6.3
1	94.6± 6.9	325.6±11.8	111.4± 9.9
10	166.7±14.1	284.0±10.9	311.6±11.3
100	374.6±10.3	210.6±12.0	178.1± 9.8

Using a modified checkerboard assay, we also demonstrated that the response to the synthetic peptides involved directed cell movement (not shown).

To study structural requirements, we analyzed the chemotactic activity of a series of synthetic $(PHG)_1$ peptides modified at the N and C terminal ends. The single subunit peptide $(PHG)_1$ was found to be chemotactic for PMNs (Table 3). The addition of a methyl group to the carboxyl end of G on this peptide resulted in a 40-50% increase in the chemotactic activity of the molecule. Substitution of the alpha amino group of P in $(PHG)_1$ with a butyloxycarbonyl (Boc) or an acetyl group decreased the chemotactic activity of the molecule by 40-50% and 90-100%, respectively.

DISCUSSION

In this communication we report that digests of bovine collagen are potent chemoattractants for human PMNs. To determine the structural requirements for chemotactic activity, we began a systematic analysis of the properties of small molecular weight synthetic polypeptides containing P, H and G, the major amino acids present in collagen. In our initial studies synthetic peptides containing P and G, $(PPG)_n$, were compared to peptides containing P, H and G, $(PHG)_n$. We found that these peptides were equipotent in inducing chemotaxis. Postlethwaite et al. (1978) reported that H is an essential constituent of the amino acid sequence recognized by the chemotactic receptor on human fibroblasts. In contrast, our results demonstrate that H is not required for PMN chemotaxis. These differences in chemotactic responsiveness may be due to differences in the cell types examined.

Peptide length appeared to play a significant role in chemotactic potency. We found that peptides containing 5 triplet sequences of PPG or PHG were more active in inducing chemotaxis than the peptides containing 10 subunits or the single subunit, $(PHG)_1$. This suggests that a critical length of the peptide may be required for maximal chemotactic activity. However, it is also possible that the longer peptides interfere with chemotactic factor receptor binding through steric hinderance.

Using substituted derivatives of $(PHG)_1$, we were able to deduce several characteristics about the PMN membrane receptor for collagen peptides. The addition of a methyl group to the carboxyl end of G to form an ester enhanced the chemotactic activity of the peptide suggesting that a free carboxyl group is not essential for chemotactic activity although it is also possible that the effects were due to an increased stability of the molecule to enzymatic degradation. Substitutions on the amino end of the molecule decreased chemotactic potency indicating that a charged group at the amino end of the tripeptide may be required for chemotactic activity.

Breakdown of interstitial connective tissue is associated with the accumulation of PMNs and monocytes at the site of injury. It has been hypothesized that this accumulation is due in part, to the generation of chemotactic stimuli generated from collagen breakdown products (Chang & Houck, 1970). Our data are consistent with the idea that the collagen molecule contains a chemotactic signal for PMNs, and that chemotactic factors are released during the process of collagen degradation.

REFERENCES

Berg RA, Kishida Y, Sakabibara S and Prockop DJ (1977). Hydroxylation of (Pro-Pro-Gly)$_5$ and (Pro-Pro-Gly)$_{10}$ by prolyl hydroxylase. Evidence for an asymmetric active site in the enzyme. Biochem 16:1615-1621.

Boyden S (1962). The chemotactic effect of mixtures of antibody and antigen on polymorphonuclear leukocytes. J. Exp Med 115:453-466.

Campbell EJ and Senior RM (1981). Cell injury and repair. Clin Chest Med 2:357-375.

Chang C and Houck JC (1970). Demonstration of the chemotactic properties of collagen. Proc Soc Exp Biol Med 13:22-26.

Laskin DL and Rovera G (1985). Stimulation of human neutrophilic granulocyte chemotaxis by monoclonal antibodies. J Immunol 134:1146-1152.

Postlethwaite AE and Kang AH (1976). Collagen- and collagen peptide induced chemotaxis of human blood monocytes. J Exp Med 143:1299-1307.

Postlethwaite AE, Seyer JM and Kang AH (1978). Chemotactic attraction of human fibroblasts to type I, II, and III collagens and collagen-derived peptides. Proc Natl Acad Sci USA 75:871-875.

Sage H and Bornstein P (1982). Preparation and characterization of procollagens and procollagen-collagen intermediates. Meth Enzymol 82:96-127.

Sakakibara S, Inouye K, Shudo K, Kishido Y, Koboyashi Y and Prockop DJ (1973). Synthesis of (Pro-Hyp-Gly)$_n$ of defined molecular weights. Evidence for the stabilization of collagen triple helix by hydroxyproline. Biochim Biophys Acta 303:198-202.

Sakakibara S, Kishida Y, Kikuchi Y, Sakai R and Kakiuchi K (1968). Synthesis of poly-(l-prolyl-L-polyglycl) of defined molecular weights. Bull Chem Soc Japan 41:1273-278.

Stecher VJ (1975). The chemotaxis of selected cell types to connective tissue degradation products. Ann NY Acad Sci 256:178-189.

CONCOMITANT EXPRESSION OF CHEMILUMINESCENCE AND BACTERIAL KILLING BY BOVINE NEUTROPHILS

Charles J. Czuprynski and Holly L. Hamilton

Department of Pathobiological Sciences, University of Wisconsin School of Veterinary Medicine, Madison, WI 53706

INTRODUCTION

Mammalian phagocytes possess both oxidative and non-oxidative systems for the killing of ingested bacteria. Although the phagocyte antibacterial machinery is remarkably effective, some bacteria have developed strategies for evading the intracellular microbicidal mechanisms of neutrophils and macrophages. These facultative intracellular pathogens are the causative agents of a number of serious diseases of both humans and domestic animals. The bovine pathogen Haemophilus somnus has been associated with a wide range of disease syndromes including respiratory infection, abortion, arthritis, and thrombomeningo- encephalitis (Stephens et al, 1981). A hallmark of the lesions produced by this organism at all these tissue sites is a vasculitis that is associated with the attraction and accumulation of large numbers of polymorphonuclear leukocytes. Little information is available as to the fate of H. somnus when it encounters the neutrophils that are attracted to infective foci in vivo. In this study we determined the events that regulate the ingestion and subsequent intracellular fate of H. somnus in the presence of bovine neutrophils. Our results suggest that H. somnus can survive within bovine neutrophils and that its intracellular survival may be related to the relatively poor chemiluminescent response that it elicits from bovine neutrophils.

MATERIALS AND METHODS

Neutrophil preparation

Adult Holstein cattle from the Dept of Veterinary Science dairy herd were used as blood donors for this study. The animals were bled by venipuncture and the neutrophils were obtained as described previously (Czuprynski and Hamilton, 1985) The neutrophil suspensions contained 95% or more neutrophils that were greater than 98% viable.

Bacteria

Haemophilus somnus and H. somnus WAHL (field isolate) were obtained from the Wisconsin State Animal Health Laboratory in Madison, Wisconsin. Haemophilus somnus strain 8025 was obtained from Dr. Ronald Schultz of the Dept of Pathobiological Sciences. Escherichia coli and Staphylococcus epidermidis were obtained from Dr. Josie Yang of the Dept. of Pathobiological Sciences.

Phagocytosis and Bacterial Killing

Phagocytosis was assessed as describing previously in detail (Czuprynski and Hamilton, 1985) by incubating 25×10^6 H. somnus and 2.5×10^6 bovine neutrophils with 10% H. somnus antiserum (titer 1:2056) for 30 min at 37° C. After extracellular bacteria were removed by washing, cytospin smears were prepared, air dried, fixed and stained with Diff-Quick. Results are expressed as the phagocytic index, as described previously. Bacterial killing was assessed by incubating 2.5×10^6 H. somnus with 2.5×10^6 neutrophils and 10% immune serum at 37° for 2 hours, followed by removal of samples for dilution and plating on chocolate agar to determine the number of viable bacteria. The results were expressed as the $\log_{10}$ reduction in bacteria as compared to the inoculum.

RESULTS

Serum Dependence of Ingestion of H. somnus by Bovine Neutrophils

In the presence of antibodies against H. somnus, bovine neutrophils ingested H. somnus in a time dependent manner. Optimal phagocytosis of H. somnus required at least 10% immune serum to be present. Uptake appeared to be mediated primarily via the Fc receptor because removal of antibody from the immune serum by absorption with formalin-killed H. somnus (titer reduced from 1:2056 to 1:20) significantly reduced phagocytosis, whereas heat-inactivation of serum complement had little effect on ingestion (Table 1). Electron microscopy confirmed the predominately intracellular location of H. somnus in our assay system.

TABLE 1. Phagocytosis of H. somnus by bovine neutrophils appears to be primarily antibody rather than complement dependent.

Serum Conditions (10%)	Mean ± SEM Phagocytic Index
Untreated immune	211 ± 14
Absorbed immune	95 ± 4
Heat-inactivated immune	197 ± 21
No serum	25 ± 6

Intracellular fate of Haemophilus somnus

When H. somnus was incubated with bovine neutrophils for 1-4 hours we consistently observed an increase in the number of viable bacteria that was similar to that in cell-free control tubes (Czuprynski and Hamilton, 1985). Similar results were obtained when bovine neutrophils were challenged with three different strains of H. somnus, including a recent field isolate obtained from the

Wisconsin Animal Health Laboratory. We can exclude the possibility that the neutrophils used in these experiments were defective in bactericidal activity, because neutrophils tested in the same experiments were readily able to kill both Escherichia coli and Staphylococcus epidermidis (Table 2).

TABLE 2. Bovine neutrophils failed to kill 3 strains of H. somnus under conditions where they killed E. coli and S. epidermidis.

Bacteria	Expts	Mean ± SEM Log_{10} Killing
H. somnus	6	-0.73 ±0.06
H. somnus 8025	4	-0.89 ±0.10
H. somnus WAHL	2	-0.86 ±0.06
E. coli	5	+1.33 ±0.15
S. epidermidis	3	+1.38 ±0.07

We next considered possible mechanisms to explain the inability of bovine neutrophils to kill H. somnus. It has been reported previously that some microbes are able to resist killing by phagocytic cells because of their ability to avoid inducing an oxidative response by the phagocyte during the process of ingestion. We chose to assess the oxidative response of bovine neutrophils to H. somnus by using luminol-dependent chemiluminescence. Our results indicated that the oxidative response of bovine neutrophils to opsonized H. somnus was reduced both in duration and maximal intensity as compared to the chemiluminescent response to opsonized E. coli. (Table 3).

TABLE 3. The maximal chemiluminescence response of bovine neutrophils to opsonized H. somnus is reduced as compared to their response to opsonized E. coli.

Stimulus	Mean ± SEM Maximal $cpm \times 10^3$
E. coli (100:1)	457 ± 12
E. coli (25:1)	290 ± 8
H. somnus (100:1)	208 ± 28
H. somnus (25:1)	88 ± 13
Unstimulated control	8 ± 2

DISCUSSION

Pathogenic microorganisms have devised various tactics for avoiding destruction with phagocytic cells. The results of this study suggest that because H. somnus does not elicit the sustained production of reactive oxygen intermediates by bovine neutrophils, it is able to survive within these cells. Other pathogens are reported to follow a similar strategy. The intracellular survival of Candida species within mouse macrophages was inversely correlated with the oxidative response that was elicited by the yeasts (Sassada and Johnston, 1980). Unopsonized Toxoplasma gondii elicits a poor oxidative response when ingested by human monocytes and it is able to survive intercellularly; however, when the organism is opsonized a more vigorous oxidative response occurs and T. gondii is killed. (Wilson et al, 1980). It has been suggested that relative differences in chemiluminescent response was associated with intracellular survival of Salmonella typhimurium (Miller et al, 1972) however others have presented evidence that the chemiluminescent response and intracellular survival were not necessarily correlated (Kossack et al, 1981). Although the present study demonstrates a clear association between chemiluminescent response and the survival of H. somnus within bovine neutrophils, at this time we cannot exclude the possibility that other mechanisms also contribute to the intracellular survival of H. somnus.

The results of this study shed new light on the host pathogen interactions that occur during H. somnus infections. When this organism broaches an epithelial barrier, the responding neutrophils will ingest but not kill the bacteria. During the initial battle it is likely that lysosomal enzymes and oxygen products of the neutrophil will be released and cause local tissue damage that may attract additional inflammatory cells, thus causing the characteristic vasculitis of H. somnus infections. Previous reports have suggested that at least some strains of H. somnus are susceptible to serum killing by antibody and complement (Simonson and Maheswaran, 1982). Our results suggest that perhaps ingestion of H.

somnus by bovine neutrophils shields it from the bactericidal effects of bovine serum and thus provides it a favorable niche from which to prolong and perhaps disseminate the infection.

In closing, we feel that the H. somnus-bovine neutrophil system may prove to be valuable for assessing the regulation of neutrophil antibacterial activity. In future experiments we plan to pretreat bovine neutrophils with various immunomodulators in hopes of identifying a defined stimulus that will enable bovine neutrophils to kill H. somnus.

REFERENCES

Czuprynski CJ, Hamilton HL (1985). Bovine neutrophils ingest but do not kill Haemophilus somnus. Infect Immun: November.

Kossack RE, Guerrait RL, Densen P, Schadelin J, Mandell GL (1981). Diminished neutrophil oxidative metabolism after phagocytosis of virulent Salmonella typhi. Infect Immun 31:674-678.

Miller RM, Carbus J, Hornick RB (1972). Lack of enhanced oxygen consumption by polymorphonuclear leukocytes on phagocytosis of virulent Salmonella typhi. Science 175:1010-1011.

Sassada M, Johnston RB (1980). Macrophage microbicidal activity. Correlation between phagocytosis-associated oxidative metabolism and the killing of Candida by macrophages. J. Exper Med 152:85-98.

Simonson RR, Maheswaran SK (1982). Host humoral factors in natural resistance to Haemophilus somnus. Amer J Vet Res 43:1160-1164.

Stephens LR, Little PB, Wilkie BN, Barnum DA (1981). Infectious thromboembolic meningoencephalitis in cattle: a review. J. Amer Vet Med Assoc 178:378-384.

Wilson CB, Tsai V, Remington JS (1980). Failure to trigger the oxidative metabolic burst by normal macrophages. Possible mechanism for survival of intracellular pathogens. J Exper Med 151:328-346.

Section VIII. Regulation and Functions of Cells With Natural Killer Activity

"Stimulation of Natural Killer and Activated Killer Cell
Cytotoxicity by Interferons and Interleukins"

J.R. Ortaldo, A. Mason, J. Langer* and R. Overton[†]

BTB, BRMP, DCT, NCI Frederick, MD, *Roche
Institute of Molecular Biology, Nutley, NJ and
[†]Program Resources Inc., NCI-FCRF, Frederick, MD

INTRODUCTION

A number of previous reports have indicated that recombinant and hybrid interferon (IFN) as well as natural IFN vary considerably in their efficacy to mediate biological activities (Ortaldo, JR, et al., 1983; Ortaldo, JR, et al., 1984; Rehberg, E, et al., 1982; Pestka, S, 1983) In addition, recent reports (Herberman, RB and Ortaldo, JR, 1983; Pestka, S., 1983) have also demonstrated that natural killer (NK) activity can be significantly augmented by natural and recombinant IFNα species and that the efficacy of the various IFNα's vary considerably. IFNαJ was found to be defective in the augmentation of NK activity after a short 2-hour pretreatment of highly purified large granular lymphocytes (LGL) effectors even at high concentrations (10,000 units/ ml). This same exposure generally resulted in maximum augmentation with other IFNα species (Herberman, RB and Ortaldo, JR, 1983). However, the lack of ability of IFNαJ to boost NK activity was not absolute, since after 18 hour exposure of effector cells to high concentrations of the IFNαJ boosting of NK activity did occur. In the present study regarding IFNs, we investigated the binding, activation of metabolic activities, as well as newly synthesized IFN proteins within NK cells in an attempt to study what mechanistic deficiency results in the delayed boosting by IFNαJ.

Interleukin 2 (IL-2) has also been reported to play a major role in many types of immune responses. This lymphokine induces proliferation of both thymus derived T lymphocytes and NK cells, the production of IFN-γ and the induction of activated killers (AK) against previously NK resistant cell preparations and cell lines (Herberman, RB and Ortaldo, JR 1983; Itoh, K, et al., 1985; Grimm, EA, et al., 1982; Grimm, EA, et al., 1983a; Grimm, EA, et al., 1983b). AK cells induced by IL-2 possibly represent a potentially unique and potent cytotoxic cells that may have an important role in immunotherapy of solid tumors. Previous reports (Grimm, EA, et al., 1983a) have indicated no specific lymphocyte markers or antibody reactivities with AK cell precursors.

Our present studies have attempted to analyze both the surface phenotype of the AK precursors by separating progenitors based on density gradient centrifugations into LGL and T lymphocytes and then by further depleting leukocyte subpopulations by the use of antibody and immunoabsorbent techniques. Secondly, effector cells were generated into activated killers as previously described (Grimm, EA, et al., 1982) from unseparated peripheral blood mononuclear cells and the effector cells, at the termination of culture, were separated into various lymphoid subsets using monoclonal antibodies.

RESULTS

Section 1. Interferon Activation

Because direct binding data using radiolabeled competition of IFNαA and IFNαJ for ^{125}I-labeled IFNα binding indicated that the lack of NK boosting was not due to a binding deficiency, (Langer, G., 1985, sub. for pub.) we investigated whether the 2'-5'A synthethase (an enzyme activated by IFN) was differentially activated in LGL by different IFN species. The kinetics of activation of 2'-5'A synthethase was considerably delayed in the IFNαJ treated LGL as compared to the levels of activity which were achieved with IFNαA. In parallel with the delayed activation of cytolytic activity, the 2'-5' synthethase activity was activated to IFNαA levels only after 18 hours of exposure with IFNαJ (data not shown). These results support the contention that one of the deficiencies in the ability of IFNαJ to activate NK cells resides in its inability to activate intracellular IFN-related events, such as the induction of 2'-5' synthethase activity.

It is our hypothesis that amino acid related structural differences are responsible for the variability seen between the various IFN molecules and directly tested this proposition by genetically constructing new IFNαJ molecules with substitutions at various amino acid positions. The details of these constructions have been published elsewhere (Pestka et al., in prep.; Rehberg, E., et al., 1982). Table 1 is a summary of the results on the ability of these IFN molecules to augment NK activity. The recombinant αA and αC demonstrated potent boosting of NK cytolytic activity. In addition, five other genetically constructed molecules of IFNαJ and/or IFNαC were compared. When IFNαJ had the 116 amino acid position changed to serine, large amounts of IFN were still required for significant boosting of NK activity. However, the J/C hybrid (with substitutions at both the 116 and 132 amino acid positions) demonstrated potent boosting of NK activity with a mean of only 7.3 IFN units. These studies directly demonstrate the importance of these amino acid substitutions to IFN activity and presumably their 3-dimensional structure.

TABLE 1. Effects of Site-specific Changes of IFNαJ on its Ability to Augment NK Activity

IFN	Amino Acids at:						Antiviral Units[*] Mean
	10	35	40	46	116	132	
A	Gly	Asp	Gln	Asn	Ser	Lys	0.8
C	Gly	Asp	Gln	Asn	Ser	Ile	1.8
J	Arg	Glu	Glu	His	Phe	Met	>30,833
J-116 (ser)	Arg	Glu	Glu	His	Ser	Met	2,170
C/J	Gly	Asp	Gln	Asp	Phe	Met	6,600
C/J-116 (ser)	Gly	Asp	Gln	Asn	Ser	Met	10,400
J/C	Arg	Glu	Gln	His	Ser	Ile	7.3

[*]Antiviral units needed to result in significant lysis with 1 hour pretreatment.

Collectively studies performed with IFNαJ indicate that this species of IFN is capable of binding to the IFN receptor on the surface of NK cells but lacks the ability to trigger postbinding events. These results are consistent with the hypothesis that the lack of post-binding activation signals is the reason that IFNαJ is incapable of causing rapid and high levels of NK activity. The results are consistant with an overall importance of the three-dimensional structure of the IFNα molecule in its interaction with the receptor, and also that binding alone is not sufficient for activation of cells. Such a three-dimensional configuration change in the molecule bound to the receptor could result in a delay in subsequent activation events such as 2'-5' oligoadenylate synthethase.

Section 2 - IL-2 Activation

In an attempt to examine progenitor and effector phenotype for IL-2 activated killer (AK) cells, leukocyte subpopulations were fractionated and then tested for their ability to generate activity after 3 to 5 days incubation with recombinant IL-2. In this first approach, populations of large granular lymphocytes (LGL) as well as T cells were prepared from mononuclear peripheral blood leukocytes. LGL were further subdivided into Leu 11 (Fcγ R) + or − populations and T cells were divided into T8 positive or negative populations. Table 2 demonstrates typical results using K562 (a human NK sensitive target cell), MBL2 (mouse NK resistant target cell) as well as fresh ovarian carcinoma cells (OV CA) (isolated from peritoneal cavity of patient with ovarian malignancy). The results from this type of progenitor experiment, demonstrated that the majority of the cytotoxic activity on a per cell basis can be generated from the LGL population. In addition, cytotoxic cells generated from the Fcγ receptor positive and negative LGL mediated significant cytotoxic effect after 3 to 5 days in culture against all 3 target cells. However, AK cells generated from unseparated peripheral blood mononuclear cells or purified T cells mediated significant cytotoxic activity, but, required substantially more effector cells to mediate similar levels of lysis. If, however, one analyzes the ability of the various subsets to mediate cytotoxicity based on the amount of total activity, different conclusions are drawn. The contribution of T cells in the generation of total lytic units population vary somewhat (depending on target cell employed) but generally they contribute between 15 and 50 percent of the total cytotoxic activity.

When experiments were performed to analyze the effector cell mediating the cytotoxic activity generated from

TABLE 2. Ability of Various Lymphoid Subsets to Mediate IL-2 Activation Against Various Tumor Targets

Cell Type	Day 0 Leu 4 % Pos	Day 0 Leu 2 % Pos	Day 0 Leu 11 % Pos	K562 LU*	K562 TLU†	MBL2 LU	MBL2 TLU	OV CA LU	OV CA TLU
PBL	89	39	10	66	66	7	7	0.5	0.5
LGL E⁻	<1	35	78	568	39	78	6	24	2
FcγR⁺LGL	<2	5	90	494	14	56	3	13	1
FcγR⁻LGL	10	65	<2	210	8	41	1	8	0.5
T cells	>95	44	<2	81	59	5	3	2	1.5
T8⁺T	>95	89	<2	<0.1	<0.1	<0.1	<0.1	<0.1	<0.1

*Lytic unit (LU) defined at 30% lysis.
†Total lytic units (TLU) based on input number of nonadherent lymhocytes.

unseparated lymphoid of cells, results similar to progenitor studies were obtained. Table 3 demonstrates results where 4 day IL-2 cultured mononuclear cells were divided into T3⁺ and T3⁻ cells or T8⁺ and T8⁻ cells. Analysis of the various cell specific markers, as well as the cytotoxic activity

TABLE 3. LAK Effector Separation*

Effector Cell Phenotype	Markers T3	Markers T8	Markers NKH1	MBL2 LU/10↑7	MBL2 TLU	OV-CA LU/10↑7	OV-CA TLU
Unsep. Lym.	95	34	7	5.8	3.8	5.9	3.8
T3 + Lym.	98	36	8	1.7	1.3	12	35
T3 − Lym.	14	11	97	108	76	60	43
T8 + Lym.	97	87	85	1	<1	<1	<1
T8 − Lym.	96	12	24	56	45	28	22

*Performed on day 4 after IL-2 activation.

against the NK susceptible K562 (not shown) and the NK insusceptible MBL2 and ovarian carcinoma cell, indicate that highest levels of cytotoxicty were seen in the $T3^-$ lymphocytes against all three targets. Furthermore, a high percentage of these T3 cells bear the NKH1 marker but only 14 percent being $T3^+$. In contrast, $T3^+$ lymphocytes demonstrated low level of cytotoxic activity. In addition, $T8^+$ lymphocytes contribute little if any cytotoxic activity against the mouse MBL-1 and ovarian carcinoma tumor cells. However, if one calculates the total contribution (TLU) of those $T3^+$ lymphocytes against fresh tumor cells (OV-CA) a significant contribution to cytotoxic activity can be seen from $T3^+$ lymphocytes.

A summary of the characteristics regarding LAK cells and NK cells are summarized in Table 4. By definition the killing by LAK cells does not occur without stimulation; however, NK cells purified using Percoll gradients have been reported to lyse fresh tumor cells (Herberman, RB and Ortaldo, JR, 1983). The target cell specificity of LAK cells and activated NK cells is very similar, both being able to kill fresh tumor cell lines, TNP modified cells and virus-infected cells. Although unseparated peripheral blood lymphocytes are very active against cultured tumor cells, virus infected cell lines, or normal thymus and bone marrow cells, the killing of fresh tumor cells is generally not seen unless NK cells are enriched by separation on Percoll density gradients.

LAK cells are stimulated mainly by IL-2 while NK cells are regulated by IL-1, IFN, as well as IL-2. The effector phenotype of NK cells have been extensively studied by a number of investigators with the major NK effector cells being negative for T3 and T8 but positive for OKT11, OKM1, Leu 11, and NKH1. The progenitors for NK cells have been studied from the bone marrow and peripheral blood (Yoda, Y, et al., 1985) and have been identified mainly in the $T3^-$, $T8^-$, $T11^-$, $M1^-$, Leu 11^- and $NKH1^-$ populations. Regarding the progenitor phenotype for LAK cells, our data is quite consistent with the earlier report of Grimm, EA, et al., 1983a. The effector phenotype of LAK cells generated from unseparated peripheral blood lymphocytes was originally reported to be $T3^+$ and $T11^+$. Our present studies have indicated that more than 1 effector cell population is involved in the activity which is denoted as LAK. Clearly a $T3^+$, T8 cell contributes a significant amount of cytotoxicity in addition to a LGL population which is $T3^-$, $T8^-$ and bears the Leu 11, NKH1 marker.

TABLE 4. Comparison of LAK and NK Activity

	LAK	NK
Unstimulated killing of:	No targets (by definition)	Tumor (fresh & cultured), virus infected lines, normal thymus cells, bone marrow cells
Stimulated by:	IL-2, lectin	IL-1, IL-2, IFN (α, β, γ)
Stimulated cells kill:	Fresh tumor (auto & allo) tumor cell lines, TNP-modified cells, virus-infected cells	Fresh tumor (auto & allo), tumor cell lines, TNP-modified cells, virus-infected cells, thymus & bone marrow cells
Effector phenotype:	T3 +/- T8 - T11 + OKM1 - Leu 11 +/- NKH1 +	T3 - T8 - T11 +/- OKM1 + Leu 11 + NKH1 +
PBL progenitor phenotype:	T3 +/- T8 - T11 - Leu11 +/- OKM1 -	T3 - T8 - T11 - Leu 11 - OKM1 -

The major LAK progenitor is very similar to the described NK progenitor. In data not shown, the kinetics of cytotoxicity generation, for these populations differ considerably. $T3^+$ cells require 3 to 5 days to generate maximal activity whereas LGL populations are activated and demonstrate high levels of killing against fresh tumor cells within 18 hours of IL-2 treatment.

As a result of these studies, we would conclude that the AK or LAK cell is generated from several different lymphocyte precursors and the cytotoxic effector cell consists of several different cell types which contribute to the overall cytotoxicity. Therefore, AK or LAK cells may not represent a unique cell population but a conglomeration of a variety of activated lymphoid killer cells.

REFERENCES

Grimm EA, Mazumder A, Zhang HZ, Rosenberg SA (1982). Lymphokine-activated killer cell phenomenon. Lysis of natural killer-resistant fresh solid tumor cells by interleukin 2 activated autologous human peripheral blood lymphocytes. J Exp Med 155:1823.

Grimm EA, Ramsey KM, Mazumder A, Wilson DJ, Djeu JY, Rosenberg SA (1983a). Lymphokine-activated killer cell phenomenon. II. Precursor phenotype is serologically distinct from peripheral T lymphocytes, memory cytotoxic thymus-derived lymphocytes, and natural killer cells. J Exp Med 157:884.

Grimm EA, Robb RJ, Roth JA, Neckers LA, Lachman LB, Wilson DJ, Rosenberg SA (1983b). Lymphokine-activated killer cell phenomenon. III. Evidence that IL-2 is sufficient for direct activation of peripheral blood lymphocytes into lymphokine-activated killer cells. J Exp Med 158:1356.

Herberman, RB, Ortaldo, JR (1981). Natural killer cells: Their role in defenses against disease. Science 214:24.

Itoh K, Tilden AB, Kumagai K, Balch CM (1985). $Leu-11^+$ lymphocytes with natural killer (NK) activity are precursors of recombinant interleukin 2 (rIL 2)-induced activated killer (AK) cells. J Immunol 134: 802-807.

Ortaldo JR, Herberman RB, Harvey C, Osheroff P, Pan YCE, Kelder B, Pestka S (1984). A species of human alpha-interferon that lacks the ability to boost human natural-killer activity. Proc Natl Acad Sci USA 31:4929.

Ortaldo JR, Mason A, Rehberg E, Moschena J, Kelder B, Pestka S, Herberman RB (1983). Effects of recombinant and hybrid recombinant human leukocyte interferons on cytotoxic activity of natural killer cells. J Biol Chem 258:15011.

Pestka S (1983). The human interferons--from protein-purification and sequence in cloning and expression in bacteria--before, between, and beyond. Arch Biochem Biophys 221:1.

Rehberg E, Kelder B, Hoal EG, Pestka S (1982). Specific molecular activities of recombinant and hybrid leukocyte interferons. J Biol Chem 257:11497.

Yoda, Y, Mathieson, BJ, Ortaldo, JR (1985 in press). Differentiation and function of natural killer (NK) cells. Acta Haematol Jap 47.

REGULATION OF VIRAL INFECTIONS BY LARGE GRANULAR LYMPHOCYTES

Raymond M. Welsh, Christine A. Biron, Jack F. Bukowski, Kim W. McIntyre, Robert J. Natuk and Hyekyung Yang
Department of Pathology, University of Massachusetts Medical School, Worcester, MA 01605

Large granular lymphocytes (LGL) are, as the name implies, lymphocytes with abundant cytoplasm containing varying numbers of azurophilic granules emanating from the Golgi (Timonen et al., 1979; Kumagai et al., 1982). These granules are thought to contain cytotoxic elements which enable LGL to lyse target cells to which they are bound and "triggered" (Millard et al., 1984; Podack and Konigsberg, 1984). Until recently, LGL were thought to be synonymous with natural killer (NK) cells, lymphocytes which mature independently of the thymus and which lyse a variety of target cells non-specifically (Welsh, 1984). However, cultured cytotoxic T lymphocyte (CTL) lines often display LGL morphology, leading to speculations that CTL may have a morphology and mechanism of cytotoxicity similar to NK cells (Podack and Konigsberg, 1984). These results with the CTL lines have nevertheless been difficult to interpret, as T cell lines can be converted to an NK cell phenotype (in regards to cytotoxic and antigenic properties) simply by exposure to high concentrations of interleukin-2-containing medium (Brooks et al., 1983). Hence, the granules in T cell lines could have been an artifact of abnormal differentiation in cell culture.

This controversy has recently been resolved by Biron, et al. (submitted), who examined T cell LGL in mice infected with lymphocytic choriomeningitis virus (LCMV), a potent inducer of CTL. The Lyt-2 antigen is a marker antigen for mouse cytotoxic/suppressor T cells and can be used to distinguish CTL from NK cells. Less than 6% of the spleen leukocytes from either control or day 7 LCMV-infected C3H/St mice were of the LGL phenotype. In uninfected mice about 95% of the LGL were in Lyt-2$^-$ populations, but in the day 7 infected mice, at the peak of the CTL response, 66% of the total LGL were $Lyt-2^+$. Only 2% of the $Lyt-2^+$ cells from control mice were LGL, whereas 21% of the $Lyt-2^+$ cells from infected mice were LGL. Up to 64% of the day 7 responding, activated, blast-size, $Lyt-2^+$ cells enriched by size separation techniques were LGL. Flow cytometry and cell sorting analyses indicated in all cases that the NK cell activity was exclusively located in the $Lyt-2^-$ population, whereas the virus-specific, H-2 restricted CTL activity was exclusively located in the $Lyt-2^+$ population. It would thus appear that T cells in a resting state do not normally have an LGL phenotype, but after activation during a virus infection they become LGL, morphologically indistinguishable but antigenically and functionally distinct from NK cells. It may well be that all cytotoxic lymphocytes have LGL morphology and kill by common mechanisms.

<u>LGL Response to Virus Infection</u>: Infection of mice intraperitoneally with LCMV results in the stimulation of several types of cytotoxic cell responses (Figure 1) (Welsh, 1978). Early in infection the virus-induced interferon activates (Welsh, 1978) and induces the blastogenesis (Biron and Welsh, 1982; Biron et al., 1984) and proliferation of NK cells (Biron et al., 1983). These cells are defined as asialo GM_1^+, NK alloantigen$^+$, $Thy^{+/-}$, $Lyt-5^+$, and $Lyt-2^-$. Both the endogenous and virus-activated NK cells and LGL have the same antigen phenotype, though subtle changes in their susceptibility to complement plus antibodies to these antigens have been noted (Yang et al., 1985). The target cell range of the activated NK cells is greatly expanded, chiefly because of an apparent amplification of the lytic process rather than a major change in target cell recognition (Targan and Dorey, 1980).

At 7-9 days postinfection there is a peak in class I H-2 antigen-restricted, virus-specific CTL activity. These CTL copurify with LGL and have the phenotype Thy^+, asialo $GM_1^{+/-}$ and $Lyt-2^+$. In C57BL/6 mice, coincidental with the virus-specific CTL response, is the appearance of alloreactive Thy^+, asialo $GM_1^{+/-}$, $Lyt-2^+$ CTL (Yang and Welsh, submitted). These alloreactive CTL can be distinguished from NK cells by injection of mice with antibodies to asialo GM_1, which eliminates NK but not CTL activity. The alloreactive CTL in the NK cell-depleted mice are distinct from the virus-specific CTL, and are likely products of polyclonal expansions, because high activity can be found in blast-size cell fractions. In contrast to activated NK cells, these alloreactive CTL do not lyse syngeneic or xenogeneic targets. These cells could easily be confused with activated NK cells or lymphokine activated killer cells if activated NK cells were not first depleted from the leukocyte preparations. C3H mice appear to make a much lower level of alloreactive CTL than do C57BL/6 mice (Yang and Welsh, submitted).

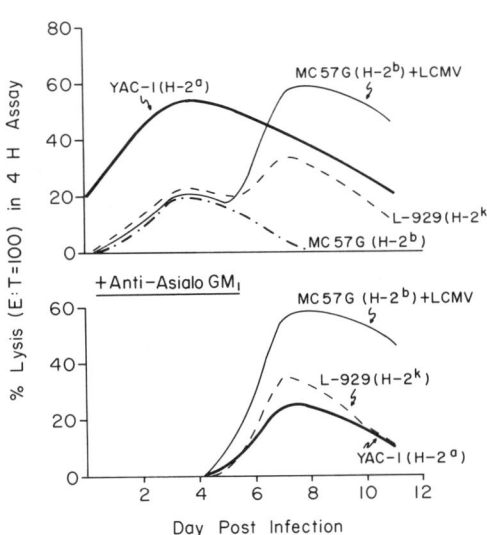

Figure 1. Cytotoxic cell response to LCMV in C57BL/6 ($H-2^b$) mice. Mice were infected intraperitoneally with 8×10^4 plaque forming units (PFU) of LCMV. Results are 4H cytotoxicity assays at effector to target ratios of 100:1. In the bottom panel, mice were injected with antibody to asialo GM_1 to eliminate NK cell activity.

Accumulation of LGL at Sites of Virus Infection.

Mice infected intraperitoneally with either of several different viruses were examined for infiltration of LGL into the peritoneum. Figure 2 shows that all virus infections tested (LCMV, mouse hepatitis virus (MHV), murine cytomegalovirus (MCMV), Pichinde virus, vaccinia virus) stimulate significant increases in peritoneal NK cell activity and LGL number. The increase in LGL number was sometimes greater than 100 fold, compared to controls. During the first 3 days of infection, virtually all NK cell activity and LGL could be eliminated by injection of mice with antibody to asialo GM_1 (data not shown).

At 7 days post LCMV infection there was a major influx of leukocytes into the peritoneum (Figure 2). This increase in cell number has been shown previously to be thymus-dependent, as this does not occur in athymic nude mice (Welsh and Doe, 1980). Correlating with this influx were high levels of virus-specific CTL activity, a decline in NK cell activity, and an increase in LGL number. Treatment with antibody to asialo GM_1 removed none of the CTL activity and less than half the LGL number, while significantly reducing the NK cell activity (data not shown). It thus would appear that NK-LGL accumulate in the peritoneum early in infection, whereas T-LGL accumulate later in the infection.

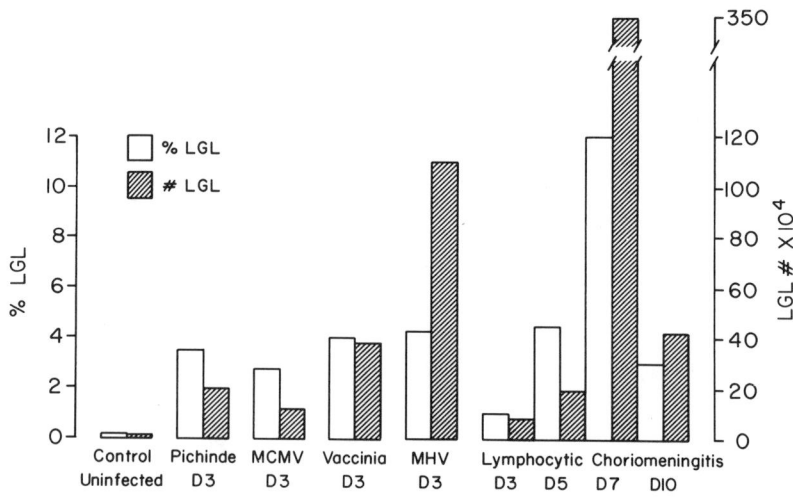

Figure 2. Accumulation of LGL in peritoneum during viral infection of mice. Peritoneal leukocytes were examined at various days postinfection for % LGL and total number (#) of LGL after infection with 1×10^5 pfu Pichinde virus, 5×10^4 pfu MCMV, 1×10^6 pfu vaccinia virus, 2×10^5 pfu MHV, or 8×10^5 pfu LCMV.

Similar results were observed in leukocytes isolated from livers (Table 1). Virus infections stimulated increases in liver LGL number and NK cell activity early in the infection. However, MHV, which causes high levels of cytopathic effect in the liver, induced a much higher accumulation than did a hepatotropic LCMV strain (WE), which is relatively non-cytopathic. Antibody to asialo GM_1 eliminated both the LGL and the NK cell activity (Table 1).

Liver leukocytes were examined at the peak of the T cell response after infection with a hepatotropic (WE) and non-hepatotropic (Armstrong) strain of LCMV (Table 2). The hepatotropic WE strain stimulated a higher leukocyte infiltrate into the liver and a higher accumulation of LGL, compared to the Armstrong strain. Whereas mice infected with the Armstrong strain had much higher levels of CTL activity in the spleen, mice infected with the WE strain had higher levels of CTL activity in the liver. It is thus again likely that the accumulation of LGL in diseased tissue late in infection is due in great part to T-LGL.

Table 1
Accumulation of NK-LGL in the Liver 3 days Postinfection

Mice	% Lysis on YAC-1*	% LGL	Total LGLx10^5
Uninfected	9.1	6	3.6
MHV	25.	10	10.
MHV + anti asialo GM_1**	2.2	2	1.5
Uninfected	13.	6	1.7
LCMV-WE	22.	14.	3.5

*-A 4 hr cytotoxicity assay with effector to target of 10:1.
**-Mice were injected with antibody to asialo GM_1 at the time of infection with virus.

Table 2
Liver LGL and CTL 7 Days Postinfection

Mice	% LGL in Liver	No. LGL X 10^5 in Liver	CTL Lytic units x 10^4*	
			Liver	Spleen
Control	4	3.8	-	-
LCMV-Armstrong	18	30.	55	240
LCMV-WE	12	71.	110	11

*-A 5 hr cytotoxicity assay on LCMV-infected MC57G cells.
Lytic units were calculated by the formula:

$$\frac{\text{Proportion of cells lysed X cell \# per organ}}{\text{Effector to target ratio}}$$

Role of LGL in Regulating Virus Infection.

T-LGL: The presence of granules implies a cytotoxic function, leading one to question whether CTL-LGL mediate resistance to virus infections. The evidence is concrete that T cells mediate resistance to LCMV and other virus infections (Volkert and Lundstedt, 1971; Zinkernagel and Welsh, 1976), but whether CTL (and thus LGL) are necessary is less clear and deserves discussion. Consistent with the concept that CTL-LGL regulate the LCMV infection are the following pieces of evidence. 1. Splenocytes taken from mice 7 days postinfection transfer adoptive immunity to recently infected recipients which bear H-2K or H-2D antigens similar to the donor cells (Zinkernagel and Welsh, 1976). These recognition molecules are required for CTL but not helper T cell activity (Zinkernagel and Doherty, 1975). 2. LCMV-specific $Lyt-2^+$ cloned CTL lines adoptively transfer immunity to recipients (Byrne and Oldstone, 1984). 3. Adoptive immunizations are exquisitely specific, as in mice dually infected with two viruses (LCMV and Pichinde virus), only the virus reactive with the specific transferred spleen cells is eliminated (McIntyre et al., 1985). This argues against nonspecific factors such as interferon-gamma being liberated by T cells as the cause of the antiviral effects. 4. As we have shown here, LGL which may be CTL accumulate in virus-infected organs just prior to elimination of the infection (Fig. 2; Table 2).

NK-LGL: A large amount of evidence indicates that NK-LGL do not provide a major role in regulating the LCMV infection. For example, mice depleted of NK activity by cyclophosphamide, antibody to asialo GM_1, or the beige mutation synthesize normal levels of LCMV (Welsh et al., 1984). In contrast, all these factors greatly elevate MCMV synthesis (Mayo et al., 1977; Bukowski et al, 1984; Shellam et al, 1981). To prove that NK cells regulate MCMV infection, Bukowski et al. (1985) transferred adult mouse splenocytes, which contain NK cell activity, into 5 day-old suckling mice, which lack NK cell activity. The transferred cells protected the recipient mice from MCMV infection. Upon fractionation, the phenotype of the leukocyte mediating protection was found to be a NK alloantigen$^+$, Thy$^-$, Ia$^-$, asialo GM_1^+, Lyt-5$^+$, nylon wool-nonadherent, low density lymphocyte. This is consistent with the phenotype of NK cells. Further, a cloned NK cell line having LGL morphology protected baby mice from MCMV (but not from LCMV) (Bukowski et al., 1985). After several months passage the NK cell clone lost its ability to lyse target cells in vitro and simultaneously lost its ability to protect baby mice against MCMV in vivo (data not shown).

Conclusions and Summary

Virus infections thus stimulate the activation and proliferation of two classes of LGL: NK cells and CTL. NK cells are stimulated early in infection and accumulate at the sites of virus infection in various tissues of the body. Later in the infection there is a decline in NK cell activity coincidental with what appears to be an infiltration of T cell LGL into the same tissues. Both NK-LGL and T-LGL may be very important in regulating virus infections, with the relative role of these two systems dependent on the particular virus infection involved.

Acknowledgements. This research was supported by USPHS grants AI-17672, CA-34461, AM-35506, AI-30727, and a Leukemia Society of America Special Fellow Award to C.B. We thank Ms. Kirsten Pedersen and Kathleen Denehy for technical assistance, and Ms. Dottie Walsh for preparation of the manuscript.

REFERENCES

Biron CA, Natuk RJ, Welsh RM (submitted). Generation of large granular T lymphocytes in vivo during viral infection.

Biron CA, Turgiss LR, Welsh RM (1983). Increase in NK cell number and turnover rate during acute viral infection. J Immunol 131:1539-1545.

Biron CA, Sonnenfeld G, Welsh RM (1984). Interferon induces natural killer cell blastogenesis in vivo. J Leukocyte Biol 35:31-37.

Biron, CA, Welsh RM (1982). Blastogenesis of natural killer cells during viral infection in vivo. J Immunol 129: 2788-2795.

Brooks CG, Urdal DL, Henney CS (1983). Lymphokine-driven "differentiation" of cytotoxic T-cell clones into cells with NK-like specificity: correlations with display of membrane macromolecules. Immunological Rev 72:43-72.

Bukowski JF, Warner JF, Dennert G, Welsh RM (1985) Adoptive transfer studies demonstrating the antiviral effects of NK cells in vivo. J Exp Med 161:40-52.

Bukowski JF, Woda BA, Welsh RM (1984). Pathogenesis of murine cytomegalovirus infection in natural killer cell-depleted mice. J Virol 52:119-128.

Byrne, JA, Oldstone MBA (1984). Biology of cloned cytotoxic T lymphocytes specific for lymphocytic choriomeningitis virus: clearance of virus in vivo. J Virol 51:682-686.

Kumagai K, Itoh K, Suzuki R, Hinuma S, Saitoh F (1982). Studies of murine large granular lymphocytes. I. Identification as effector cells in NK and K cytotoxicities. J Immunol 129:388-394.

Mayo DR, Armstrong JA, Ho M (1977). Reactivation of murine cytomegalovirus by cyclophosphamide. Nature 267:721-723.

McIntyre KW, Bukowski JF, Welsh RM (1985). Exquisite specificity of adoptive immunization in arena-virus infected mice. Antiviral Res in press.

Millard PJ, Henkart MP, Reynolds CW, Henkart PA (1984). Purification and properties of cytoplasmic granules from cytotoxic rat LGL tumors. J Immunol 132:3197-3024.

Shellam GR, Allan JE, Papadimitriou JM, Bancroft GJ (191). Increased susceptibility to cytomegalovirus infection in beige mutant mice. Proc Nat Acad Sci 78:5104-5108.

Targan S, Dorey F (1980). Interferon activation of "prespontaneous killer" (Pre-SK) cells and alteration in kinetics of lysis of both "Pre-SK" and active SK cells. J Immunol. 124:2157-2161.

Timonen T, Ranki A, Saksela E, Hayry P (1979). Human natural cell-mediated cytotoxicity against fetal fibroblasts. III. Morphological and functional characterization of the effector cells. Cell Immunol 48:121-132.

Volkert M, Lundstedt C (1971). Tolerance and immunity to the lymphocytic choriomeningitis virus. Ann NY Acad Sci 181:183-195.

Welsh RM (1978). Cytotoxic cells induced during lymphocytic choriomeningitis virus infection of mice. I. Characterization of natural killer cell induction. J Exp Med 148: 163-181.

Welsh RM (1984). Natural killer cells and interferon. CRC Crit Rev Immunol 5:55-93.

Welsh RM, Biron CA, Bukowski JF, McIntyre KM, Yang H (1984). Role of natural killer cells in virus infection of mice. Surv Synth Path Res 3:409-431.

Welsh RM, Doe WF (1980). Cytotoxic cells induced during lymphocytic choriomeningitis virus infection of mice. III. Natural killer cell activity in cultured spleen leukocytes concomitant with T cell dependent immune interferon production. Infect and Immun 30:473-483.

Yang H, Welsh RM (submitted). Induction of alloreactive T cells by acute virus infection of mice.

Yang H, Yogeeswaran G, Bukowski JF, Welsh RM (1985). Expression of asialo GM_1 and other antigens and glycolipids on NK cells and spleen leukocytes in virus-infected mice. Nat Immun Cell Growth Regul 4:21-39.

Zinkernagel RM, Doherty PC (1975). H-2 compatibility requirement for T cell-mediated lysis of target cells infected with lymphocytic choriomeningitis virus. Different cytotoxic T cell specificities are associated with structures coded for in H-2K or H-2D. J Exp Med 141: 1427-1436.

Zinkernagel RM, Welsh RM (1976). H-2 compatibility requirement for virus-specific T cell-mediated effector functions in vivo. I. Specificity of T cells conferring antiviral protection against lymphocytic choriomeningitis virus is associated with H-2K and H-2D. J Immunol. 117: 1495-1502.

NK SUSCEPTIBILITY OF HUMAN CELLS MAY BE REGULATED BY GENES IN THE HLA REGION OF CHROMOSOME 6

Annick Harel-Bellan, Anne Quillet, Carmen Marchiol, Robert De Mars and Didier Fradelizi

Laboratoire d'Immunologie Institut Gustave Roussy 94805 Villejuif France (A.H.B., C.M., D.F.) and Genetic building, University of Wisconsin, Madison Wisconsin 53706 USA (R. D. M.)

INTRODUCTION

A decisive advance in the understanding of the function of Natural Killer (NK) cells would be the identification of the exact characteristics of the target cells. In fact, NK cells are able to kill in vitro targets that are mainly of tumoral but also of normal origin. The nature of the molecule(s) responsible for the binding of effector to target cells and for the triggering of the killing mechanism is still controversial.

One attractive hypothesis would be that the susceptible cells are those lacking Major Histocompatibility Complex (MHC) antigen expression on their surface. This hypothesis is sustained by several lines of evidences (Stern, 1980; Kiessling, 1984). We report here results about variants of a human B lymphoblastoid cell line in wich the loss of HLA expression at the cell surface was accompanied by the acquisition of NK susceptibility.

RESULTS

LCL 721 is an Epstein-Barr Virus -transformed human B cell line, which expresses normally the HLA class I and class II molecules. We studied variants 721. 84.5 and 721.134 (referred to as .84 and .134 below), both of which had been derived from an intermediate variant clone, .45, from which one entire haplotype had been physically deleted. Mutant .84 does not express DR and DQ antigens because it has homologous deletions of DR and DQ genes (Auffray, 1983). Mutant .134 has normal expression of the class II antigens but has greatly reduced expressions of the HLA-A and -B antigens (De Mars, 1984).

The susceptibility of these cell lines to lysis by NK cells in a long term (18h) ^{51}-chromium release assay was measured and results of a typical experiment are shown in Table 1. Lysis of LCL 721 by normal human PBL was not significantly above the background. The variant lacking HLA-DR and DQ expression (.84) was significantly but slightly lysed by the same effector cells. The variant showing perturbation in the expression of class I antigen (.134), on the contrary, was highly susceptible to NK lysis. Positive (K 562) and negative (Priess) controls are also shown. 721.134, however, was lysed to a highly significant amount by Lymphokine Activated Cells (LAK) (Table 1), showing that this cell line is not resistant to lysis in general.

TABLE 1. Susceptibility of the different cell lines to lysis by NK and LAK cells

Targets	% of lysis by			
	NK cells (a)		LAK cells (b)	
	100/1 (c)	50/1	100/1	50/1
K562 (d)	82	68	88	81
721-LCL	0.2	0	40	34
721.134	49	23	52	54
721.84.5	18	11	66	58
Priess (e)	0	0.5	38	27

a) Normal human (Peripheral Blood Lymphocytes) PBL were depleted of adherent cells by a one hour plastic adherence step
b) Normal human PBL were activated with a crude human PHA-activated PBL supernatant during 48 h.
c) Effector to target ratio
d) Positive control
e) Negative control

In order to test if the different susceptibility to NK lysis were associated with significant differences in the ability of target cells to bind effector cells, Large Granular Lymphocytes (LGL) were purified from PBL on a Percoll density gradient and incubated with target cells. The conjugation of the LGL cells to the targets was then assessed microscopically. Table 2 shows that NK resistant LCL-721 bound LGL as efficiently as the NK sensitive K 562 positive control.

Table 2. Target binding assay using Percoll gradient purified LGL and the different cell lines.

Target	% of conjugates (a)	
	Donor 1	Donor 2
K 562	18	23
721	21	20.9
.134	34	23
.84	17	37
CTL-L2 (b)	7	5.8

(a): LGL from PBL depleted of adherent cells were purified on Percoll and used as effectors for the target binding assay. The % of conjugated LGL (LGL in conjugates/total LGL) was estimated using an hemacytometer.
(b): CTL-L2 is a mouse IL2 dependent T cell line used here as a negative control.

Cold target inhibition experiments were also performed. Graded numbers of unlabeled K 562, LCL 721, .84, .134 and Priess cells were added during the cytolysis tests to fixed numbers of PBL and ^{51}Chromium -labeled K 562, .84 or .134. In the three systems, unlabeled LCL 721 cells were not able to inhibit the lysis of the susceptible targets, indicating that the 721 cells do not express the target molecule(s) present on the surface of .84, .134 and K 562 cells. Cross inhibition results obtained with K 562 cells on the three systems and lack of reverse inhibition by .134 or .84.5

mutants on K 562 can be interpreted in two ways which are discussed elsewhere (Manuscript in preparation).

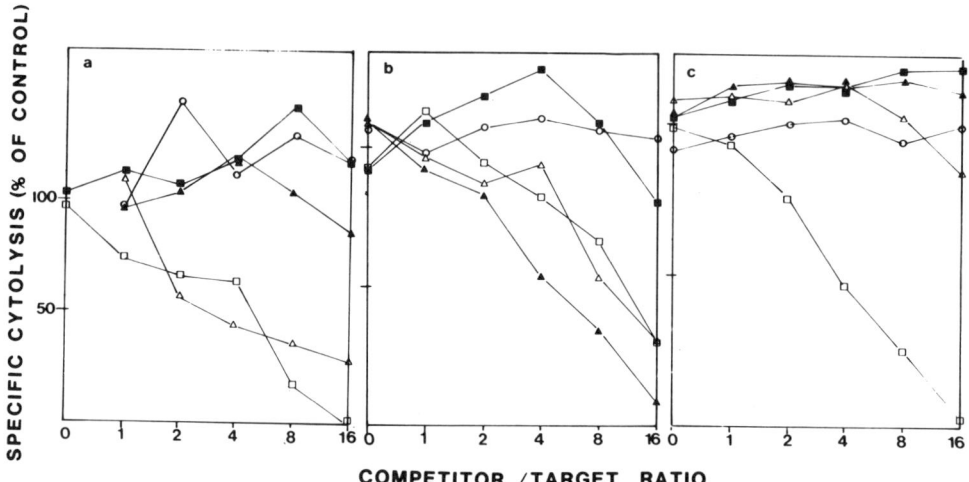

Figure 1. Cold target inhibition by unlabelled K 562 (□), 721.LCL (■), 721.134 (△), 721.84 (▲) and Priess (○) cells on the NK lysis of ^{51}Cr labelled 721.134 (a), 721.84 (b) and K 562 (c).

Treatment with interferon, has been shown to protect target cells against NK lysis (Trinchieri, 1978) and simultaneously to enhance the expression of HLA molecules at the cell surface (Fellous, 1979). We therefore tested the effect of interferon on the susceptibility of .134 to NK lysis. K 562 and .134 cells were treated with interferon and then submitted to FACS analysis and to NK lysis. K 562 expressed very low levels of HLA class I and class II molecules and interferon enhanced the expression of class I molecules on these cells (data not shown). Coordinately, interferon induced protection of these cells against NK lysis, since maximum specific lysis dropped from 62% to 28% However, interferon neither modified the level of expression of HLA class I molecules on the variant (data not shown) nor it's susceptibility to NK lysis (52% compared to 54%). A similar study with .84 cells gave identical results (data not shown).

DISCUSSION

A role for murine class I molecules in NK susceptibility has been discussed. Decreased expression of H-2 was accompanied by increased NK susceptibility in variants of mouse Lymphoma RBL5 (Kiessling, 1984). Furthermore, treatment of target fibroblasts with interferon resulted in a loss of sensitivity to NK lysis (Welsh, 1981) and enhanced expression of MHC antigens (Fellous, 1982). However, opposite results have been described in the mouse system. Variants from the highly susceptible mouse YAC-1 cell line, selected for reduced expression of H-2 molecules, were relatively insensitive to lysis in general and to NK lysis in particular (Dalianis, 1981). Loss of H-2 expression also resulted in decreased susceptibility to activated killer cells in a variant thymoma cell line (Lattime, 1982).

In the human cell system described here, susceptibility to NK lysis seems to be related to reduced expression of HLA antigens. It remains possible that susceptibility to NK lysis is caused by altered expression of a non-class I molecule, as a direct result of mutation in the MHC or as an indirect effect of reduced class I antigen expression. While the involvement of mutations outside the MHC cannot be totally excluded, the chance of such involvement is remote (R. De Mars, submitted for publication).

The mechanism by which reduction in class I antigen expression results in NK lysis susceptibility is not understood. Target binding assays indicate that LCL 721 expresses the molecule necessary to bind effector cells. However, results from cold target inhibition experiments indicate that the expression of the lytic target molecule is difficult to detect in 721 cells relative to the two variants. We propose one model to explain these two results. The various target cells bind the effector cells to the same extent via binding structures. Once bound, interaction between the effector and a molecule on the target cell (possibly HLA molecules) would decide whether the target cell is lysed or not. If HLA molecules are intact on the surface, the target would not be lysed and the effector cells would be recycled. If class I antigen expression is sufficiently reduced, the targets would be lysed. This mechanism could be ancestral to that of the CTL system, in which the <u>induction</u> of specific cytolytic T cells results from their recognition of allogeneic class I amino-acid sequence differences or of autologous class I antigens that are modified as a result of viral infection. In fact, HLA molecules could be a sign of cellular integrity, a "good health" signal for cells.

REFERENCES

AUFFRAY C, KUO J, DE MARS R, STROMINGER J L (1983). A minimum of four human class II α-chain genes are encoded in the HLA region of chromosome 6. Nature 304: 174-177.

DALIANIS T, AHRLUND-RICHTER L, MERINO F, KLEIN E, KLEIN G (1981). Reduced humoral and cellular cytotoxicity sensitivity in major histocompatibility variants of the YAC (Moloney) lymphoma. Immunogenetics 12: 371-380.

DE MARS R, CHANG C C, SHAW S, RERTNAUER P J, SONDEL P M (1984). Homozygous deletion that simultaneously eliminate expression of class I and class II antigens of EBV-transformed B-lymphoblastoid cells. Hum Immunol 11: 77-97.

FELLOUS M, KAMOUN M, GRESSER I, BONO R (1979). Enhanced expression of HLA-antigens and β_2-microglobulin on interferon-treated human lymphoid cells Eur J Immunol 9: 446-449.

FELLOUS M, NIR U, WALLACH D, MERLIN G, RUBINSTEIN M, REVEL M (1982). Interferon dependant induction of mRNA for the major histocompatibility antigens in human fibroblasts and lymphoblastoid cells. Proc Natl Acad Sci USA 79: 3082-3086

KIESSLING R (1985). What do NK cells recognize on the surface of tumor cells and hematopoïetic normal target cells? Symposium communication at the "Reunion de la societe francaise d'immunologie" Hopital Necker -PARIS.

LATTIME E C, PECORARO G E, STUTMAN O (1982). Target cell recognition by natural killer and natural cytotoxic cells in "NK Cells and Other Natural Effector Cells" Ed. HERBERMAN, B (Academic Press) p 713-718.

STERN P, GIDLUND M, ORN A, WIGZELL H (1980). Natural killer cells mediate lysis of embryonal carcinoma cells lacking MHC Nature 285: 341-342.

TRINCHIERI G, SANTOLI D (1978). Enhancement of human natural killer activity by interferon and antagonistic inhibition of susceptibility of target cells to lysis. J Exp Med 147: 1314-1333.

WELSH R M, KARRE K, HAUSSON M, KUNKEL L A, KIESSLING R W (1981). Interferon mediated protection of normal and tumor target cells against lysis by human natural killer cells J Immunol 126: 219-225.

ACTIVATION OF ALVEOLAR MACROPHAGE INTRACELLULAR MICROBICIDAL ACTIVITY BY A PREFORMED LGL CYTOKINE

Arnold H. Greenberg, Jose Gomez, Bill Pohajdak, Shane O'Neill and John Wilkins
Departments of Pediatrics (A.H.G.,B.P.), Medicine (J.G.,S.O., J.W.), University of Manitoba, Winnipeg, Canada R3E 0V9

INTRODUCTION

Although it is generally thought that NK cells play a central role in resistance to tumors and viral infections, it is now becoming apparent that they may also have important immunoregulatory functions. This could take at least two forms; a direct one in which sensitive progenitor or regulatory cells are killed or growth inhibited, and indirectly through the release of cytokines, such as interferon (IFN)-γ and IL1 and possibly IL2 (see Ortaldo & Herberman, 1985). We recently reported that NK cells can synergize with macrophages to stimulate oxidative metabolism (Pohajdak et al, 1984) and may do so through a soluble factor released by large granular lymphocytes (LGL). The activation of macrophages by lymphokines has been demonstrated in the context of intracellular lysis of microbial pathogens, some of which utilize an oxygen dependent mechanism of kill. We will describe below a cytokine which is rapidly released by LGL after contact with tumor cells. This cytokine enhanced alveolar macrophage intracellular kill of <u>Staphylococcus aureus</u>.

RESULTS

Activation of Alveolar Macrophage Microbicidal Activity

Utilizing a recently described double isotope assay (O'Neill et al, 1984), we examined supernatants obtained from Percoll fractionated LGL after a 15-30 min. incubation with the NK sensitive K562 tumor line for their ability to enhance phagocytosis and intracellular killing of S. aureus. While no effect was detected on phagocytosis, the supernatants consistently activated rat and human alveolar macrophage intracellular kill (Fig. 1). When intracellular microbicidal activation was attempted with supernatants obtained from LGL incubations using the NK resistant L5178Y lymphoma or from LGL, K562 or L5178Y incubated alone for the same time period, enhanced microbial kill could not be detected. Supernatants from 10^7 LGL were optimally active at a concentration of 1/20 or greater, 50% of maximum at 1/40 and undetectable at 1/80. Cytokine release was extraordinarily rapid with maximal activity detected in supernatants obtained within 5 minutes of the initiation of LGL contact with K562. This rapid release together with the insensitivity of the LGL to pretreatment with Actinomycin D and cycloheximide treatment (Fig. 2) suggested that it was preformed and released on tumor activation of the LGL. Furthermore, an intact secretory apparatus was required since the carboxylic ionophore monensin inhibited cytokine release and this drug is known to interrupt traffic of Golgi derived vesicles and block NK lytic activity.

Phenotype of the Cytokine-Producing Mononuclear Cell

Cytokine production by peripheral blood mononuclear cells fractionated on Percoll gradients indicated that maximal macrophage microbicidal kill was detected when supernatants were taken from cells in the fraction showing peak lytic activity and HNK-1 fluorescence, but not from T cell rich fractions. Following isolation of LGL on Percoll gradients, cells were treated with HNK-1 and FITC-labelled goat anti-mouse IgM F(ab')$_2$. HNK-1$^+$ and HNK-1$^-$ cells were FACS sorted and cytokine production of each population evaluated. This experiment clearly demonstrated that the cells releasing the factor were in the HNK-1$^+$ fraction while supernatants derived from HNK-1$^-$ cells were consistently inactive (Fig. 2). Fractionation of T cells from NK cells in the LGL was also accomplished by E-rosetting at 29°C, a condition where NK cells do not form rosettes. The cells responsible for active supernatants were contained exclusively within the lytic, non E-rosetting LGL fraction (Fig. 3). The additional observation that an NK^s tumor (K562), but

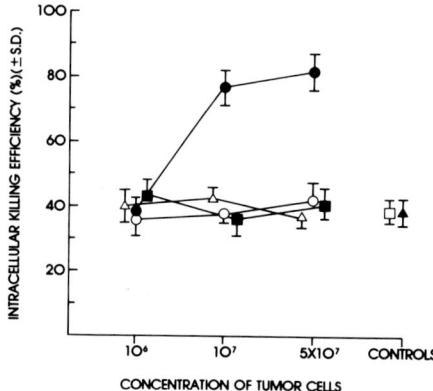

Figure 1. Stimulation of rat alveolar macrophage Staphylococcidal activity. Supernatants from LGL incubated with increasing numbers of K562 (●) or L5178Y (○) tumor cells, compared to K562 (△), L5178Y (■) or LGL (▲) incubated on their own and saline control (□).

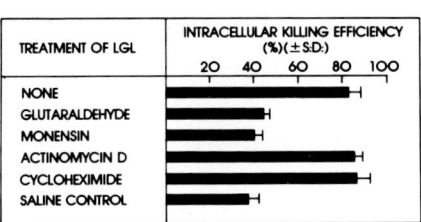

Figure 2. The influence of pretreatment of LGL on the release of MAF. Supernatants were inactive when LGL were either fixed with gluteraldehyde (0.25%) or incubated with the carboxylic ionophore monensin (10 μg/ml). Neither Actinomycin D (5 μg/ml) nor cycloheximide (28 μg/ml) pretreatment affected factor production.

not NK^R lines (L5178Y, P815), could stimulate cytokine production (Fig. 1) would favor an NK cell rather than a T cell origin of the factor. Although it is still possible that a small T cell subset bearing the HNK-1 marker can be a cytokine producer, on the basis of these results we think this is unlikely.

Characteristics of the Macrophage Activating LGL Cytokine

Characterization of the LGL derived macrophage activating cytokine suggests that it is a small protein. It was inactivated at 100°C for 5 min. but not at 56°C for 30 min. Activity was also lost at pH 2.0 or 10.0. Treatment of the cytokine with insolubilized trypsin, chymotrypsin and non-specific protease completely abolished activity while RNase was without effect. Supernatants from 1.5×10^8 LGL stimulated with K562 were

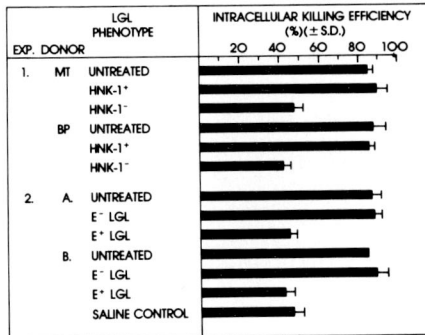

Figure 3. Characterization of the LGL producing the macrophage activating factor. HNK-1$^+$ LGL isolated by FACS sorting, and E$^-$ LGL isolated by rosetting with sheep erythrocytes at 29°C, produced active supernatants.

concentrated from 15 ml to 3 ml using a UM10 Diaflo membrane and then applied to a 60 x 1.7 cm AcA44 column. Activity was detected only in two pools from the 10-20,000 Dalton range.

Several laboratories have identified IFN-γ as the lymphokine that activates macrophage antimicrobial activity. The possibility that the LGL-MAF described here is IFN-γ was considered, however, we believe that this is unlikely for a number of reasons. Secretion of IFN-γ requires more than 18 hrs. of stimulation and both RNA and protein synthesis are necessary for its production while LGL-MAF release is rapid and is resistant to Actinomycin D and cycloheximide. In addition IFN-γ displays an apparently high molecular weight on gel filtration of 50,000 and this is considerably more than LGL MAF described here (10-20,000). We were unable to find anti-viral activity in highly concentrated LGL cytokine preparations (<.01 U/ml), and purified human IFN-β and recombinant human IFN-γ (2000 U/ml) failed to stimulate rat alveolar microbicidal activity. Although these are strong arguments against the cytokine being an IFN, it is possible that the microbicidal assay can detect levels of IFN-γ below the sensitivity the viral plaque assay. Furthermore IFN-γ has been shown to synergize with non-IFN macrophage activators at extremely low levels (Hamann & Krammer, 1985), so the participation of IFN-γ cannot be completely excluded at this point.

DISCUSSION

The results of this study demonstrate that human NK cells (LGL) release a factor that augments intracellular

microbicidal activity of alveolar macrophages. The
process occurs during the ingestion of microorganisms
without enhancing phagocytosis. Whether cytokine induced
macrophage activation requires the presence of bacteria
or their products is not known, however triggering of
IFN-γ treated macrophages by bacterial lipopolysac-
charide has been well described and the process may be
similar.

It has been widely argued that a secretory process
is part of the NK lytic mechanism and recently it was
found that the contents of cytoplasmic granules are
rapidly exocytosed on tumor contact (Podack & Dennert,
1983). These granules contain a cytolysin thought to
mediate the lethal hit (Henkart et al, 1984). Although
there is no direct evidence that LGL granules contain
immunoregulatory cytokines, other cells, in particular
mast cells, have granules which are rich in mediators of
inflammation. Our observations raise the intriguing
possibility that LGL granules may also store cytokines
which are capable of rapidly enhancing macrophage
activity.

The notion that NK cells may participate in resistance to microbial pathogens is not new. Preferential NK
lysis of virally infected cells (Santoli et al, 1978)
destruction of Trypanosoma cruzi (Hatcher & Kuhn, 1982)
and, Cryptococcus neoformans (Murphy & McDaniel, 1982)
have all been documented. Less is known about NK
participation in resistance to facultative microorganisms, although it has been suggested that the NK cell
may mediate an antibody-dependent cell-mediated anti-
bacterial activity (Tagliabue et al, 1984). All of these
studies have considered only the direct lytic effect of
NK cells on microorganisms. In view of our observations
one may now consider an indirect immunoregulatory
role for NK cells in which the rapid release of a
preformed cytokine can enhance macrophage microbicidal
activity.

ACKNOWLEDGEMENTS

This work was supported by the MRC and NCI of Canada.

REFERENCES

Hamann U, Krammer PH (1985). Activation of macrophage tumor cytotoxicity by the synergism of two T cell-derived lymphokines: immune interferon (IFN-) and macrophage cytotoxicity inducing factor 2 (MCIF2). Eur J Immunol 15:18-24.

Hatcher FM, Kuhn RE (1982). Destruction of Trypanosoma cruzi by natural killer cells. Science 126:295-269.

Henkart PA, Millard PJ, Reynolds CW, Henkart MP (1984). Cytolytic activity of purified cytoplasmic granules from cytotoxic rat large granular lymphocyte tumors. J Exp Med 160:75-93.

Murphy JW, McDaniel DO (1982). In vitro reactivity of natural killer (NK) cells against Cryptococcus neoformans. J Immunol 128:1577-1583.

O'Neill S, Lesperance E, Klass DJ (1984). Rat lung lavage surfactant enhances bacterial phagocytosis and intracellular killing by alveolar macrophages. Am Rev Respir Dis 130:225-231.

Ortaldo JR, Herberman RB (1984). Heterogeneity of NK cells. Am Rev Immunol 2:359-394.

Podack ER, Dennert G (1983). Assembly of two types of tubules with putative cytolytic function by cloned natural killer cells. Nature (Lond.) 302:442-445.

Pohajdak B, Gomez JL, Wilkins JA, Greenberg AH (1984). Tumor activated NK cells trigger monocyte oxidative metabolism. J Immunol 133:2430-2436.

Santoli D, Trinchieri G Lief FS (1978). Cell mediated cytotoxicity against virus infected cells in humans. I. Characterization of the effector lymphocytes. J Immunol 121:526-531.

Tagliabue A, Nencioni L, Vitta L, Keren DF, Lowell GH, Boraschi D (1984). Antibody-dependent cell mediated anti-bacterial activity of intestinal lymphocytes with secretory IgA. Nature 306:184-186.

ROLE OF LAMININ AND LAMININ RECEPTORS IN NATURAL KILLER CELL RECOGNITION OF TUMOR METASTASES.

John C. Hiserodt, Dan M. Hyder, Katherine A. Laybourn and James Varani
Department of Pathology, University of Michigan
Ann Arbor, Michigan 48109

INTRODUCTION

Natural Killer (NK) and Natural Cytotoxic (NC) lymphocytes comprise a subpopulation of cytotoxic effector cells capable of spontaneously lysing (i.e., without prior sensitization) a variety of virally infected and tumor target cells in vitro. Recent evidence has clearly demonstrated that NK/NC cells are the major effectors in controlling metastatic spread of tumors via the hematogenous route. Because of this, NK/NC cells have been proposed to be important in natural immunosurveillance mechanisms against the development and spread of neoplasia.

Although NK and NC cells recognize and lyse tumor cells in a non-MHC restricted manner (contrary to cytotoxic T cells (CTL)) and are operationally nearly identical to CTL, neither the NK/NC recognition structures nor target "antigens" are known.

EVIDENCE FOR LAMININ/LAMININ RECEPTORS IN NK RECOGNITION

We have recently demonstrated the presence of laminin receptors on target cells recognized by NK/NC cells (1). These receptors were demonstrated by 125-I-laminin binding and laminin induced cell-cell aggregation. That laminin receptors were important in NK/NC recognition of the target cells was shown by the ability of exogenous laminin to block NK/NC binding without affecting the binding by other killer cells such as CTL. Furthermore, when sensitive targets were pretreated with laminin they were reduced in their ability to bind to NK cells (in a single cell assay) and were impaired in their ability to cold target compete for untreated NK sensitive targets.

These findings led us to propose that NK/NC cells may express cell surface laminin-like structures which serve as a ligand for the binding to the laminin receptors on susceptible tumor cells. Using highly specific anti-laminin antibodies, together with immunoperoxidase, flow cytometry and complement (C') dependent lysis we could indeed show that NK cells express laminin-like structures on their surface (2). Furthermore, the data indicate that this laminin is important in NK recognition of tumor cells.

Immunoperoxidase staining (Figure 1) and flow cytometric analysis revealed that the frequency of laminin positive cells was very close to the frequency of both asialo GM_1 and NK 2.1 positive cells and correlated well with NK activity in different lymphoid organs (PBL > spleen > lymph node > thymus). Laminin was not detected on the surface of CTL or thymocytes. The presence of laminin on the surface of NK cells was proven by the ability of anti-laminin antibodies to inactivate NK function in the presence of C'. We found that even in the absence of C', laminin pretreated NK cells were reduced in their cytolytic activity due to reduced target binding (Table 1). However, although anti-asialo GM_1 could also eliminate NK activity in the presence of C', it did not affect NK activity in the absence of C'. Thus, laminin and asialo GM_1 appear to occupy functionally distinct sites on the surface of the NK cell. The fact that anti-laminin also affected NC binding whereas anti-asialo GM_1 did not suggest that NC cells also express surface laminin.

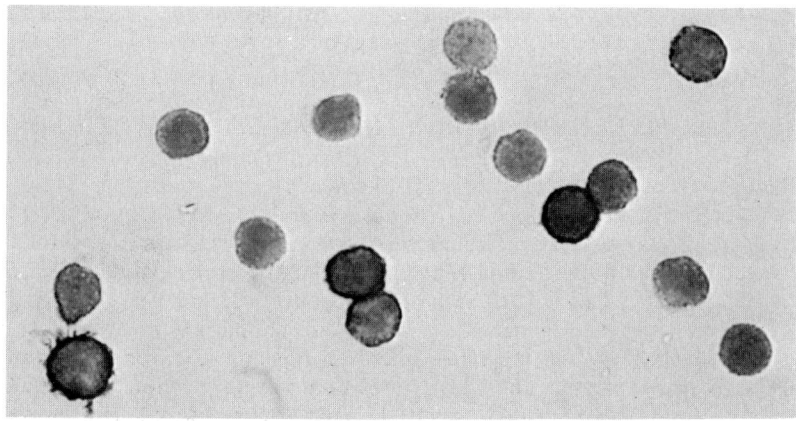

Figure 1: Anti-laminin immunoperoxidase staining of C57B1/6 peripheral blood mononuclear cells (ABC Method).

RECOGNITION OF TUMOR TARGET CELLS BY NK CELLS: INFLUENCE ON METASTASIS.

A. In vitro recognition of NC targets by NK cells.

A number of studies have demonstrated the involvement of NK cells in control of metastasis. Factors which augment NK activity reduce metastasis by the hematogenous route and factors which suppress NK activity promote metastasis. Additionally, animals with intrinsically low NK activity demonstrate a greater propensity for metastasis than do animals with intrinsically higher activity. Resistance to metastasis in animals with low NK activity can be potentiated by adoptive transfer of NK cells from high-responding animals (3). In spite of this, it has not yet been convincingly shown that differences in metastatic activity among heterogeneous tumor cell lines are related to differences in NK sensitivity. While some studies have

Table 1. Anti-laminin pretreated NK/NC cells but not CTL are reduced in their abiltiy to bind and lyse target cells

Pretreatment of Killers		Target	% Binding to Targets	Cytotoxicity 100:1	10:1
(NK)[a]	NRS	YAC-1	15±2	38±2	-
	αLaminin	YAC-1	4±1	14±1	-
	αAsialo GM$_1$	YAC-1	14±1	34±3	-
(NC)[b]	NRS	1.0/Anti-B^r	17±2	22±2	-
	αLaminin	1.0/Anti-B^r	7±2	9±2	-
(CTL)[c]	NRS	P815	26±4	-	54±4
	αLaminin	P815	22±2	-	51±3

[a,b] Normal C57BL/6 spleen cells; [c] day 10 C57BL/6 anti P815 peritoneal exudate lymphocyte (PEL).

shown that metastatic tumors are more NK-resistant than the primary tumors from which they arose, other studies have shown no consistent pattern (4-6). In a recent study (1), we compared the NK sensitivity and NC sensitivity of highly-malignant murine fibrosarcoma cell lines and low-malignant lines isolated from the same parent tumors. The highly-malignant cells were resistant to killing in both the 4-hour assay for NK activity and in the 18-hour assay for NC activity. The low-malignant cells were highly-sensitive to killing in the 18-hour assay but were resistant to killing in 4-hours. Treatment of the effector cells with anti-asialo GM_1 had no effect on killing although this treatment completely inhibited killing of Yac-1 targets by the same effector cells. These findings strongly imply that the low-malignant fibrosarcoma cells are sensitive to NC but not NK cells.

Although the low-malignant fibrosarcoma cells are resistant to NK-mediated killing *in vitro*, there is evidence to indicate that these cells are recognized by NK cells. This evidence comes from studies in which the fibrosarcoma cells were used to cold-target compete for the killing of Yac-1 cells in a 4-hour assay. The unlabeled fibrosarcoma cells were mixed with 51-Cr-labeled Yac-1 cells and incubated with nonadherent mouse spleen cells. The presence of the low-malignant fibrosarcoma cells inhibited Yac-1 killing in a concentration-dependent manner. Unlabeled Yac-1 cells also inhibited killing but the presence of P815 cells (a known NK-resistant line) did not (Table 2). These studies are not the first to document cross competition between NC and NK targets (7). However, our studies provide a clue to structures on the target cells responsible for this competition. The low-malignant fibrosarcoma cells, like many other murine tumor cells, express receptors for the laminin molecule (8). That the expression of laminin receptors by these fibrosarcoma cells might facilitate their recognition by NK cells is suggested by the finding that when they are preincubated with laminin, their ability to act as cold target competitors for the killing of Yac-1 cells is decreased (Table 1). This is not to imply that the laminin receptor is the only structure in common between NK and NC targets. There may be several. However, if the presence of laminin-like structures on the NK cell surface does, in fact, play a role in NK recognition, then it would seem reasonable to find the corresponding moiety (i.e., the laminin receptor) on the cells recognized by these effector cells.

B. NK recognition of NC cells *in vivo*: Effects on metastasis.

Does the ability of NK cells to recognize targets which they are, apparently, unable to kill in the standard

Table 2. Inhibition of Yac-1 killing by control and laminin-treated fibrosarcoma cells

Cold-Target Competitor	% Yac-1 Lysis
None	33± 1
Yac-1	4± 1
1.0/anti-B^r	13± 3
1.0/anti-B^r (laminin-pretreated)	24± 4
P815	31± 1

The ^{51}Cr-release assay was carried out using standard procedures. The effector:target ratio was 50:1 and the cold:hot ratio was 20:1. The laminin pretreated, low-malignant fibrosarcoma cells (1.0/anti-B^r) were preincubated with laminin (200 μg per 2 x 10^6 cells) for one hour and then washed.

in vitro assays have any in vivo relevance? In an attempt to answer this question, we injected the low-malignant fibrosarcoma cells into syngeneic (C57BL/6) mice which had been pretreated with anti-asialo GM$_1$ serum. The treatment of animals with anti-asialo GM$_1$ has been shown to almost

Table 3. Lung tumor formation in normal and anti-asialo GM$_1$-treated mice.

Tumor Line	Treatment	Median Number of Lung Tumors	Range
1.0/anti-B^r	Control	9	3-29
	Anti-asialo GM$_1$	131	125->300
1.1/anti-B^r	Control	18	13-26
	Anti-asialo GM$_1$	84	83-95

The animals were treated with anti-asialo GM$_1$ one day prior to intravenous injection with these low-malignant fibrosarcoma cells. Lung tumors were counted 30 days later.

completely eliminate circulating NK activity and spleen NK activity while having minimal effect on macrophage function (9-12). Using our injection protocol, we found that the spleen lymphocytes from the treated animals were completely deficient in their ability to kill Yac-1 targets in a 4-hour assay but were unaffected in their capacity to kill the fibrosarcoma cells in 18 hours. In spite of this, the anti-asialo GM_1 treated animals that were injected with the fibrosarcoma cells developed many more pulmonary metastases than did the control animals (Table 3). This suggests that even though NK cells cannot kill the low-malignant fibrosarcoma cells in vitro, they may play an important role in regulating their behavior in vivo.

If NK cells do, in fact, influence the behavior of the fibrosarcoma cells in vivo and, if laminin receptors/laminin do play a role in NK recognition of these cells, then it might be expected that preincubation of the target cells with laminin would increase their metastatic potential. Previous studies have shown that when the low-malignant fibrosarcoma cells are treated with laminin prior to injection, many more tumors develop than in control animals injected with the same number of untreated cells (8). We had originally postulated that the increased tumor formation seen with the laminin-treated cells reflected their enhanced ability to interact with basement membranes. While this hypothesis is still valid, the data is also consistent with the idea that increased tumor formation by the laminin-treated cells results from their ability to avoid the host's natural defense system. Certainly the two ideas are not mutually exclusive.

REFERENCES

1. Hiserodt J, Laybourn K, Varani J. Laminin inhibits the recognition of tumor target cells by murine natural killer (NK) and natural cytotoxic (NC) lymphocytes. Am J Path (in press).
2. Hiserodt J, Laybourn K, J. Varani (1985). Expression of a laminin-like substance on the surface of murine natural killer cells and its role in NK recognition of tumor cells. J Immunol 135:1484.
3. Hanna N (1982). Role of natural killer cells in control of cancer metastasis. Cancer Metastasis Rev 1:45-64.

4. Gorelik E, Fogel M, Feldman M, Segal S (1979). Difference in resistance of metastatic tumor cells and cells from local tumor growth to cytotoxicity of natural killer cells. J Nat Cancer Inst 63:1397-1404.
5. Poupon M, Judde J, Pot-Deprun J, Sweeney F, Lespinats G (1983). Variable susceptibility to NK activity of cloned cell lines derived from a primary rat rhabdomyosarcoma: Relationship to metastatic potential. Br J Cancer 48:75-82.
6. Hanna N, Fidler I (1981). Relationship between metastatic potential and resistance to natural killer cell-mediated cytotoxicity in three murine tumor systems. J Nat Cancer Inst 66:1183-1190.
7. Stutman O, Dien P, Wisun R, Picoraro G, Lattime E (1980). Natural cytotoxic (NC) cells against solid tumors in mice: Some target cell characteristics and blocking of cytotoxicity by D-mannose. In: Natural Cell-Mediated Immunity Against Tumors. R.B. Herberman (ed.) Academic Press, New York, p. 949-961.
8. Malinoff H, Varani J, McCoy J, Wicha M (1984). Metastatic potential of murine fibrosarcoma cells correlates with endogenous surface-receptor bound laminin. Int J Cancer 33:651-655.
9. Wiltrout R, Santoni, Peterson E, Knott D, Overton W, Herberman R, Holden H (1985). Reactivity of anti-asialo GM_1 serum with tumoricidal and non-tumoricidal mouse macrophages. J Leuk Biology 37:597-614.
10. Saijo N, Ozaki A, Beppu K, Takahashi K, Fujita J, Sasaki Y, Nomori H, Kimata M, Shimizu E, Hosh A (1984). Analysis of metastatic spread and growth of tumor cells in mice with depressed natural killer activity by anti-asialo GM_1 antibody or anti cancer agents. J Cancer Res Clin Oncol 107:157-163.
11. Keller R, Bachi T, Okumura K (1983). Discrimination between macrophages - and NK-type tumoricidal activities via anti-asialo GM_1 antibody. Exp Cell Biol 51:158-164.
12. Wiltrout R, Herberman R, Zhang S, Chirigos M, Ortaldo J, Green K, Talmadge J (1985). Role of organ-associated NK cells in decreased formation of experimental metastases in lung and liver. J Immunol 134:4267-4275.

Section IX. Tumor-Host Interactions

TUMORIGENESIS AND IMMUNE SURVEILLANCE

Zvi Grossman

School of Mathematical Sciences, Tel Aviv University, Tel Aviv, Israel and National Cancer Institute, Frederick Cancer Research Facility, Frederick, MD 21701

INTRODUCTION

The notion of immune surveillance against cancer has known several ups and downs since it was proposed (Thomas, 1959; Burnet, 1964, 1971). According to that hypothesis the immune system recognizes tumor-associated antigens and destroys cells that express them. The range of effector cells proposed for this activity now includes not only T and B cells but also cells that mediate "natural immunity" such as the natural killer (NK) cells and macrophages. The observation that immuno-suppression may increase the frequency and spread of certain tumors is considered to support the concept of immuno-surveillance. It has been more difficult to directly demonstrate the immunogenicity of tumor cells as a general phenomenon. In this communication an alternative mode of surveillance is put forward. It is suggested that a major function of the immune system is to assist in regulating the differentiation of a variety of normal cells. Thus, tumor escape from surveillance may imply escape from regulatory differentiation pressures.

"SNEAKING-THROUGH" OF ANTIGENIC TUMORS

A simple mathematical model was described for the interactions between a tumor and a part of the cell-mediated immune response, namely, the activation of cytotoxic T-lymphocytes (Grossman and Berke, 1980). We studied non-monotonic growth patterns of tumors and in particular the sneaking-through phenomenon, where small amounts of experimentally transplanted immunogenic tumor cells grow progressively, medium-sized amounts are rejected, and large ones break through again. In the model, the strength of the immune response was determined by an interplay between tumor-induced expansion of the specific CTL population on the one hand, and blocking of these cells by tumor-shed antigen on the other. An initially small tumor induced only a slow expansion of CTL and led to a quasi-steady state of CTL-tumor coexistence. This state allowed for a progressive blocking of the CTL and consequently a progressive tumor growth. In contrast, an initially medium-sized tumor induced an overshooting wave of specific CTL that eliminated the tumor.

Our model represented only some aspects of the anti-tumor response and was meant as a paradigm for the analysis of tumor escape mechanisms. In particular, other ways by which the tumor could exert negative influence on the immune system may be suggested. For instance, imbalance between the initial rates of growth of responding versus helper cells upon interaction with a small tumor could eventually cause exhaustive differentiation of high-affinity responding cells (Grossman 1982, 1984). Aiming to pinpoint the minimal requirements for the occurrence of the sneaking-through phenomenon, De Boer and Hogeweg (1985) analyzed a series of models derived, by successive modifications, from the Grossman and Berke model. These can still demonstrate the sneaking-through-type kinetics.

The sneaking-through phenomenon was linked to the induction of "low-zone tolerance" by repeated stimulation with small antigen concentrations (Grossman and Berke, 1980; Grossman, 1982). In general, the strength of the immune response depends not on the magnitude of the challenge but rather on the associated gradients. The typical rise and fall in the number of effector cells in response to a sudden challenge is characteristic of a transient phenomenon. Persistent or gradually changing antigenic stimulation appears to select low-affinity lymphocyte populations that cannot easily be depleted by terminal differentiation or blocked by specific factors. The analysis shows that it may be quite possible for a potentially immunogenic tumor to develop in the presence of an intact immune system. Instead of mounting a destructive response, the immune system may adapt, through a process of selection, to the tumor growth. It has even been suggested that the positive selection of low-affinity proliferating lymphocytes in the vicinity of a parasite population may provide protection of the parasite from more effective clones (Grossman et al, 1985). These considerations, and the uncertainty concerning the potential immunogenicity of many physiologically occurring tumors, call for examining alternative explanations for the observed association between immuno-suppression and tumor promotion.

TUMOR DEVELOPMENT: THE EXAMPLE OF CML

Chronic myelocytic leukemia (CML) starts as an overproduction of mature granulocytes in the marrow, related to an expansion of the progenitor populations. It is usually associated with a typical chromosomal aberration, the Philadelphia chromosome (Ph^1). Later it develops into the malignant blastic phase, or crisis, characterized by the dominance of immature blast cells. The cell-population changes appear to involve successive cellular alterations. The generally accepted hypothesis is that the cell-population changes, and in particular the blastic crisis, are caused by the cellular alterations. These alterations, in turn, are believed to reflect intrinsic genetic instability of the leukemic cells (Foulds, 1969; Nowell, this issue).

An alternative view has recently been proposed (Grossman 1985a, 1985b). Cellular and tissue alterations develop dynamically in a network of causal relations. The initiating event may be assumed to be a DNA modification in an early hemopoietic progenitor, but even this is not certain (Rubin, 1984).

More explicitly, the new hypothesis proposes that the relative rates of self-renewal and differentiation of mitotic cells in the hemopoietic tissue are regulated by microenvironmental and feedback inter-cellular interactions. The differentiation pressures increase with the size of the mature cell compartment (feedback). Self-renewal capacity is a measure of the cell's resistance to differentiation pressures; normally, it declines as the cells undergo a series of changes in their patterns of gene expression - a process called maturation - heading towards the stage of terminal differentiation. At steady state, the feedback differentiation pressure is such that the most primitive cells are replicating and differentiating at the same rate, while the more differentiated cells have a higher probability of maturation.

The rule that hemopoietic cells become more responsive to differentiation signals as they mature makes maturation an autocatalytic process. This, together with the feedback assumption, ensure the stability of the hemopoietic hierarchy (Grossman, 1985a), namely, of the normal phenotypic profile. It is postulated, however, that cell replication is also potentially autocatalytic: the force that drives replication tends to endow the cell with a slowly increasing capacity for self-renewal or, equivalently, decreasing inducibility to differentiation. The two opposing forces are balanced at the level of the most primitive cells, endowing them with "stemness." For more differentiated cells the autocatalytic circuit of differentiation is normally dominant. Certain perturbations of the tissue can weaken the differentiation feedback loop, leading to a self-driven cascade of interrelated changes in the growth characteristics of the hemopoietic cells and in the microenvironment and eventually to malignancy.

The assumption that the growth characteristics of hemopoietic cells are subject to adaptive changes in both directions, and not only to down-regulation of the self-renewal capacity with differentiation, is indirectly supported by several observations (Grossman, 1984b): External influences can change the self-renewal capacity (e.g., Spooncer et al, 1984; Chang and McCulloch, 1981); DNA methylation may have a role in regulating blast cell self-renewal (Motoji et al, 1985); striking heterogeneities exist in the capacity of cells belonging to the same "compartment" to form colonies (McCulloch et al, 1982); cultured cell lines and clones often undergo gradual loss of differentiative capacities and of responsiveness to various inducers (Rubin, 1985; Brooks et al, 1983); some growth factors can regulate the expression and affinity of their own receptors (Smith and Cantrell, 1985).

Cell crowding, with the associated distortion of the population balance in the tissue, is indicated as a perturbation which can destabilize the normal cell configuration (Grossman, 1985b). A mathematical model supported the following scenario: (1) Genomic, heritable event in an early hemopoietic cell reduces the responsiveness of the clone to feedback. (2) Consequently, the clone expands to maintain the balance between self-renewal and maturation of stem cells. (3) Cell crowding arises and also the beginning of a selection in favor of blast cells and against (non-dividing) mature cells and (slowly dividing) primitive cells. This is the chronic stage of CML. If crowding exceeds a certain threshold, the following happens: (4) Blast cells adapt to the distorted microenvironmental conditions by increasing their self-renewal capacity. As a result, the balance among mature and immature cell populations is distorted even further. (5) This is a positive feedback loop – a snowball-like process of slipping control – leading eventually to blast cell dominance. Alternative scenarios have also been proposed (Grossman, 1985b).

IMMUNE SURVEILLANCE WITHOUT ANTIGENICITY

How does this view of leukemogenesis relate to the notion of immune surveillance? The hypothesis did not define the range of mature cells which affect the differentiation of earlier hemopoietic cells. It has become clear that T cells are a direct source of factors affecting a wide range of lymphoid and hemopoietic cells (reviewed: Schrader, 1983). Although generally associated by immunologists with antigen presentation, Ia antigens may play another role in the regulation of hemopoiesis (Schrader, 1983). They may be involved in Ia-restricted communication with regulatory T-cells. The recognition that the levels of histocompatibility antigens on progenitor cells are influenced by external factors may indicate such a role of MHC products in hemopoiesis. In addition to T cells, NK cells and related large granular lymphocytes, in their capacity as "natural helper" cells (Grossman and Herberman, 1982), may be involved in similar regulatory functions. Moreover, a growing body of evidence indicates the existence of reciprocal communication between the immune system and several other cell systems. For instance, the immune and neuroendocrine systems appear to share a common set of hormones and their receptors (Blalock, this issue). In general, lymphokines and MHC antigens are obvious potential channels of communication.

Generalizing the CML-blastic crisis scenario, it may be conjectured that lymphoid cells are an important component of the regulatory cell population which generates maturation pressures in some tissues. Since maintenance of these pressures is proposed to be essential for the cell population balance in the tissue and for the stability of its phenotypic profile, this conjecture defines a new mode of immune surveillance. Thus, "tumor escape from surveillance" may represent reversal of the feedback circuit of differentiation pressures, involving suppression of some regulatory lymphocytic populations as part of the change in the composition of the tissue. It may be sufficient for this suppression to be only local and limited in time, to allow for the acquisition of the malignant, differentiation-resistant phenotype.

It is likely that lymphocytes are more central to the regulation of lymphoid and hemopoietic tissues than to that of other cell systems. This is consistent with the observation that immmuno-suppression is more often associated with lymphomas and leukemias than with other cancers.

A prediction of the new concept of surveillance is that, even when disruption of the immune system is not an apparent cause of the disease, observable changes in the distribution and phenotype of T cells and NK cells may accompany the tumorigenic process. Situations in which a preleukemic state exists, or when there are predictable switches in the state of malignancy over time, may provide an opportunity to identify such changes and correlate them to the progression of the tumor. Such studies would optimally consist of a combination of multivariate flow cytometry and functional assays. An example of such a situation is the development of secondary acute leukemia in patients with multiple myeloma. An attempt to develop an animal model of this progression, to be studied along these lines, is presently underway (I. Witz, personal communication).

REFERENCES

Brooks, C. G., Urdal, D. L. and Henney, C. S. (1983). Lymhokine-driven "differentiation" of cytotoxic T-cell clones into cells with NK specificity: correlations with display of membrane macromolecules. Immunol Rev 72:43-72.
Burnet, F. M. (1964). Immunological factors in the process of carcinogenesis. Br Med Bull 20:154-158.
Burnet, F. M. (1971). Immunological surveillance in neoplasia. Transplant Rev 7:3-25.
Chang, L. J-A. and McCulloch, E. A. (1981). Dose-dependent effects of a tumor promotor on blast cell progenitors in human myeloblastic leukemia. Blood 57:361-367.
De Boer, R. J. and Hogeweg, P. (1985). Tumor escape from immune elimination: simplified precursor bound cytotoxicity models. J Theor Biol 113:719-736.

Foulds, L. (1969). Neoplastic Development. Academic Press, New York.

Grossman, Z. and Berke, G. (1980). Tumor escape from immune elimination. J Theor Biol 83:267.

Grossman, Z. and Herberman, R. B. (1982). Hypothesis on the development of natural killer cells and their relationship to T cells. In: Herberman, R. B. (Ed.), NK Cells and Other Natural Effector Cells, Academic Press, New York, pp. 229-238.

Grossman, Z. (1982). Recognition of self, balance of growth and competition: horizontal networks regulate immune responsiveness. Eur J Immunol 12:747-756.

Grossman, Z. (1984). Recognition of self and regulation of specificity at the level of cell populations. Immunol Rev 79:119-138.

Grossman, Z., Greenblatt, C. and Cohen, I. R. (1985). Parasite immunology and lymphocyte population dynamics. J Theor Biol, in press.

Grossman, Z. (1985a). On the nature of the dynamic processes leading to blast cell dominance in chronic myelocytic leukemia. Int J Mathematical Modelling, in press.

Grossman, Z. (1985b). A new approach to the evolution of the blastic crisis from chronic myelocytic leukemia: interplay of cellular alterations and a changing microenvironment. Submitted.

McCulloch, E. A., Smith, L. J. and Minden, M. D. (1982). Normal and malignant hemopoietic clones in man. Cancer Surv 1:279-298.

Motoji, T., Hoang, T., Tritchler, D. and McCulloch, E. A. (1985). The effect of 5-azacytidine and its analogues on blast cell renewal in acute myelocytic leukemia. Blood 65:894-901.

Rubin, H. (1984). Mutations and oncogenes - cause or effect. Nature 309:518.

Rubin, H. (1985). Cancer as a dynamic developmental disorder. Cancer Res 45:2935-2942.

Schrader, J. W. (1983). CRC Crit Rev Immunol 4:197-277.

Smith, K. A. and Cantrell, D. A. (1985). Interleukin 2 regulates its own receptors. Proc Natl Acad Sci USA 82:864-868.

Spooncer, E., Boettiger, D. and Dexter, T. M. (1984). Continuous *in vitro* generation of multi-potential stem cell clones from src-infected cultures. Nature 310:228-230.

Thomas, L. (1959). Reactions to homologous tissue antigens and relation to hypersensitivity. In: Cellular and Humoral Aspects of the Hypersensitive States (H. S. Lawrence, ed.). Hoeber, New York, pp. 529-532.

CYTOSTATIC FACTORS PRODUCED BY LYMPHOCYTES IN RESPONSE TO TUMOR CELLS

T.J. Sayers, J.H. Ransom,* A.C. Denn, III,
H.M. Shepard,° R.B. Herberman, and J.R. Ortaldo.
BTB, BRMP, DCT, NCI-FCRF, Frederick, MD 21701,
Litton Bionetics Inc.,* Rockville, MD 20850-4373,
and Genentech/Inc.,° San Francisco, CA 94080

INTRODUCTION

In recent years much interest has centered on proteins isolated from activated leukocytes which possess cytostatic activities against tumor cells in vivo and in vitro. Interferons (IFNs) (Gresser et al., 1978; Blalock et al., 1980), lymphotoxin (LT), (Evans and Heinbaugh, 1981), tumor necrosis factor (TNF), (Carswell et al., 1975) (TNF) and leukoregulin (LRG), (Ransom et al.,1985) have all been reported to exhibit growth inhibitory activity against various tumor cell lines. Furthermore, combinations of lymphokines can act synergistically giving greater growth-inhibition than either lymphokine alone (Williams and Bellanti, 1983).

We were interested in investigating whether cytostatic factors were released after the co-incubation of human lymphocytes with tumor cells. A cytolytic factor natural killer cell cytotoxic factor (NKCF), has been reported to be released during incubation of lymphocytes with tumor cell lines (Wright et al., 1983). However, as yet little information is available on whether other cytotoxic molecules are released in such cultures.

The cloning of the genes for IFNα, IFNγ, TNF, and LT into Eschericia coli has resulted in the availability of highly purified protein preparations which appear to have the biological activity identical to that of the natural material and are completely devoid of traces of other lymphokines. The availability of highly purified recombinant LT (rLT), TNF (rTNF), and IFN (rIFN) together with specific neutralizing antibodies allowed us to directly assess the growth inhibitory effects of these lymphokines and to investigate the array of factors released in the mixed tumor-lymphocyte cultures.

METHODS

Tumor-Lymphocyte Supernatants(TLS)

5×10^6 lymphocytes (nylon and plastic non-adherent) plus 1×10^5 K562 cells/ml were cultured for 24 hours at 37°C in Iscoves media supplemented with transferin, insulin, selenium and BSA. Supernatants were collected, filtered, concentrated, dialysed and stored frozen at -70°C.

Growth Inhibition Assay

1×10^4 cells per well plus dilutions of lymphokines were added together in Iscoves media plus supplements. Cells were cultured for 48 hours, and pulsed labeled with ^{3}H-thymidine (0.5uCi/well) for the last 8 hours.

TABLE 1. A Comparison of the Cytostatic Activities of Various Lymphokine Preparations Against a Range of Tumor Cells

Lymphokine preparation	Growth inhibition units*					
	K562	L929	Molt-4	MBL-2	YAC	RAJI
TLS	160	15	120	80	>135	24
LRG	800	11	80	20	>135	nd
r-LT	<5	3×10^6	<5	<5	<5	<5
r-TNF	<5	1×10^6	<5	<5	<5	<5

* The reciprocal of the dilution which gives 50% inhibition of ^{3}-H thymidine incorporation in the growth inhibition assay.

TABLE 2. Distinction of the Growth Inhibitory Effects of TLS and LRG from Those of IFNs.

Lymphokine preparation	Concentration	Antibody* to IFNα	IFNγ	%Cytostasis#
TLS	1:40	−	−	80
	1:40	+	+	76
IFNα	5000U/ML	−	−	42
	5000U/ML	+	−	26
	500U/ML	−	−	25
	500U/ML	+	−	2
IFNγ	5000U/ML	−	−	23
	5000U/ML	−	+	0

*Antibodies at a final concentration of 1000 neutralizing units/ml.
#Inhibition of ^{3}H-thymidine incorporation.

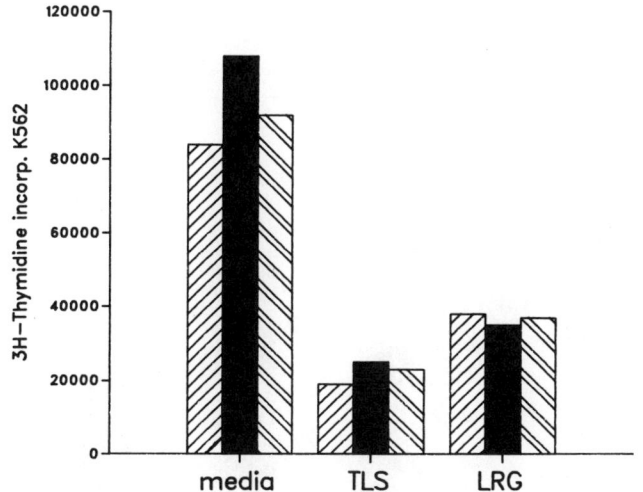

Fig.1. Effect of anti-LT and anti-TNF on TLS and LRG. TLS (1:20) and LRG (1:40) were pre-incubated for 1hr. with medium (▨), anti-LT (10 neutralizing units/ml.), (■), or anti-TNF (100nu/ml.) (▧).

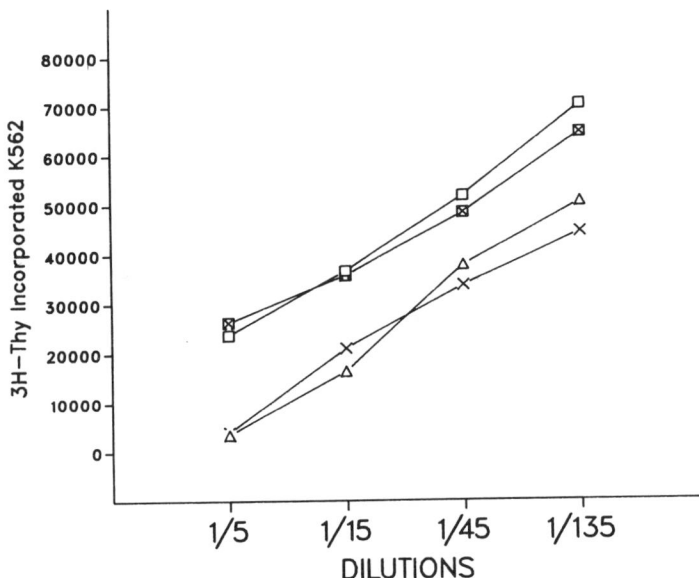

Fig.2. Effect of mannose-PO4 on LRG or TLS. TLS was pre-incubated with medium (X-X) or 10mM mannose PO4 (△-△) LRG was also pre-incubated with medium (□-□) or 10mM mannose PO4 (⊠-⊠).

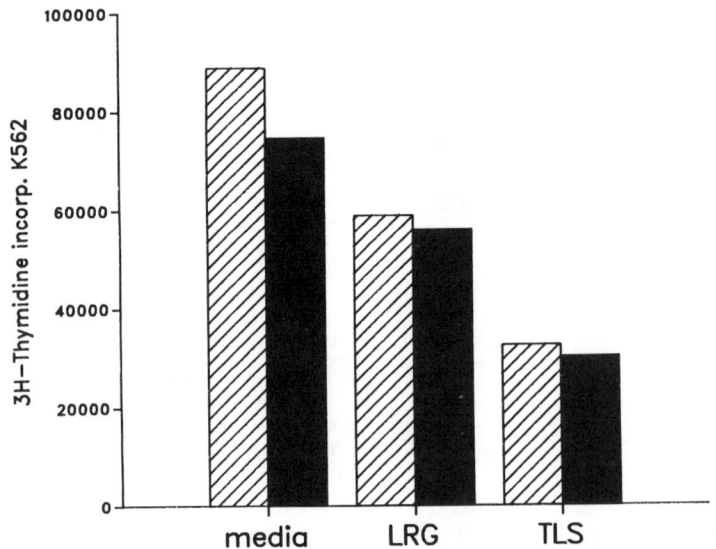

Fig.3. Inhibition by TLS or LRG after treatment with medium (▨) or anti-granule antibody (1:20) (■).

RESULTS

As shown in Table 1, K562, Molt-4, Raji, MBL-2 and YAC tumor cell lines were sensitive to growth inhibition by TLS or LRG preparations but were completely resistant to the effects of rLT or rTNF. In contrast, L929 were extremely sensitive to even very low levels of rLT or rTNF and relatively resistant to the effects of TLS or LRG. The growth inhibition observed was not due to IFN since K562 cells are only susceptible to very high levels of IFNs and antibodies to IFNs block the anti-proliferative effects of IFNs, but do not affect those of TLS or LRG (Table 2).

Since neutralizing antibodies to LT or TNF have no effect on the growth inhibitory activity of TLS or LRG (Fig.1) it seems that LT or TNF play no role either directly or indirectly in the anti-proliferative effects of TLS or LRG. Further, mannose-6-PO_4 or antibodies to rat cytolytic granules, both of which have been reported inhibit NKCF (Ortaldo et al., in press) have no effect on the cytostatic activity of TLS or LRG (Figs 2 and 3). Consequently NKCF is not involved in this cytostasis.

SUMMARY

Co-incubation of tumor cells with non-adherent lymphocytes leads to the production of factors which are cytostatic to a variety of tumor cell lines. IFNs, LT and TNF play no role in this growth inhibition since they appear to have a different spectrum of cytostatic activity and neutralizing antibodies to these lymphokines do not block the anti-proliferative effects of TLS. Furthermore, agents which are reported to inhibit NKCF are also without effect, ruling out an involvement of this factor in the observed cytostasis. However, in terms of target cell specificity, the observed cytostasis resembles that of the recently described lymphokine leukoregulin.

REFERENCES

Carswell EA, Old LJ, Kassel RL, Green S, Fiore N, Williamson B (1975). An endotoxin-induced serum factor that causes necrosis of tumors. Proc Natl Acad Sci USA 72:3666-3670.

Blalock JE, Georgiades JA, Langford NF, Johnson HM (1980). Purified human immune interferon has more potent anticellular activity than fibroblast or leukocyte interferon. Cell Immunol 49:390-394.

Evans CH, Heinbaugh JA (1981). Lymphotoxin cytotoxicity, a combination of cytolytic and cytostatic cellular responses. Immunopharmacol 3:347-359.

Gresser I, Tovey MG (1978). Antitumor effects of interferon. Biochim Biophys Acta 516:231-247.

Ortaldo JR, Blanca I, Herberman, RB.(in press). Studies of human natural killer cytotoxic factor (NKCF): Characterization and analysis of its mode of action. In: Mechanisms of Cytotoxicity by NK Cells. Orlando: Academic Press.

Ransom JH, Evans CH, McCabe RP, Pomato N, Heinbaugh JA, Chin M, Hanna MG (1985). Leukoregulin, a direct-acting anticancer immunological hormone that is distinct from lymphotoxin and interferon. Cancer Res 45:851-862.

Williams TW, Bellanti JA (1983). In vitro synergism between interferons and lymphotoxin: Enhancement of lymphotoxin-induced target cell killing. J Immunol 130:518-520.

Wright SC, Weitzen ML, Kahle R, Granger GA, Bonavida B (1983). Co-culture of human PBL with NK sensitive or resisant cell lines stimulates release of natural killer cell cytotoxic factors (NKCF) selectively cytotoxic to NK-sensitive target cells. J Immunol 130:2479-2483.

THE ROLE OF CYTOTOXINS IN MONOCYTE/MACROPHAGE TUMOR CYTOTOXICITY IN VITRO

Jim Klostergaard
Department of Tumor Biology, University of Texas,
M.D. Anderson Hospital and Tumor Institute,
Houston, Texas 77030

INTRODUCTION

The role that macrophages play in host defense against tumors was probably first noted by Gorer about 30 years ago (Gorer, 1956). Since then much evidence has been rendered from numerous investigators to support this role. Macrophages have been observed histologically infiltrating tumor allografts, chemical carcinogen-induced tumors, and tumor metastasis (Den Otter, 1972; Evans, 1972; Eccles and Alexander, 1974). Furthermore, suppression of host macrophage function increases the susceptibility to tumor induction or to tumor grafts (Allison et al., 1966; Keller, 1976; Nelson and Nelson, 1978). More recently it has been demonstrated in the rodent that in situ activation of macrophages, may prevent or eradicate metastatic lesions (Fidler, 1980; Lopez-Berestein, et al., 1984). Thus, macrophages may participate in a surveillance role against tumors, and are amenable to manipulation for immunotherapy of metastatic disease.

At the cellular level, the murine in vitro macrophage-mediated, nonspecific tumoricidal reaction may be divided into two distinct phases (Marino and Adams, 1980; Adams et al., 1982). The first involves recognition of and binding to the target cell by the effector. This is presumably mediated by a macrophage membrane receptor recognizing unique constituents or topographical distributions of components on the target plasma membrane. Aside from the selection of tumor targets in preference to normal targets, this recognition-binding phase appears to trigger the subsequent cascade of events, including further effector cell activation, manifest in the second phase of cytolysis:target-injury.

The cytotoxic interaction between activated macrophages and conjugated targets has been examined by a number of laboratories at the ultrastructural level. There are great discrepancies in these reports (Chambers and Weiser, 1972; Snodgrass and Hanna, 1973; Keller et al., 1976; Steward et al., 1976; Dingemans et al., 1981; Bucana et al., 1983), and only some have observed membrane destabilization and target vacuolation near the zone of contact with the effector cell. The latter are suggestive of effector cell deposition of a toxic substance on the target.

A number of molecular mechanisms have been proposed to account for the macrophage-mediated tumoricidal reaction. These differ in their requirements for effector-target conjugation during cytolysis. They include reductive cell division of the target (Kaplan et al., 1978), macrophage lysozomal exocytosis (Hibbs, 1974), inhibition of target cell mitochondrial respiration (Granger et al., 1980; Kilbourn et al., 1984), and a variety of secreted mediators: arginase(s) (Currie, 1978), oxygen metabolites (Nathan et al., 1979), thymidine (Stadecker et al., 1977), C3a (Ferluga et al., 1976), tumor necrosis factor (Carswell et al., 1975), neutral proteases (Adams et al., 1980; Reidarson et al., 1982a; Klostergaard et al., submitted), and several other cytotoxic factors (Matthews, 1981; Hammerstrom, 1982; Drysdale et al., 1983; Zacharchuk, 1983; Sone et al., 1984).

In attempting to resolve the cytolytic mechanism, a number of criteria can be utilized to implicate a particular mediator. The mediator should appear under conditions known to be associated with macrophage activation for cytolysis, and not appear when macrophages are incapable of cytolysis. Known inhibitors of the direct macrophage-mediated reaction should be used to probe their effects either on the appearance of or the activity of the candidate mediator. Conversely, inhibitors of the mediator, such as specific antibody, or inhibitors of its production or release offer probes for the direct cell-mediated reaction, with the understanding that the inhibitors may be ineffective for number of reasons under complex culture conditions or may be unable to influence events occuring in the space between the effector and conjugated target. A correlation between genetically controlled modulation of macrophage tumoricidal function and the level of the mediator may also provide evidence for its participation. Finally, effects of the mediator on tumor target cells should be correlated with the effects on target cells following coculture with activated macrophages.

It is imperative to recognize that even if a mediator plays a role, even the principal role, in the target-injury phase of cytolysis, its effects when delivered to the target via the fluid-phase (supernatant) may contrast with those observed in coculture (direct). Since the fluid-phase route entails a "bolus" and global exposure of the target to the mediator, this is clearly distinct from the solid-phase route operative in coculture, where the macrophage may present the mediator to the conjugated target in a circumscribed contact zone, and in a protracted and continuing fashion ("flux").

RESULTS AND DISCUSSION

Murine Macrophages

We have previously described (Reidarson, et al., 1982a,b) a lytic moiety, termed macrophage cytotoxin (MCT), obtained from inflammatory or alloimmune macrophages further triggered *in vitro*. MCT was rapidly released after triggering, and was bound to and lysed tumor cells in preference to normal cells *in vitro*, and in the presence of serum. Native MCT had an apparent molecular weight of ∽150kd as determined by molecular sieving, and its lytic activity could be blocked by inhibitors of trypsin like-proteases.

Earlier Adams and coworkers (Adams, et al., 1980) had reported similar results regarding a cytolytic factor (CF) or cytolytic protease (CP) derived from triggered inflammatory or BCG-activated macrophages. CP had a preferential lytic effect on tumor cells compared to normal cells, and was inhibited by a panel of neutral protease inhibitors. However, important distinctions between MCT and CP were noted in that the latter had a molecular weight of 40kd and its lytic activity could by blocked by serum in the lytic assay medium.

More recently, we have employed the BCG-activated macrophage as a model (Klostergaard, et al., submitted). These effector cells may be triggered by LPS, MDP derivatives, and PMA to rapidly release a cell-toxin termed cytolytic factor (CF). Synthesis/release of CF depended on transcription, translation, and an intact secretory apparatus. CF in our hands, in contrast to the reports of Adams and coworkers, had an apparent molecular weight of ~150kd, and its lytic activity was expressed to the same extent in medium containing fetal calf serum or in the medium of Neumann-Tytell. The lytic activity of CF could be blocked by reversible and inversible inhibitors of neutral proteases. Thus, MCT and CF appeared to be very similar biochemically and functionally and distinct from the CP reported by Adams with respect to molecular weight and activity in serum.

The recent cloning of murine TNF will allow a thorough comparison of it to MCT, CF, and a number of other cytotoxic mediators at the serological, peptide, and mRNA levels. Our own interets are to use antibody probes to CF and TNF to further characterize their possible role(s) in direct macrophage mediated tumor cytolysis at the level of blocking killing and to analyze the mechanism of lesion formation by immunoelectromicroscopy.

Over the past few years, Granger and collegues (Granger, et al., 1980; Granger and Lehininger, 1982) have extensively characterized one possible mechanism of macrophage-mediated tumor cytolysis involving inhibition of the function of the electron transport chain (ETC) of the target. We have recently described (Kilbourn, et al., 1984) a monokine, termed respiration inhibitory factor (RIF) which appears to mimick the macrophage itself in inflicting specific lesions in the ETC. RIF was heterogeneous with respect to molecular weight, with two species appearing at 55 and 80kd. Our results suggest that if CF and RIF are relevant to the cytotoxic reactions occuring in coculture, then it is possible to have a CF dependent pathway for lysis independent of inhibitory effects on the ETC; similarly, RIF-mediated effects on the ETC involve primarily cytostasis, and not cytolysis. Thus, these important cytotoxic pathways may be under distinct control by the macrophage.

Human Monocytes

The tumoricidal mechanism of human peripheral blood monocytes has been studied extensively; a number of laboratories have reported that these effector cells, when activated to a level at which they display cytotoxic functions in coculture, can release cytotoxic factors (Reed and Lucas, 1975; Matthews, 1981; Hammerstrom, 1982; Cameron, 1983; Sone, et al., 1984).

In our studies of the tumoricidal mechanism of peripheral blood monocytes, we have employed monocytes isolated by counterflow elutriation from normal donors undergoing plateletapheresis (Klostergaard, et al., submitted). These monocytes are isolated under conditions of exacting control for endotoxin contamination, are highly purified (>95% nonspecific esterase staining), and are functionally intact by a number of criteria (Lopez-Berestein, 1983). Adherent monocytes isolated from donors subjected to apheresis for the first time release moderate levels of toxin(s) when exposed for 4 hours to LPS, MDP derivatives or PMA. Synthesis/release of toxins could be blocked by actinomycin D, cycloheximide, and monensin. Further maturation with or without recombinant IFN-γ (rIFN-γ) lead to decreased LPS-responsiveness. In marked contrast, donors which had been subjected to recent apheresis were initially poorly responsive to LPS; responsiveness could be increased greatly by maturation in vitro for several days, followed by rIFN-γ treatment for 24 hr. Our interpretation is that apheresis involves demargination of the immature, rIFN-γ responsive monocytes, and that monocytes matured normally in vivo or immature monocytes matured in vitro with rIFN-γ are essentially equivalent with regard to tumor cytotoxicity and toxin production. Furthermore, the toxin produced by either type of monocyte is principally a beta form (60-70 kd) as determined by conventional or HPLC molecular sieving. The beta-toxin does not appear to be a neutral protease, nor is H_2O_2 or superoxide anion produced during target cell lysis. This toxin is cytotoxic for a number of human and murine tumor target cell lines in vitro.

Further characterization of the beta toxin suggests that it is serologically related to but distinct from recombinant human TNF (rHuTNF); the toxin is completely neutralized by an antiserum raised against rHuTNF, but much higher levels of serum are required than can neutralize an equivalent number of units of rHuTNF. Moreover, initial immunoprecipitation analysis employing an antiserum against rHuTNF reveals a major peptide in the 60-70 kd region, and no signal corresponding to the 17kd rHuTNF peptide is evident. Characterization of the beta-toxin is being continued.

Studies similar to those described above for the murine system on the role of TNF and the beta-toxin in human monocyte mediated tumor cytotoxicity are underway. Immunoelectronmicroscopic characterization of the localization of these mediators in the tumor cell, as well as biochemical characterization of the lytic lesion itself, should greatly deepen our understanding of the tumoricidal mechanism of human monocytes.

ACKNOWLEDGEMENTS

The author wish to thank Angelina Jones for her assistance in preparing this manuscript.

REFERENCES

Adams DO, Johnson WJ, Marino PA (1982). Mechansims of target recognition and destruction in macrophage-mediated cytotoxicity. Fed Proc 41:2212-2221.

Adams DO, Kao K-J, Farb R, Pizzo, SV (1980). Effector mechanisms of cytolytically activated macrophages. II. Secretion of a cytolytic factor by activated macrophages and its relationship to neutral protesses. J Immunol 124:293-300.

Allison AC, Harington JS, and Birbeck MJ (1966). An examination of the cytotoxic effects of silica on macrophages. J Exp Med 124:141.

Bucana C, Hoyer LC, Hobbes B, Bressman S, McDaniel M, Hanna MG Jr (1976). Morphologic evidence for the translocation of lysosomal organelles from cytotoxic macrophages into the cytoplasm of tumor target cells. Cancer Res 36:4444-4458.

Cameron, DJ (1983). Purified human macrophage secretions suppress tumor growth in the mouse. J Reticuloendothel Soc 34:45-52.

Carswell EA, Old LJ, Kassel RL, Green S, Fiore N, Williamson B (1975). An endotoxin-induced serum factor that caused necrosis of tumors. Proc Natl Acad Sci 72:3666-3670.

Chambers VC, Weiser RS (1972). The ultrastructure of sarcoma I cells and immune macrophages during their interaction in the peritoneal cavities of immune C57BL/6 mice. Cancer Res 32:413-420.

Currie GA (1978). Activated macrophages kill tumor cells by releasing arginase. Nature 273:758-759.

Den Otter W, Evans R, Alexander P (1972). Cytotoxicity of murine peritoneal macrophages in tumor allograft immunity. Transplantation 14:220-227.

Dingemans KP, Pels E, Den Otter W (1981). Destruction of murine lymphoma cells by allogeneic immune peritoneal macrophages in vitro: An ultrastructure study. J Natl Cancer Inst 66:67-74.

Drysdale B -E, Zacharchuk CM, Shin HS (1983). Mechanism of macrophage-mediated cytotoxicity: Production of soluble cytotoxic factor. J Immunol 131:2362-2365.

Eccles SA, Alexander P (1974). Macrophage content of tumors in relation to metastatic spread and host immune reaction. Nature 250:667-670.

Evans R (1972). Macrophages in syngeneic animal tumors. Transplantation 14:468-476.

Fergula J, Schorlemmer HU, Baptista LC, Allison AC (1978). Production of the complement cleavage product, C3a, by activated macrophages and its tumorlytic effects. Clin Expl Immunol 31:512-517.

Fidler IJ (1980). Therapy of spontaneous metastases by intravenous injection of liposomes containing lymphokines. Science 208:1469-1471.

Gorer PA (1956). Some recent work on tumor immunity. Adv Cancer Res 4:149-180.

Granger DL, Lehninger AL (1982). Sites of inhibition of mitochondrial electron transport in macrophage-injured neoplastic cells. J Cell Biol 95:527-538.

Granger DL, Taintor RR, Cook JL, Hibbs JB Jr (1980). Injury of neoplastic cells by murine macrophages leads to inhibition of mitochondrial respiration. J Clin Invest 65:357-370.

Hammerstrom J (1982). Soluble cytostatic factor(s) released from human macrophages. Scand J Immunol 15:311-318.

Hibbs JB Jr (1974). Heterocytolysis by macrophages activated by bacillus Calmette-Guerin: Lysosome exocytosis into tumor cells. Science 184:468-471.

Kaplan AM, Brown J, Collins JM, Morahan PS, Snodgrass MJ (1978). Mechanisms of macrophage-mediated tumor cell cytotoxicity. J Immunol 121:1781-1789.

Keller R, Bregnard A, Gehring WJ, Schroeder HE (1976). Morphologic and molecular changes in target cells during in vitro interaction with macrophages. Exp Cell Biol 44:108-120.

Keller R, (1976). Susceptibility of normal and transformed cell lines to cytostatic and cytocidal effects exerted by macrophages. J Natl Cancer Inst 56:369-374.

Kilbourn RG, Klostergaard J, Lopez-Berestein G (1984). Activated macrophages secrete a soluble factor that inhibits mitochondrial respiration of tumor cells. J Immunol 133:2577-2581.

Lopez-Berestein G, Milas L, Hunter N, Mehta K, Hersh EM, Kurahara CG, Vanderpas M, Eppstein DA (1984). Prophylaxis and treatment of experimental lung metastasis in mice after treatment with liposome-encapsulated 6-0-stearoyl-N-acetylmuramyl-L-α-aminobutyryl-D-isoglutamine. Clin Exp Metastasis 2:127-137.

Lopez-Berestein G, Reuben J, Hersh EM, Kilbourn RG, Hester JP, Bielski M, Talpaz M, Mavligit GM (1983). Comparative functional analysis of lymphocytes and monocytes from plateletapheresis. Transfusion 23:201-206.

Marino PA, Adams DO (1980). Interaction of bacillus Calmette-Guerin-activated macrophages and neoplastic cells in vitro II. The relationship of selective binding to cytolysis. Cell Immunol 54:26-35.

Matthews N (1981). Production of anti-tumor cytotoxin by human monocytes. Immunology 44:135-142.

Nathan CF, Silverstein SC, Brukner LH, Cohn ZA (1979). Extracellular cytolysis by activated macrophages and granulocytes. II. Hydrogen peroxide as a mediator of cytotoxicity. J Exp Med 149:100-113.

Nelson M, Nelson DS, (1978). Macrophages and reistance to tumors. Influence of agents affecting macrophages and delayed-type hypersensitivity on resistance to tumors inducing concomitant immunity. Aust J Exp Biol Med Sci 56:211-218.

Reed WP, Lucas ZJ (1975). Cytotoxic activity of lymphocytes. V. Role of soluble toxin in macrophage-inhibited culture of tumor cells. J Immunol 115:395-404.

Reidarson TH, Granger GL, Klostergaard J (1982a). Inducible macrophage cytotoxins. II. Tumor lysis mechanism involving target cell-binding proteases. J Natl Cancer Inst 69:889-894.

Reidarson TH, Levy WE, Klostergaard J, Granger GA, (1982b). Inducible macrophage cytotoxins. I. Biokinetics of activation and release in vitro. J Natl Cancer Inst 69:879-888.
Stadecker M, Calderon J, Karnovsky M, Unanue E, (1977). Synthesis and release of thymidine by macrophages. J Immunol 119:1738-1743.
Steward CC, Adles C, Hibbs JB Jr (1975). Interactions of macrophages with tumor cells. Adv Exp Med Biol 73B:423-430.
Sone S, Tachibana K, Ishii K, Ogawara M, Tsubura E (1984). Production of a tumor cytolytic factor(s) by activated human alveolar macrophages and its action. Cancer Res 44:646-651.
Snodgrass MJ, Hanna MG Jr (1973). Ultrastructural studies of histiocyte-tumor cell interactions during tumor regression after intralesional injection of Mycobacterium bovis. Cancer Res 33:701-712.
Zacharchuk CM, Drysdale BE, Mayer MM, Shin HS (1983). Macrophage mediated cytotoxicity:Role of soluble macrophage cytotoxic factor similar to lymphotoxin and tumor necrosis factor. Proc Natl Acad Sci USA 80:6341-6345.

CHEMOIMMUNOTHERAPY OF ADVANCED MURINE RENAL CARCINOMA

R.R. Salup and R.H. Wiltrout*

Program Resources Incorporated, Frederick Cancer Research Facility and Biological Therapeutics Branch*, Biological Response Modifiers Program, DCT, NCI, Frederick, MD 21701

To date the application of immunotherapy to the treatment of human cancer has achieved only modest success. This may be partially a result of experimental tumor models which often bear little similarity to the progression and anatomical distribution of clinical malignancies. However, there is now conclusive evidence that adoptive immunotherapy with specific (Cheever, MA, et al., 1981) or non-specific (Mulé, JJ, et al., 1984) cytotoxic cells can be successful for the treatment of microscopic metastatic cancer. Therefore, it is imperative to investigate the therapeutic potential of adoptive immunotherapy in an experimental animal tumor model which mimicks as closely as possible the natural history and stage progression of clinical human cancer. The present study presents our experience with adoptive chemoimmunotherapy of a murine renal carcinoma (Renca), which grows progressively in a manner analogous to the clinical course of adult type human renal carcinoma.

MATERIALS AND METHODS

Animals

Inbred male and female BALB/C mice were obtained from the Animal Production Area, NCI-Frederick Cancer Research Facility, Frederick, MD, and were routinely used at 7 to 10 weeks of age.

Tumor Cell Lines

A renal adenocarcinoma of spontaneous origin (Renca) in BALB/C mice (7) was kindly provided to us by Drs. E.J. Pontes and G.P. Murphy (Roswell Park Memorial Institute, Buffalo, NY). The tumor was maintained in vivo by serial intrarenal passage and single cell suspensions obtained as previously described (Salup, RR, et al., 1985a). Renca was routinely injected under the capsule of the left kidney. Tumor growth and metastases formation were monitored and confirmed histologically at various intervals thereafter. YAC-1 was used as the reference target for NK activity and was maintained in continuous in vitro culture in complete medium (Wiltrout, RH, et al., 1984).

Reagents

Doxorubicin hydrochloride (DOX) was purchased from Sigma Chemical Co. (St. Louis, Mo.). The in vitro sensitivity of Renca to DOX was assessed as previously described (Salup, RR, Wiltrout, RH, 1985b). Human recombinant interleukin 2 (rIL-2) was kindly provided by Dr. J. Schindler of Biogen, Inc. (Cambridge, MA) and contained 8.5×10^5 units of IL-2/mg of protein (units defined by ^{3}H-thymidine incorporation into the CTLL-2 cell line).

Generation of Effector Cells

Cytotoxic lymphocytes were obtained by incubation of unseparated splenocytes for 24 hours with various concentrations of rIL-2, at 2.5×10^6 cells/ml in RPMI 1640 medium (M.A. Bioproducts, Walkersville, MD), supplemented with 10% fetal calf serum, 5×10^{-5}M 2-mercaptoethanol, 1 μm sodium pyruvate (Gibco Laboratories, Grand Island, NY), 0.1 mM of nonessential amino acids (Gibco), 300 μg/ml L-glutamine, 50 μg/ml gentamycin (Schering Co., Kenilworth, NJ). Aliquots of these rIL-2-stimulated cytotoxic lymphocytes (CL) were routinely tested for cytotoxicity in vitro.

Experimental Design and Statistics

All experimental groups consisted of at least 10 mice. The observation time was at least three months after completed therapy. Each experiment was performed at least two times. Statistical analyses were performed by chi-square test.

RESULTS

Growth and Stage Progression of Intrarenal Renca.

Inoculation of 1×10^5 tumor cells under the capsule of the left kidney gave consistent and predictable numbers of metastases to abdominal lymph nodes, liver and lungs. As shown in Table 1, the progression of Renca can be classified by stages which mimick those of clinical, adult type renal carcinoma (Glenn, JF, 1979). The tumor remains contained by the organ capsule during the first 14 days post inoculation (stage I), then invades through the renal capsule into the

Table 1: Progression of Tumor Growth Following Intrarenal Implantation of Renca*

Days post tumor inoculation	Locoregional invasion	Lymph node metastases	Organ metastases	Stage
< 14	−	−	−	I
> 15	+	−	−	II
> 21	+	+	−	III
> 24	+	+	+	IV

*Tumor inoculation consisted of injection of 1×10^5 Renca cells under the capsule of the left kidney.

perirenal tissue (third week, stage II). The first microscopic lymph node metastases can be detected about 21 days after tumor inoculation (stage III) and, finally, the first distant metastases can be detected histologically by 24 days (stage IV). Without therapy, the mean survival time of Renca-bearing mice is 46 $\pm$ 3 days. This progression of Renca through distinct stages makes intrarenal Renca an extremely relevent and therapeutically challenging experimental model for renal cancer.

Therapy of Established (stage I) Renca:

In order to evaluate the therapeutic potential of adoptive immunotherapy (AIT) and/or chemotherapy in this tumor model, we first attempted to treat mice bearing one week old, stage I Renca. As shown in Fig. 1, i.v. chemotherapy with DOX alone cured only 17% of the tumor-bearing mice. Similarly, adoptive immunotherapy with rIL-2 activated CL administered i.v. together with rIL-2 only moderately increased the mean survival time, but did not cure Renca-bearing mice. In contrast, the combination of i.v. DOX and AIT with activated CL and rIL-2 (ACIT) significantly ($p<0.01$) increased the incidence of cures to 67%.

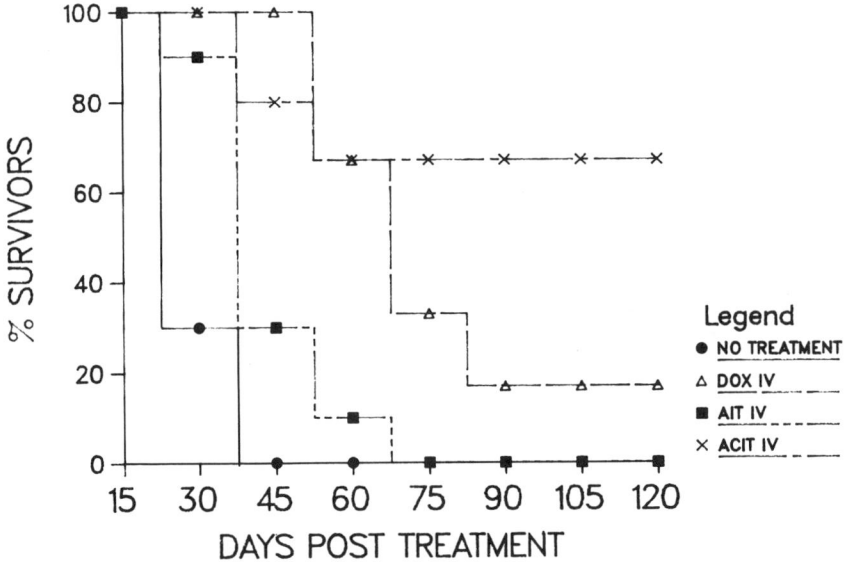

Figure 1. Therapy of stage I Renca. DOX (8 mg/kg B.W.) was administered i.v. on the 7th day following intrarenal tumor cell inoculation. AIT, consisting of 3.5×10^7 CL and 10.000 UrIl-2 were administered i.v. daily from day 8 to day 10.

Therapy of Invasive (stage II) Renca

Based on the encouraging results of ACIT for stage I Renca, we applied the same i.v. ACIT protocol to mice with 15 day old, stage II disease. Although we obtained some prolongation in mean survival time, this therapy regimen failed to cure mice bearing stage II Renca, with many mice exhibiting extensive carcinomatous growth in the peritoneal cavity upon autopsy (data not shown). Since, stage II Renca consists of a fairly large primary tumor (average diameter 11 mm) and invasive growth in the perirenal tissue, we postulated that the efficacy of ACIT might be enhanced by performing nephrectomy (N.E.) of the tumor bearing organ prior to initiation of the ACIT. We also administered ACIT intraperitoneally (i.p.) in order to control post-surgical minimal residual peritoneal disease. As shown in Fig. 2, N.E. followed by bicompartmental (i.v. plus i.p.) ACIT cured 80% of mice with stage II Renca. In contrast N.E. followed by

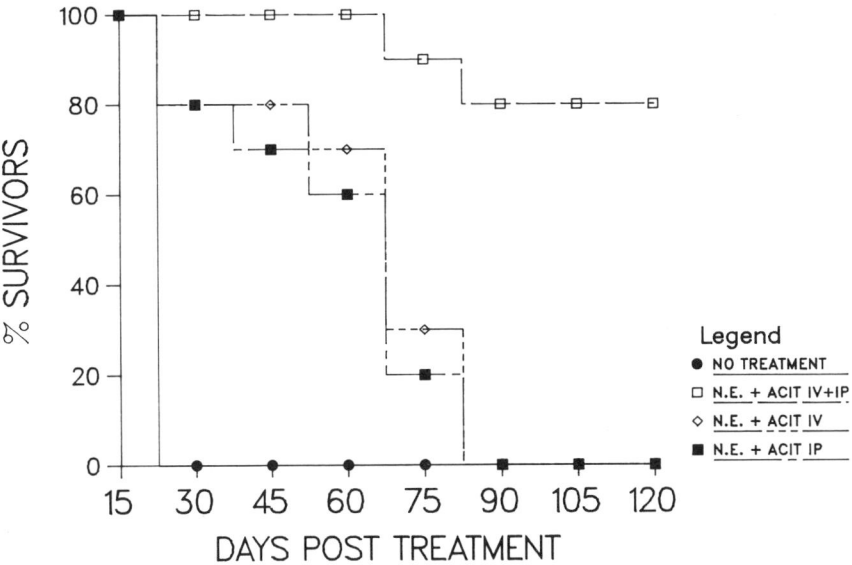

Fig. 2. Therapy of stage II Renca. Nephrectomy and chemotherapy (i.v. and/or i.p.) were performed on day 15 following tumor inoculation. AIT was administered i.v. and/or i.p. on day 16 to 18.

either i.v. or i.p. ACIT as well as bicompartmental i.v. and i.p. ACIT in the absence of N.E. failed to cure the mice (data not shown). Therefore, tumor reductive surgery, together with ACIT administration to local, regional or disseminated tumor foci can provide cures for invasive (stage II) Renca.

DISCUSSION

Recent evidence that natural cell-mediated cytotoxicity against tumors can be augmented by BRMs, and that these BRMs can have antitumor effects in experimental animals, have focused interest on the therapeutic potential of cell-mediated antitumor immunity against tumors (Herberman, RR, 1982). Similarly, progress in the methodology of in vitro generation and/or expansion of nonspecific (Mulé, JJ., et al., 1984) and specific (Cheever, MA, et al., 1981, Eberlein, TJ, et al., 1982.) CL has raised the possibility that the adoptive transfer of such cells into tumor bearing animals may be useful in treating established tumors. The availability of large amounts of pure rIL-2 has allowed the generation of sufficient numbers of CL for initiation of adoptive immunotherapy protocols in experimental animals (Mulé, JJ, et al., 1984). Minimal local or metastatic cancer can be controlled by adoptive transfer of specific (Cheever, MA, et al., 1981, Eberlein, TJ, et al., 1982) or non-specific (Mulé, JJ, et al., 1984) CL. Further, simultaneous administration of exogeneous IL-2 significantly improved the therapeutic success rate of both specific or nonspecific AIT (Cheever, MA, et al., 1982, Mulé, JJ, et al., 1984). We have extended these findings by utilizing nonspecific AIT in conjunction with chemotherapeutic drugs for the therapy of murine renal cancer. This model has the advantage of not being dependent on tumor specific antigens, which have not been clearly demonstrated in humans. Further, the association of AIT with chemotherapy and surgery is more analogous to the treatment of cancer in humans. In addition, these therapeutic modalities can be applied to various stages of tumor growth which mimick disease progression in humans (Glenn, JF, 1979).

Previous studies have demonstrated that Renca is lysed by NK cells from mice treated by biological response modifiers (BRMs) and modulation of the hosts' NK activity significantly influences metastasis formation following intrarenal inoculation of tumor cells (Salup, RR, et al., 1985a). Similarly, unsensitized splenocytes became quite cytotoxic for Renca following culture in rIL-2 (Salup, RR, et al., 1985b). In the present studies we have shown that the I.V. administration of such CL into mice bearing one week old, established intrarenal Renca, was curative for most (67%) of the mice only when preceeded by i.v. chemotherapy (Fig. 1). These data support previous observations that AIT is most efficient against minimal disease (Cheever, MA, et al., 1981, Cheever, MA, et al., 1982, Eberlein, TJ, et al., 1982, Mulé, JJ, et al., 1984). Therefore, we conclude that for established stage I tumors ACIT is an effective form of therapy. The need for tumor reduction prior to adoptive immunotherapy is illustrated by our experience with stage II, loco-regional, Renca. At this stage, cytoreductive surgery (N.E.) is imperative prior to successful ACIT. Furthermore, since stage II cancer includes extrarenal tumor in the abdominal cavity, inclusion of the i.p. compartment in the ACIT administration protocol is necessary to assure cure of the disease. These results demonstrate that successful treatment of disseminated cancer requires the delivery of ACIT to all tumor foci. We are currently evaluating the potential of this therapeutic concept for advanced stages (III and IV) of murine renal carcinoma, and studying the mechanism by which AIT and chemotherapeutic drugs complement each other in cancer treatment.

REFERENCES

Cheever, MA, Greenberg, PD, Fefer, A (1981). Specific adoptive therapy of established leukemia with syngeneic lymphocytes sequentially immunized in vivo and in vitro and unspecifically expanded by culture with interleukin 2. J Immunol 126:1318-1322.

Cheever, MA, Greenberg, PD, Fefer, A, Gillis, S (1982). Augmentation of the anti-tumor therapeutic efficacy of long-term cultured T lymphocytes by in vivo administration of purified interleukin 2. J Exp Med 155:968-980.

Eberlein, TJ, Rosenstein, M, Rosenberg, SA (1982). Regression of a disseminated syngeneic solid tumor by systemic transfer of lymphoid cells expanded in interleukin 2. J Exp Med 156:385-397.

Glenn, JF (1979). Renal tumors. In "Campbell's Urology, 4th Edition," Philadelphia: W.B. Saunders Co., pp. 967-1009.

Herberman, RB (1982). "NK Cells and Other Natural Effector Cells." New York: Academic Press.

Mulé, JJ, Shu, S, Schwarz, SL, Rosenberg, SA (1984). Adoptive immunotherapy of established pulmonary metastases with LAK cells and recombinant interleukin 2. Science 225:1487-1489.

Murphy, GP, Hrushesky, WJ (1973). A murine renal cell carcinoma. JNCI 50:1013-1025.

Salup, RR, Herberman, RB, Wiltrout, RH (1985a). Role of natural killer activity in development of spontaneous metastases in murine renal cancer. J. Urol. In press.

Salup, RR, Wiltrout, RH (1985b). Role of NK cells and IL-2 generated activated killer cells in prophylaxis and therapy of murine renal carcinoma. Proceedings of AACR, 1250.

Wiltrout, RH, Mathieson, BJ, Talmadge, JE, Reynolds, CW, Zhang, SR, Herberman, RB, Ortaldo, JR (1984). Augmentation of organ-associated NK activity by biological response modifiers: J Exp Med 160:1431-1449.

TUMOUR-INDUCED SUPPRESSION OF CELL-MEDIATED IMMUNITY: SELECTIVE EFFECTS ON LYMPHOKINE PRODUCTION AND LYMPHOCYTE TRANSFORMATION AND INDEPENDENCE OF CYCLOPHOSPHAMIDE-SENSITIVE SUPPRESSOR CELLS

Lesley C. McIntosh, Lora M. Morrice, Yasuhiro Udagawa and Angus W. Thomson

Department of Pathology, University of Aberdeen, Aberdeen Royal Infirmary, Foresterhill, Aberdeen AB9 2ZD, Scotland, G.B.

INTRODUCTION

Tumour development and related soluble products have been shown to depress various aspects of cell-mediated immunity (CMI) including delayed-type hypersensitivity (DTH) responses (Nelson et al., 1981). This depression may occur by induction of suppressor cells including the T suppressor (T_s) cell (Naor, 1979), the precursors of which may be eliminated by high dose cyclophosphamide (Cy; Turk and Parker, 1982). Whilst tumour induced splenic T_s cells may mediate inhibition of interleukin production (Burger et al., 1984), there is little published information on the influence of tumour carriage on production of lymphokines affecting macrophage behaviour. We have previously reported the ability of the Landschütz ascites carcinoma (LAC) to inhibit various macrophage responses in vivo and in vitro (McIntosh et al., 1982; McIntosh and Thomson, 1984).

The present study was initiated to determine whether suppression of DTH by tumour carriage (1) is independent of Cy-sensitive suppressor cells, (2) is also found in normal animals upon administration of soluble tumour-associated factors, (3) is mediated through inhibition of lymphocyte transformation and (4) involves altered production of the lymphokines macrophage procoagulant-inducing factor (MPIF) and lymphocyte-derived chemotactic factor (LDCF).

MATERIALS AND METHODS

DTH responses in saline or Cy-pretreated, (200 mg/kg, i.p., day -2) CD1, female mice to sheep red blood cells (SRBC) and ovalbumin were determined as described previously (Thomson et al., 1983 a,b). At the time of immunisation (day 0) appropriate groups also received either saline or 10^6 LAC cells (lactate dehydrogenase-elevating virus and mycoplasma free) i.p. Some antigen preparations for foot-pad challenge also contained various concentrations of cell-free ascitic fluid (AF), day 11 tumour-bearer serum (TBS) or normal mouse serum (NMS).

Pooled spleen cell populations were obtained from mice that had been immunised with 10^6 SRBC 4 days previously. The ability of these cells to respond to various mitogens (see Fig. 1 legend) was assessed by their ability to incorporate $[^3H]$-thymidine and to produce the lymphokines MPIF and LDCF. The following stimulants were used for the indicated period of time, in order to produce lymphokine-containing spleen culture supernatants: concanavalin A (Con A, 2 µg/ml, 24 h); phytohaemagglutinin (PHA, 10 µg/ml, 48 and 72 h) and SRBC (4 and 6%, 72 h). Results of MPIF-induced procoagulant activity expressed in thromboplastin units (U) as the mean ± 1S.D. of triplicate cultures in the 1-stage clotting assay. LDCF activity (at 33% dilution) was expressed as the total number of migrated macrophages on the lower surface of the filter, per 10 fields of vision (using x 400 overall magnification), with mean ± 1S.D. for triplicate wells. Endotoxin-activated mouse serum (EAMS) was used as a positive control in the microchemotaxis system. Peritoneal exudate cells (PEC), obtained 5 days after 1.4 mg killed C.parvum i.p., were used as indicator cells in the MPIF and LDCF assay. Experimental details of these procedures can be found elsewhere (Thomson et al., 1983 c).

RESULTS

In both saline and Cy-pretreated mice the presence of growing tumour or tumour-associated products (50% dilution of AF and 20% TBS) significantly depressed the DTH reaction to antigen (SRBC and ovalbumin) at 24 and 48 h (60-100% inhibition, $p < 0.01$ using the Mann Whitney U-test). NMS exhibited no suppressive effects at these concentrations.

This inhibition was evident despite an enhanced DTH response (> 2.5 fold at 48 h, p < 0.01) following Cy treatment of normal animals.

A marked decrease in the proliferative responses to all stimulants was demonstrated by splenic lymphocytes from tumour-bearing mice pretreated with saline (36-74% depression, comparing group B with A) or Cy (26-61% depression, comparing group D with C) as shown in Fig. 1. The observed differences are outwith the 9% intra-experimental variation inherent in the assay.

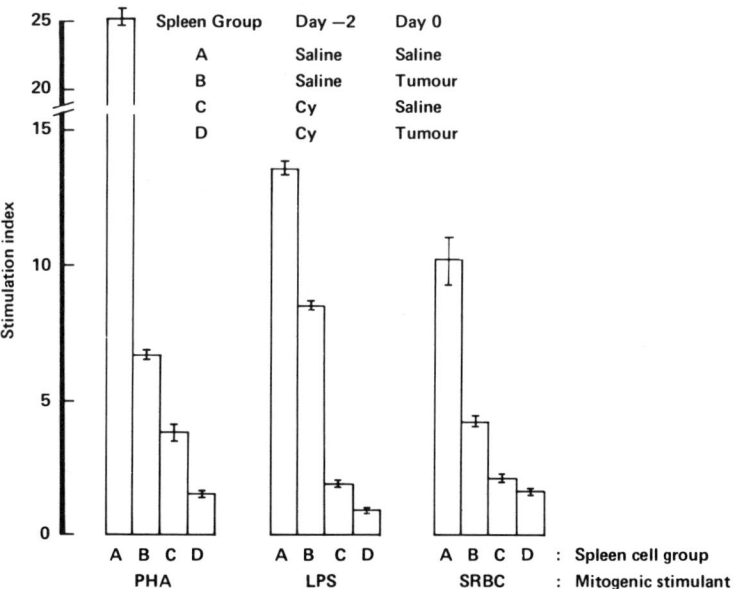

Figure 1. Mitogenic response of SRBC-sensitised mouse spleen cells to PHA (5 μg/ml), E.coli-lipopolysaccharide (LPS; 10 μg/ml) and SRBC (2%).

The suppressive effect of the growing tumour on MPIF production was evident in saline (14-43% reduction; comparing group B with A) and Cy-pretreated (30-42% reduction; comparing group D with C) mice (Fig. 2). The observed differences are outwith the 4% intraexperimental variation inherent in the assay.

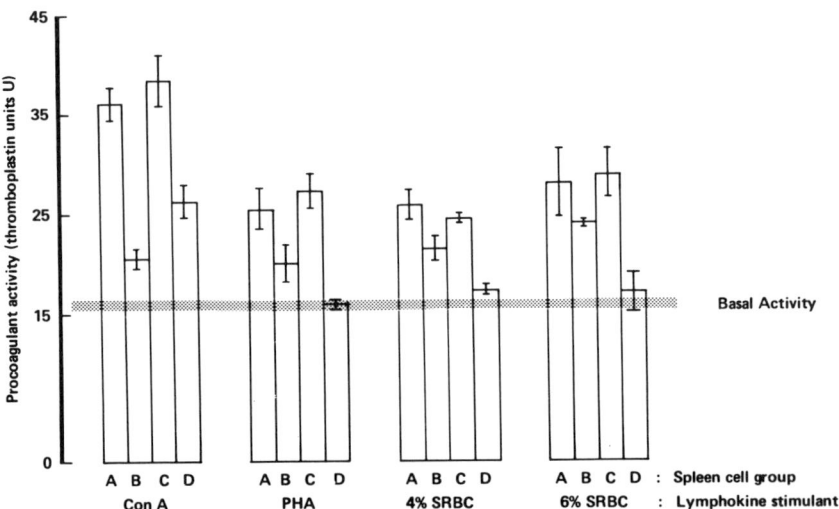

Figure 2. MPIF-induced procoagulant activity of washed PEC after incubation with lymphokine supernatants (20%, 4 x 10^6 cells/ml, 37°C, 4 h) produced by spleen cells of normal (A, C) and tumour-bearing (B,D) mice. Groups C and D received Cy. Basal activity indicates the response of washed PEC following incubation with medium containing no lymphokine.

In saline-pretreated animals, the tumour did not affect production of LDCF by spleen cells stimulated with PHA and indeed increased lymphokine activity (> 2 fold, compared to mice receiving saline alone) was observed with Con A as the stimulant. In contrast, the tumour did reduce the amount of lymphokine produced in response to immunising antigen (25-30% reduction). This finding is contrary to the suppressive effect of the tumour on both lymphocyte transformation and the production of MPIF to all stimulants tested.

In Cy-pretreated, tumour-bearing mice however, inhibition of LDCF production (17-46% reduction, comparing Group D with C) was evident with both mitogen (Fig. 3a) and antigen (Fig. 3b). As observed with the other lymphokine, MPIF, unstimulated cells produced no LDCF activity in the culture supernatant and Cy pretreatment alone (group C) had no effect on production of this lymphokine when compared to saline pretreatment (group A). The observed differences are outwith the 8% intraexperimental variation inherent in the assay.

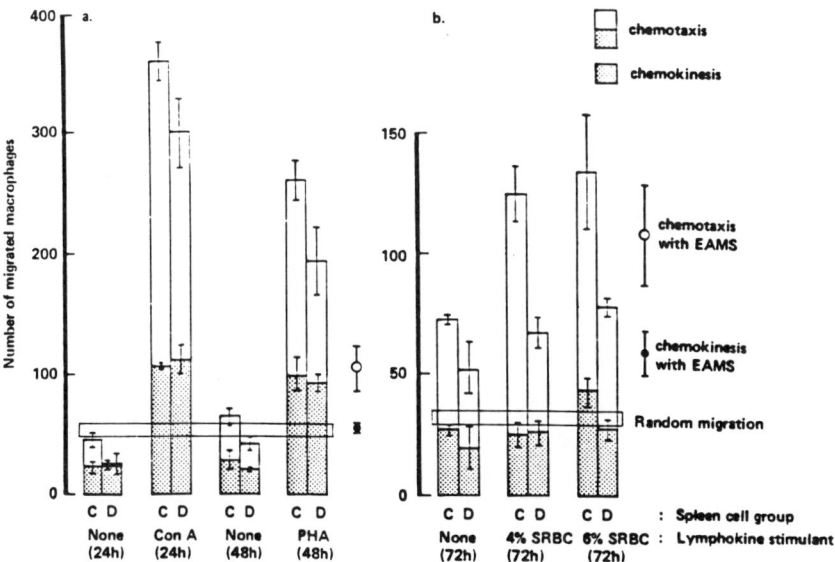

Figure 3. LDCF activity of 24-72 h culture supernatants from SRBC-sensitised spleen cells from mice pretreated with Cy also receiving saline (C) or tumour (D).

CONCLUSIONS

In this study we have shown that, at a time when DTH responses were suppressed in tumour bearing mice, splenic T lymphocytes exhibited decreased proliferative responses to antigen and mitogen and compromised production of the lymphokines LDCF and MPIF. The capacity of B cells to respond to LPS was also impaired. These observations were made both in animals with an intact immune system at the time of immunisation and in those in which suppressor cell precursors had been eliminated by high dose Cy. The only departure from this phenomenon was the failure of tumour carriage in normal mice to impair LDCF production in response to non-specific mitogens.

Our results imply that impaired production/function of lymphokines affecting macrophage behaviour may play a key role in tumour-induced suppression of CMI and that this inhibition is independent of Cy-sensitive suppressor cells. The role and nature of soluble tumour-associated factors in these events requires to be further investigated.

REFERENCES

Burger CJ, Elgert KD, Farrar WL (1984). Interleukin 2 (IL-2) activity during tumour growth: IL-2 production kinetics, absorption of and responses to exogenous IL-2. Cell Immunol 84: 228-239.

McIntosh LC, Pugh-Humphreys RGP, Fraser RA, Thomson AW (1982). Inhibition by the Landschütz ascites carcinoma of the granulomatous inflammatory response to C.parvum. Br. J Cancer 45: 598-612.

McIntosh LC, Thomson AW (1984). Effects of soluble mediators generated during growth of the Landschütz ascites carcinoma on the chemotaxis of normal and Corynebacterium parvum-stimulated peritoneal leucocytes. Br J exp Path 65: 441-451.

Nelson DS, Nelson M, Farram E, Inoue Y (1981). Cancer and subversion of host defences. Aust J exp Biol Med Sci 59: 229-262.

Naor D (1979). Suppressor cells: permitters and promotors of malignancy? Adv Cancer Res 29: 45-125.

Thomson AW, Nelson DS, Moon DK (1983a). Augmentation of delayed-type hypersensitivity reactions to ovalbumin by cyclophosphamide in the mouse: strain variability, antigen specificity and nature of the suppressor cell. Annal Immunol 134: 267-275.

Thomson AW, Moon DK, Nelson DS (1983b). Suppression of delayed-type hypersensitivity reactions and lymphokine production by cyclosporin A in the mouse. Clin exp Immunol 52: 599-606.

Thomson AW, Moon DK, Geczy CL, Nelson DS (1983c). Cyclosporin A inhibits lymphokine production but not the responses of macrophages to lymphokines. Immunol 48: 291-299.

Turk JH, Parker D (1982). Effects of cyclophosphamide on immunological control mechanisms. Immunol Rev 65: 99-113.

Section X. Thymocyte Development

PHENOTYPIC PROPERTIES AND IN VITRO GROWTH OF IMMATURE Lyt-2⁻/L3T4⁻ THYMOCYTES

Rh. Ceredig and H.R. MacDonald

John Curtin School of Medical Research, Canberra Australia (Rh.C) and Ludwig Institute for Cancer Research, Lausanne, Switzerland (HRMcD).

INTRODUCTION

The mouse thymus initially develops as an aggregation of ectodermal and endodermal epithelial elements derived from the third pharyngeal pouch. By about the 11th day of fetal development, this epithelial structure is colonized by blood-bourne hematopoietic cells which then start to proliferate and differentiate to generate the various subpopulations of thymocytes seen in the adult animal (Owen et al., 1981).

Using a combination of flow microflurometry (FMF) and monoclonal antibodies (mAb) to Lyt-2 and L3T4, we have identified at least four subpopulations of thymocytes in the mouse and have determined their ontogenic appearance in the developing thymus (Ceredig et al., 1983). The majority (80%) express both Lyt-2 and L3T4 (Lyt-2⁺/L3T4⁺) being comprised of 20% large cycling and 60% small non-cycling cells. Some (15%) thymocytes share phenotypic properties with peripheral T cells and express either Lyt-2 (Lyt-2⁺/L3T4⁻, 5%) or L3T4 (Lyt-2⁻/L3T4⁺, 10%) in a mutually exclusive fashion. A rare subpopulation (2-3%) express neither Lyt-2 nor L3T4 (Lyt-2⁻/L3T4⁻). Based on the fact that such Lyt-2⁻/L3T4⁻ cells are the first to appear in the developing thymus (Ceredig et al., 1983), can differentiate to Lyt-2⁺/L3T4⁺ cells in vitro (Fowlkes et al., 1984, Ceredig et al., 1985) and can reconstitute in vivo all other thymocyte subpopulations, it was decided to study their phenotypic and in vitro growth requirements in further detail.

Using FMF and a panel of mAb to mouse cell surface antigens Lyt-2$^-$/L3T4$^-$ cells, obtained by negative selection using a cocktail of αLyt-2 and αL3T4 IgM mAb plus complement, were clearly heterogeneous. Whereas all cells were H-2K bright and T200$^+$, only 85% were Thy-1$^+$. Expression of Lyt-1 was heterogeneous with 15% being Lyt-1 bright. With Mel-14 (Gallatin et al., 1983), 80% stained at levels comparable to so-called Mel-14 high thymocytes, a phenotype originally thought to be characteristic of cells about to migrate from the thymus (Reichert et al., 1984). Biphasic staining was obtained with two other mAb, namely M1-69 (Springer et al., 1978) directed at the heat stable antigen present on most hematopoietic cells and anti-Pgp-1 (Trowbridge et al., 1982), an antigen normally found on bone marrow cells and B lymphocytes.

We (Ceredig et al., 1985a) and others (Raulet 1985, Takacs 1984) have recently observed that about 50% of Lyt-2$^-$/L3T4$^-$ thymocytes stained with mAb directed against the IL-2 receptor. Although it was recently reported that such cells proliferated when cultured in purified IL-2 (Raulet 1985) we have failed to confirm this. The lack of proliferation of cells cultured in IL-2 alone was not surprising in view of the finding that the affinity for ligand of the IL-2 receptor on Lyt-2$^-$/L3T4$^-$ thymocytes was 5-10-fold lower than that on T cell clones and polyclonally-activated T cells (Ceredig et al., 1985a).

Since only Lyt-2$^-$/Lt34$^-$ thymocytes spontaneously expressed IL-2 receptors, the anatomical location of such cells within the thymus could be determined. Thus by immunoperoxidase staining, positive cells were scattered throughout the thymus being found in subscapular, cortical and medullary areas (Ceredig et al., 1985a). The apparently random distribution of IL-2-receptor positive Lyt-2$^-$/L3T4$^-$ cells throughout the thymus confirmed our previous unpublished immunohistochemical studies of normal thymuses stained with αLyt-2 or αL3T4 mAb in which a distinct subcapsular zone of cells lacking Lyt-2 or L3T4 was not found. Furthermore, in an immunohistochemical study of the regenerating thymus in radiation bone marrow chimeras (Ceredig et al., 1984), early donor-derived cells were found distributed throughout the thymus. The conclusion from all these studies was that the anatomically-related, subcapsular → cortical → medullary pathway of thymocyte differentiation (Weissman, 1973) must be incorrect.

Recently, we have been studying the in vitro growth requirements of Lyt-2⁻/L3T4⁻ thymocytes in more detail. As shown in Table 1, microcultures initially containing 3×10^4 freshly isolated cells proliferated well in the presence of both PMA and the calcium ionophore Ionomycin, with or without added IL-2.

TABLE 1. Proliferation of Adult Lyt-2⁻/L3T4⁻ Thymocytes

	^{3}H-Thymidine Incorporated (10^{-3} x cpm)		
Additions	IL-2 (100 u/ml)	PMA (1 ng/ml)	Ionomycin (300 ng/ml)
0	1.3	0.5	0.2
IL-2	-	4.9	6.5
PMA	-	-	258.2
PMA + IONO	343.7	-	-

3×10^4 cells/well, 72 hr culture

Addition of Con-A in the presence or absence of IL-2 resulted in very poor proliferation (not shown). The proliferation seen with PMA + Ionomycin in the absence of added IL-2 suggested that these two signals alone were sufficient for the growth of Lyt-2⁻/L3T4⁻ thymocytes. Interestingly, supernatants from such bulk cultures of stimulated cells contained significant titres of IL-2 suggesting, but not proving, that their growth was IL-2 dependent.

In conclusion, Lyt-2$^-$/L3T4$^-$ thymocytes are a heterogeneous population of cells whose in vitro growth requirements we are beginning to understand. Therefore, with this in vitro approach to T cell growth and differentiation, a detailed molecular analysis of a number of interesting aspects of T cell development should be amenable to further investigation.

REFERENCES

Ceredig Rh, Dialynas DP, Fitch FW MacDonald HR (1983). Precursors of T cell growth factor producing cells in the thymus: Ontogeny, frequency and quantitative recovery in a subpopulation of phenotypically mature thymocytes defined by monoclonal antibody GK-1.5. J Exp Med 158: 1654.

Ceredig Rh, Schreyer M (1984). Immunohistochemical localization of host and donor-derived cells in the regenerating thymus of radiation bone marrow chimeras. Thymus 6: 15-26.

Ceredig Rh, MacDonald HR (1985). Intrathymic differentiation: some unanswered questions. Surv immunol Res 4: 87-95.

Ceredig Rh, Lowenthal JW, Nabholz M, MacDonald HR (1985a). Expression of Interleukin-2 receptors as a differentiation marker on intrathymic stem cells. Nature 314: 98-100.

Fowlkes BJ (1984). Characterization and differentiation of thymic lymphocytes in the mouse. PhD Thesis. George Washington University Graduate School of Arts and Sciences.

Fowlkes BJ, Edison L, Mathieson BJ, Chused TM (1984). Differentiation in vitro of an adult precursor thymocyte. In: Regulation of the Immune System, UCLA Symosia on Molecular and Cellular Biology. Sercarz E, Cantor H, Chess L, editors. Alan R Liss Inc., New York, p 275.

Gallatin WM, Weissman IL, Butcher EC (1983). A cell-surface molecule involved in organ-specific homing of lymphocytes. Nature (Lond) 304: 30-34.

Owen JJT, Jenkinson EJ (1981). Embryology of the lymphoid system. Progr Allergy 29: 1-27.

Raulet D (1985). Embryonic and immature adult thymocytes express IL-2 receptors and respond to IL-2 *in vitro*. Nature 314: 101-103.

Reichert RA, Gallatin WM, Butcher EC, Weissman IL (1984). A homing receptor-bearing cortical thymocyte subset: implications for thymus cell migration and the nature of cortisone-resistant thymocytes. Cell 38: 89-95.

Springer T, Galfre G, Secher DS, Milstein C (1978). Monoclonal xenogeneic antibodies to murine cell surface antigens: identification of novel leukocyte differentiation antigens. Europ J Immunol 8: 539-545.

Takacs L, Osawa H, Diamenstein T (1984). Detection and localization by the monoclonal anti-interleukin 2 receptor antibody AMT-13 of IL-2 receptor-bearing cells in the developing thymus of the mouse embryo and in the thymus of cortisone-treated mice. Europ J Immunol 14: 1152-1156.

Trowbride IS, Lesley J, Schulte R, Hyman R, Trotter J (1982). Biochemical characterization and cellular distribution of a polymorphic, murine cell-surface glycoprotein expressed on lymphoid tissues. Immunogenetics 15: 299-305.

Weissman IL (1973). Thymus cell maturation. Studies on the origin of cortisone-resistant thymic lymphocytes. J Exp Med. 137: 504-510.

Index

Aconitase
  in Krebs cycle, 270-271
  macrophage inhibition of, 266-267, 269-274
Acquired immune deficiency syndrome. *See* AIDS
ACTH
  in lymphocyte function modification, 213
  thymosin effect on, 190-193
  in viral infection, 200
Actinomycin D, 419, 420
Acute lymphocytic leukemia, 157-158
Acute myelogenous leukemia, 160-161
Acute myelomonocytic leukemia, 161
Acute promyelocytic leukemia
  chromosomal translocations in, 160-161
  gene amplification in, 161-162
ADCC, 302, 305
Adenylate cyclase activation
  immunoglobulin binding proteins in, 243-250
  neutrophil, 374, 377
  prostaglandin in, 243
Adjuvants
  for enhancement of vaccines, 338, 342-343
  lipoprotein, 338
  tripalmitoyl pentapeptide, 338-343
Adoptive immunotherapy, 457-463
Adrenocorticotropic hormone. *See* ACTH
AIDS
  immune response modulation in, 175-183
    cytotoxicity, 179-181
    HTLV-III effect on, 181-182
    mitogen response, 176-177
    monocyte activation in, 179
    natural killer cells in, 179
    prostaglandin synthesis in, 179
    soluble suppressor factor in, 178-179
  met-enkephalin therapy for, 210
AIDS related virus, 175
Allergic reactions
  basophils in, 347
  eosinophilia with, 357
  mast cells in, 347
Anaphylaxis, 352
Angiogenesis, 350
Animal models
  for adoptive immunotherapy evaluation, 457
  chickens, 69-73
  hamsters, 347-348
  mice. *See* Mice
  pig
    sodium influx in T cell proliferation, 123-129
    T cell activation regulation, 137-142
  rats
    cell surface markers of T lymphocytes of, 47
    mast cell heterogeneity in, 347-349
    pulmonary fibrosis of, 351
    for thymic epithelial matrix recombination, 12-17
Antibodies. *See also* Immunoglobulins
  adjuvant-antigen induction of, 340-342
  autoantibodies, 328
  clonotypic, 331-336
  monoclonal. *See* Monoclonal antibodies
Antibody dependent cellular cytotoxicity, 302, 305
Antigen presenting cells, thymic, 23-24
Arachidonic acid
  as eicosanoids, 365
  eosinophil metabolism of, 360
  neutrophil metabolism of, 367-369

platelet metabolism of, 366, 367
  thrombin and collagen effect on, 369
Arginase, 448
Asbestosis, 349
Astrocytes
  interleukin effect on, 221-225
  prostaglandin effect on, 222, 224
Autacoids, 365
ATPase in lymphocyte proliferation, 123-129
Autoimmunity
  autoreactive T cell clones in, 328
  defects in nonspecific suppressor mechanisms with, 69, 73
  interleukin-2 and, 69-73
Autonomic nervous system
  in immune system modulation, 227
  in tear gland innervation, 230-231

B cell leukemias and lymphomas
  chromosomal translocations in, 156-158
  tropomyosin synthesis in, 172
B lymphocytes
  adjuvant stimulation of, 338
  in AIDS, 176, 182
  bacterial lipoprotein stimulation of, 337
  differentiation of
    interleukin-1 in, 115
    interleukin-2 in, 109, 110, 221
    macrophage Fc receptor in, 243
  interleukin-1 receptors on, 115-119
  interleukin-2 as growth factor for, 109-113
  natural killer cell susceptibility of transformed lines of, 411-416
  tumoricidal activity of, 433
Bacterial adjuvants,
Bacterial toxins, 373-378
Basophils
  in allergic and hypersensitivity reactions, 347
  histamine effect on chemotactic response of, 351
BCG in interleukin-1 secretion, 330
Bone marrow
  interleukin-3 induction of stem cells of, 131
  mast cells derived from, 348

pulmonary alveolar macrophage independence from, 307-310
  retroviral infection of cells of, 275-280
  T lymphocyte precursors from, 51
Bone marrow transplants
  immune function with, 17
  macrophage growth factor therapy for, 239
Bromocryptine, 213-218
Burkitt's lymphoma
  c-myc gene expression in, 155-156, 163
  chromosomal translocations in, 155-156

Calcium
  chemoattractant receptors and, 377
  in interferon release, 78-79
  interleukin effect on, 76-77, 131-136
  in lymphocyte activation, 135
  in neutrophil receptor regulation, 377
Callus formation, 349
Cancer. See also Tumors
  adoptive immunotherapy for, 457-463
  chemotherapy for, 457-463
  development of. See Oncogenesis
  immune surveillance against, 433-438
  Landschütz ascites, 465
  leukemia. See Leukemia
  lung, 209-210
  lymphoma. See Lymphoma
  macrophage growth factor therapy for, 239
  met-enkephalin therapy for, 209-210
  renal, chemoimmunotherapy for, 457-463
  surgical therapy for, 461-463
Candida, 389
Carcinogenesis. See Oncogenesis
Cell growth
  glial, immunoregulatory molecules modulating, 221-225
  self-renewal capacity in, 435
  terminal differentiation with, 435
  in tumors, 168, 436-437
Central nervous system
  in chronic inflammation, 225
  immune system and, 188, 193-194, 197
  mast cell role in, 352
  opioid peptides of, 206

thymosin effect on, 193
Chemotaxis and collagen, 379-383
Chemotherapy for renal carcinoma, 460-463
Chicken models for interleukin-2 hyperproduction, 69-73
Chloroquine, 326
Chondroitin sulfate, 350
Chromosomes. *See also* DNA
    gain or loss of, in leukemia and lymphoma, 161-162
    Philadelphia, 154, 158-160
    translocations of
        in B cell tumors, 156-158
        in lymphocytic tumors, 155-156
        in nonlymphocytic tumors, 159-161
        in T cell tumors, 158-159
Chronic lymphocytic leukemia, 162
Chronic myelogenous leukemia
    blastic phase of, malignant, 435
    chromosomal abnormalities of, 154, 158-160
    crowding of cells in, 436-437
    development of, 435-437
    granulocyte production in, 435
    immune surveillance in, 437-438
    lymphoid cells in, 437
Cimetidine, 351
Colchicine, 377
Collagen
    amino acid composition of, 379
    chemotactic properties of, 379-384
    in platelet-neutrophil interactions, 369
Collagenase, 379, 380
Colony stimulating factors
    genomic cloning for, 235
    interleukin-3. *See* Interleukin-3
    macrophage. *See* Macrophage growth factor
Complement, 351
Concanavalin A
    in c-*myc* gene expression, 85
    capping phenomenon in response to, 373, 376
    in lymphocyte proliferation, 124-125
    in T cell antigen receptor stimulation, 40
    in thymocyte differentiation, 475

Cordecypin, 66
Corticosteroids as tumor promoter, 170
Corticosterone
    in immune response, 198, 199
    thymosin effect on, 190, 191
    in tumor cell response, 202
Cortisol
    thymosin effect on, 190
    in viral infection, 200
Crohn's disease, 349
Cryptococcus neoformans, 421
CSF-1. *See* Macrophage growth factor, CSF-1
Cyanide bromide, 380
Cycloheximide, 418
Cyclosporine, 104-106
Cytolytic factor, 449-450
Cytomegalovirus, 405
Cytotoxins in tumoricidal reaction, 449-450

Dendritic cells, thymic
    as antigen bearing cells, 23, 24
    MHC antigens of, in T cell development, 23-25
Diacylglycerol
    in interferon transcription regulation, 79
    in phosphorylation of protein kinase C substrate, 77
    in protein kinase C activation, 76
Dinorphins, 205-206
Disodium chromoglycate, 349
DNA. *See also* Chromosomes
    colony stimulating factor, cloning of, 235
    interleukin-3, cloning of, 235
    lymphocyte repair of strand breaks in, 127-129
    macrophage growth factor
        amino acid sequence of, 236
        characterization of clones of, 236-238
        production of, 236
    macrophage inhibition of synthesis of, 261
    transforming, in oncogenesis, 167
DNA viruses, 171
Doxantrazole, 349

482   Index

Eicosanoid pathway
  cell-cell interactions in, 366
  definition of, 365
  platelet-neutrophil interactions in, 367–370
Endocrine system
  hormones in. *See* Hormones
  immune system in relation to, 188
    activated immune cell mediation, 202
    feedback circuits, 197–203
    glucocorticoid circuit, 198–202
    hypothalamus-pituitary-adrenal axis immunoregulation, 198–202
    insulin circuit, 202
    thymosin modulation of hormones, 188–194
    thyroxin circuit, 202
Endorphin
  localization of, 206
  in lymphocyte function modification, 213
  mast cell responsiveness to, 348, 349
  precursor for, 205
  structure of, 205
  thymosin effect on, 191–193
Enkephalinase, 206
Enkephalins
  leu-enkephalin, 205, 206
  localization of, 206
  methionin. *See* Methionin-enkephalin
  precursor for, 205
  structure of, 205
Enzyme-linked immunosorbent assay
  of adjuvant-antigen induced antibodies, 340–342
  of interleukin-2 receptor, 95–96, 101
Eosinophil-differentiating factor, 358
Eosinophil stimulation promoter, 358–360
Eosinophilia, 357
Eosinophils
  arachidonic acid metabolism in, 360
  function of, 357
  heparin effect on, 350
  histamine effect on, 351
  larval helminth cytotoxicity of, 360–361
  lymphokine effect on, 358
  monoclonal antibodies to, 361–362

  in nematode infection, 350
  proteins of, basic granular, 361
  in schistosome egg destruction, 360
Epithelial cells, thymic
  cortical vs medullary, 26
  ectodermal vs endodermal-derived, 22
  isolation and purification of, 11–13
  lymphohematopoietic cell interaction with, 11
  MHC antigens of, in T cell development, 22–23
  recombination grafts of
    immunodeficient mouse models for, 12
    repopulating lymphohematopoietic cells from, 13–14
    splenic reconstitution in, 14–17
    T lymphocytes from, 16–17
    thymocytes from, 14
  thymocyte interaction with, 7–8
Epstein Barr virus
  in AIDS, 176, 179–180, 182
  B lymphocytes transformed by
    interleukin-1 receptors on, 115–119
    natural killer cell susceptibility in, 411–416
Erythrocytes
  macrophage phagocytosis of, 262, 263
  monocyte cytotoxicity against, 302
Escherichia coli
  cytostatic factor gene cloning in, 441
  lipoprotein from cell wall of, in B cell stimulation, 337
  neutrophil killing of, 388

Fibroblasts
  chemotactic receptor on, 383
  collagen chemotaxis for, 379
  histamine effect on, 351
  monocyte conjugation to, 302
Fibrosarcoma, 350
  laminin treatment of, 428
  natural killer cell influence on, 425–428
Forskolin, 377

Genes. *See also* Chromosomes, DNA
  macrophage growth factor, 238

oncogenes. See Oncogenes
Genetics
  of autoreactive T cell clones, 327
  of interleukin-2, 57-67
  of leukemia, 153-163
  of natural killer cell susceptibility of human cells, 411-416
  of thymic stromal cells in T cell development, 26-27
  of thymocyte T cell receptors, 29, 30-32, 34
Glucocorticoid increasing factor, 199-200
Glucocorticoids
  activated immune cell products mediation of, 199-200
  in immune cell function control, 198
  during immune response, 198-199
  immunoregulatory circuit of, 201
  in interleukin inhibition, 201
  in lymphocyte differentiation and regulation, 194
Graft-vs-host disease, 349
Growth hormone, 188
GTP-binding proteins, 373-378

Haemophilus somnus, 385-389
Hamster models of mast cell heterogeneity, 347-348
Harderian gland, 227-232
Hemopoiesis, 437
Heparin, 350
Histamine
  actions of, 351
  cimetidine block of, 351
  mast cell synthesis of, 347
  psychological conditioning for secretion of, 351
Hormones
  glucocorticoids. See Glucocorticoids
  growth hormone, 188
  immune system regulation of, 188, 194
  insulin, 200-201
  luteinizing hormone, 188, 189
  prolactin
    gonadotropin levels in relation to, 218
    macrophage inhibition from pharmacologic blockade of, 213-218

  thymosin modulation of, 188-189
  tumor cell inoculation effect on, 201
  testosterone, 201
HTLV-III
  in AIDS, 175, 181-182
  B cell infection by, 176
  carriers of, 176
  HTLV-I and HTLV-II vs, 175
Hypereosinophilic syndrome, 357
Hypersensitivity reactions
  basophils in, 347
  eosinophils in, 357
  mast cells in, 347
  tumor suppression of, 465-470
Hypoxia, pulmonary, 349

IDS, 83, 86-88
IgE in allergic and hypersensitivity reactions, 347
Immune system
  in AIDS, 175-183
    cytotoxicity, 179-181
    HTLV-II effect on, 181-182
    mitogen response, 176-177
    monocyte activation, 179
    natural killer cells in, 179
    prostaglandin synthesis in, 179
    soluble suppressor factor in, 178-179
  adaptation of, to tumor, 434-435
  autonomic nervous system effect on, 227
  central nervous system and, 188, 194, 197
  endocrine system in relation to, 188
  function of, 315
  in hormonal regulation, 188, 194
  luteinizing hormone effect on, 189
  lymphocytes in. See Lymphocytes
  lymphokines in. See Lymphokines
  macrophages in. See Macrophages
  natural killer cells in. See Natural killer cells
  prolactin effect on, 189
  tumor-associated antigen recognition by, 433
Immunoglobulins
  adjuvant-antigen induction of, 340-342
  macrophage Fc receptors for, protein binding of, 243-250

adenylate cyclase activation with, 245-246
calmodulin effects on, 247
EGTA effects on, 246-247
liposomal insertion of proteins with, 244
isolation and fractionation of proteins in, 244
membrane effects of, 246
protein kinase activity with, 247-248
of tears, plasma cell production of, 227

Immunotherapy
adoptive, 457
macrophage growth factor therapy for, 239
met-enkephalin therapy for, 209-210
for renal carcinoma, 457-463
success of, 457

Inflammation
GTP-binding proteins in, 377
macrophage proliferation in, 316
mast cells in, 350
monocyte influx in, 316

Inositol trisphosphate, 76
Insulin, 202-203

Interferon
in AIDS, 179, 180, 182
of autoreactive T cell clones, 326
gene cloning for, 441
histamine effect on synthesis of, 351
inhibition of, tumor-induced, 465
in initiation of interleukin-2 activity, 75, 76
in MHC antigen expression, 415
in macrophage antimicrobial activity, 420
macrophage growth factor effect on, 239
in macrophage-parasite interaction, 317-322
in monocyte activation, 287
in natural killer cell stimulation, 393-396
in natural killer lysis susceptibility, 414, 415
in post-transcription gene expression modulation, 257
release of, interleukin-2 in, 78-79, 89
transcription regulation of, 78-79

in tumor growth, 441, 443

Interleukin-1
accessory cell signals from, 137
in astrocyte growth, 221, 222
as autocrine signal, 115-119
of autoreactive T cell clones, 326
BCG effect on, 330
corticosterone blood levels with, 200, 201
forms of, 118
function of, 221
glucocorticoid effect on, 201
immunological cross-reactivity of, 115-116
macrophage growth factor effect on, 239
molecular weight of, 115
monocyte synthesis of, 285
monocyte-derived, 115-119
in natural killer cell regulation, 398
properties of, in EBV-B cell lines, 115-116
receptors for, 115, 116-119
in T lymphocyte activation, 140-142

Interleukin-2
in adoptive immunotherapy, 460
in astrocyte growth, 222
autoimmunity and, 69-73
of autoreactive T cell clones, 326
in B cell differentiation and proliferation, 109-113, 221
biochemical mechanisms of, 75-81
in c-*myc* gene expression, 84, 85, 89, 93
calcium mobilization with action of, 76-77, 131-136
clonotypic antisera effect on, 333-334
corticosterone blood levels with, 198
cyclosporine inhibition of, 104-106
function of, 221
gene expression for, 57-67
biologically active mRNA formation with, 58-60
cordycepin effect on, 66
cycloheximide effect on, 61-64
DRB inhibition of, 58, 61
de novo transcription, 61, 64
functional half-life of mRNA from, 59, 61
irradiation effects on, 66-67

labile protein repressor effect on, 57,
    58, 63, 65–66
repression mechanisms in, 63–64
superinduction of, 57–58, 60–64
transcriptional control of, 58
translocational control of, 59–60
glucocorticoid effect on, 199
hyperproduction of, in obese strain
    chickens, 69–73
initiation of activity of, 75
in interferon release, 78–79, 89
in lipoxygenase pathway activation, 89
met-enkephalin effect on, 209, 211
monoclonal antibodies to, 103
in natural killer cell stimulation,
    393–394, 396–400
in oligodendrocyte growth, 222, 225
in oncogene stimulation, 80
phosphatidylinositol turnover and,
    76–77
potassium conductance with stimulation
    of, 89
in protein kinase C activation, 76–77, 89
protein synthesis patterns with, 89–93
in T lymphocyte conversion to natural
    killer cell, 403
in T lymphocyte lineage mapping, 52
in T lymphocyte proliferation, 83–88
T lymphocyte proliferation independent
    of, 103–108
thymocyte receptors for, 48
in transcription regulation, 78–80
in transferrin receptor induction, 89, 93
tumor promoters and, 76
Interleukin-2 receptor
    in AIDS, 182
    on B lymphocytes, 109–113
    cellular activation for expression of, 95
    identification and characterization of,
        95–102
        cell cultures and cell lines for, 96, 99
            101
        enzyme linked immunosorbent assay
            for, 95–96, 101
    induction of, interleukin-2, 89, 93
    molecular weight estimation for,
        96–97, 99, 100
    monoclonal antibodies to

in B lymphocyte activation, 110
in T lymphocyte activation independent of interleukin-2, 103–107
recombinant ligand effects on, 134
Tac, 75, 76
    in interleukin-2 independent proliferation of T cells, 104–106
    monoclonal antibodies to, 95
    phosphorylation of, 77
    as protein kinase C substrate, 77
    in T lymphocyte activation, 95, 101
on thymocytes, 107, 474
in tumor response, 101
Interleukin-3
    in blood cell differentiation, 235
    calcium mobilization with action of, 76,
        77, 131–136
    function of, 221
    genomic cloning for, 235
    in mast cell growth and differentiation,
        348
    as multi-colony stimulating factor, 131
    in protein kinase C activation, 76–77
Interstitial lung disease, 349
Ions
    calcium
        chemoattractant receptors and, 377
        in interferon release, 78–79
        interleukin effect on, 76–77, 131–136
        in lymphocyte activation, 135
        in neutrophil receptor regulation,
            377
    potassium
        interleukin-2 effect on conductance
            of, 89
        in lymphocyte proliferation, 124–127
    sodium
        in lymphocyte proliferation, 123–129
        in repair of lymphocyte DNA strand
            breaks, 128
Iron
    in macrophage cytotoxicity, 262–267
    in mitochondrial electron system, 266

Kaposi's sarcoma, 175, 176
    natural killer cell activity in, 179
    T lymphocyte response to mitogens in,
        176

Keloids, 349, 351

Lacrimal gland nerve and plasma cell association, 227–232
Laminin
  on natural killer cell surface, 424
  in tumor cell recognition by natural killer cells, 423–428
  tumor growth with, 428
Landschütz ascites carcinoma, 465
Large granular lymphocytes
  alveolar macrophage activation by cytokine of, 417–421
  function of, 403
  in lysis susceptibility of target cells, 413
  natural killer cells and, 403, 404
  from resting T lymphocytes, 404
  in viral infection regulation, 403–408
LAV in AIDS, 175
Leishmania major, 316–322
Leukemia
  acute lymphocytic, 157–158
  acute myelogenous, 160–161
  acute myelomonocytic, 161
  acute promyelocytic, 160–162
  B cell
    chromosomal translocations in, 156–158
    tropomyosin synthesis in, 172
  chromosomal gain or loss in, 161–162
  chromosomal translocations in, 155–161
    for lymphocytic tumors, 155–159
    for nonlymphocytic tumors, 159–161
  chronic lymphocytic, 162
  chronic myelogenous. *See* Chronic myelogenous leukemia
  genetic changes in, 153–163
  immunosuppression and, 438
  interleukin-2 receptor in, 95, 101
  multiple myeloma and, 438
  T cell
    chromosomal translocations in, 158–159
    interleukin-2 receptor in, 101
    trisomy in, 162
    tropomyosin synthesis in, 172–174
Leukocyte function associated-1 antibodies, 301–305

Leukocytes. *See also* specific cells
  eicosanoid pathways of, 366
  in viral infection, 406
Leukoregulin in tumor growth inhibition, 441–445
Leukotrienes
  arachidonate oxygenation to, 367, 368
  in lymphocyte proliferation inhibition, 350
  mast cell synthesis of, 347, 350
  neutrophil-derived, 367
  platelet-derived, 368
Lipoprotein immunoadjuvants, 338–343
Listeria monocytogenes, 331–336
Luteinizing hormone, 188, 189
Lymphadenopathy associated virus, 175
Lymphadenopathy syndrome, 176
  natural killer cell activity in, 179
  T lymphocyte response to mitogens in, 176
Lymphocyte-derived chemotactic factor, 465, 468, 469
Lymphocytes
  B. *See* B lymphocytes
  calcium in activation of, 135
  in hemopoietic tissue regulation, 438
  heparin inhibition of, 350
  hnRNP complexes in lectin-stimulated, 143–150
    acetylation of, 147, 149
    amount of core proteins in, 143, 144
    assembly control of, 143–144
    in vitro reconstitution of, 150
    metabolic effects on, 144
    methylation of, 145–146
    multiple charge isomers of, 147
    phosphorylation of, 147
    snRNP complexes in association with, 144–145
    as substrates for protein kinase, 149
  large granular. *See* Large granular lymphocytes
  natural cytotoxic, 423–428
  neurotransmitter receptors on, 227
  prolactin receptors on, 213
  repair of DNA strand breaks in, 127–128
  sodium influx in proliferation of, 123–129

substance P effect on, 227
T. See T lymphocytes
of tear gland, 231
tropomyosin synthesis in, 172–173
tumor-induced cytostatic factors produced by, 441–445
Lymphocytic choriomeningitis virus, 403–408
Lymphocytic leukemia
chromosomal translocations in, 157–158
trisomy 12 in, 162
tropomyosin synthesis in, 172
Lymphokine activated killer cells
human cell susceptibility to, 412
interferon effect on, 393–396
interleukin effect on, 396–400
progenitor for, 400
Lymphokines
in eosinophil activity, 358, 361
in glial cell growth, 221
IDS, 83, 86–88
interferon. See Interferon
interleukin. See Interleukin
in macrophage-parasite interactions, 316–322
tumor-induced suppression of, 465–470
Lymphoma
B cell
chromosomal translocations in, 156–158
tropomyosin synthesis in, 172
Burkitt's
c-*myc* gene expression in, 155–156, 163
chromosomal translocations in, 155–156
chromosomal gain or loss in, 161–162
chromosomal translocations in, 155–157
genetic changes in, 153
immunosuppression and, 438
tropomyosin synthesis in, 172
Lymphotoxin
genome cloning for, 441
in tumor growth inhibition, 441, 442, 445

Macrophage growth factor, CSF-1
amino acid sequence of, 236
characterization of, 237
function of, 235, 238–239
genomic clones of
isolation of, 236–237
structure of DNA and mRNA of, 237–238
production of, induced, 236
therapeutic uses for, 239
Macrophage procoagulant-inducing factor, 465, 467–469
Macrophages
in aconitase inhibition, 226–267, 269–274
alveolar
cytokinetic behavior of, 307–312
preformed LGL cytokine activation of, 417–421
bacterial killing by, 385
bromocryptine effect on, 213–218
in candidiasis, 389
cell line establishment via bone marrow cell infection, 275–280
cytotoxins in tumor cytotoxicity of, 447–457
in environmental integrity preservation, 315
in erythrocyte phagocytosis, 262, 263
Fc receptors of, protein binding of, 243–250
adenylate cyclase activation with, 245–246
calmodulin effects on, 247
EGTA effects on, 246–247
liposomal insertion of proteins with, 244
isolation and fractionation of proteins in, 244
membrane effects of, 246
protein kinase activity with, 247–248
heterogeneity of, 295–300
in induction of antimicrobial effector reactions, 315–322
in inflammatory reactions, acute, 316
interferon effect on antimicrobial activity of, 420
iron effects on cytotoxicity of, 262–267
Landschütz ascites carcinoma inhibition of, 465
lymphokines and, in parasitic infection, 316–322

in metabolic inhibition of tumor target cells, 261-262
in mitochondrial respiration inhibition, 265-267, 269, 448
molecular bases for activation of, 253-258
monoclonal antibodies to varying stages of development of, 289-293
in NADH-coenzyme Q reductase inhibition, 266, 269
natural killer cell interaction with, 417-421
in parasitic infection, 316-317
    intracellular killing, 319-322
    resistance to infection, 317-319
pergolide effect on, 213-218
phenotypic changes with differentiation of, 289, 295
prolactin release blockade in inhibition of, 213-218
prostaglandin synthesis by, 243
resident, bone marrow independence of, 307-312
secretory products of, 315, 316
in succinate-coenzyme Q reductase inhibition, 266, 269
surface antigen analysis of, 295-300
thymic, 11
thymocyte interactions with, 52
tumor infiltration of, 447
tumoricidal activity of, 433
    cytolysis, 448
    molecular mechanisms for, 448
    target cell recognition in, 447-448
Mast cells
in allergic and hypersensitivity reactions, 347
in asbestosis, 349
in callus and scar formation, 349
as central nervous system-inflammatory response link, 352
chondroitin sulfate of, 350
in Crohn's disease, 349
disodium chromoglycate effect on, 349
doxantrazole effect on, 349
environmental effects on differentiation of, 348
in eosinophil cytotoxicity, 361
in fibrosarcoma, 350
in graft-vs-host disease, 349
heparin of, 350
heterogeneity of, intraspecies and interspecies, 347-348
histamine synthesis of, 347, 351
histochemical staining of, 348
hyperplasia of, 349-350
in hypoxia, 349
in inflammatory process, 350
interleukin-3 effect on, 348
in interstitial lung disease, 349
leukotriene synthesis in, 347, 350
in nematode infection, 350
in nerve repair, 350
in neurofibromata, 349
neurohumoral regulation of, 351
in osteoporosis, 349
peritoneal vs intestinal mucosal, 348-349, 350
platelet-activating factor synthesis in, 347
prostaglandin synthesis in, 350
psychological conditioning for secretion of products of, 351
quercetin effect on, 349
in rheumatoid arthritis, 350
in scleroderma, 350
in ulcerative colitis, 349
Melanoma
cellular adhesion molecules associated with, 302
monocyte conjugation to cells of, 301-305
trisomy 7 in, 162
Metastasis
adoptive immunotherapy for, 457
macrophage role in, 447
natural killer cell influence on, 425-428
Methionin-enkephalin
for AIDS, 210
immunological effects of, 205-211
in interleukin 2 production, 209
in lung cancer therapy, 209-210
lymphocyte receptors for, 206-207
mechanism of action of, 210
natural killer activity with, 207
for pre-AIDS, 210

surface antigens of lymphocytes affected by, 207–209
therapeutic uses for, 211
Mice
alveolar macrophage cytokinetic behavior in, 307–312
B lymphocyte activation by interleukin-2 in, 109–113
bone marrow cell infection of, 275–280
cell surface markers of thymocytes and T cells of, 47, 48
fibroblast line NIH3T3 from, 168–169
listeriosis of, clonotypic antisera for, 331–336
macrophage differentiation in, 289–293
macrophage-mediated tumoricidal reaction in, 447, 449–450
mast cell heterogeneity in, 347–348
mycobacterial infection of, T cells derived from, 325–330
renal carcinoma chemoimmunotherapy for, 457–463
T lymphocyte antigen receptors of, 37–43
in thymic epithelial matrix recombination studies, 12–17
Mitogens
in AIDS, 176
accessory cell signals and, 137, 138
in c-*myc* gene expression, 85
cation pump site increase with, 123
histamine effect on, 351
interleukin-1 effect vs, 140
in T lymphocyte activation, 137–143
in T lymphocyte antigen receptor stimulation, 40, 43, 85
tripalmitoyl pentapeptide, 337, 338
Monensin, 418
Monoclonal antibodies
to antigen presenting cells, 23
to dendritic cells, thymic, 23, 26
to eosinophil, 361–362
to interleukin-1, 115–116
to interleukin-2 receptor
in B lymphocyte activation, 110
in T lymphocyte activation, 95, 101
in T lymphocyte activation independent of interleukin-2, 103–107

to laminin, 424
to macrophages at different stages of development, 289–300
met-enkephalin effect on, 207–208
in monocyte ADCC inhibition, 305
to monocyte-associated cellular adhesion molecules, 301–305
in monocyte-melanoma cell conjugate formation inhibition, 304
to stromal cells, thymic, 25
to T lymphocyte antigen receptors, 37, 38, 41
to thymocyte receptors for T lymphocytes, 32
in thymocyte subset identification, 473, 474
to transferrin receptors, 85–86
Monocytes
activation of
nonspecific, 284, 285
specific, 285
in AIDS, 179
beta toxin in tumoricidal reactions of, 451–452
cellular adhesion molecules associated with, 301–305
collagen chemotaxis for, 379
connective tissue breakdown and, 383
cytotoxins in tumor cytotoxicity of, 447–457
fibroblast conjugation to, 302
functional differences among, 285
heterogeneity of, 283–287
histamine inhibition of complement synthesis by, 351
in inflammatory reactions, acute, 316
interleukin-1 derived from, 115–119
MHC class II molecules of, 284
macrophage growth factor effect on, 238
maturation stage expression of, 283–287
melanoma cell conjugation to, 301–305
physical properties of, 285
in resident macrophage maintenance, 307, 312
splenectomy effects on kinetics of, 310
prolactin receptors on, 213
Monokines
in eosinophil cytotoxicity, 361

in glial cell growth, 221
respiratory inhibitory factor, 450
Mouse. *See* Mice
Multiple myeloma, 438
Mycobacterium bovis, 325–330
Mycobacterium leprae, 336
Myelogenous leukemia
   acute, 160–161
   chronic. *See* Chronic myelogenous leukemia
Myelomonocytic leukemia, 161

NADH-coenzyme Q reductase, 266, 269
Naloxone, 206, 207
Natural cytotoxic lymphocytes, 423–428
Natural killer cell cytotoxic factor, 441
Natural killer cells
   in AIDS, 179, 183
   genetics of human susceptibility to, 411–416
   HLA antigen expression and lysis susceptibility by, 415–416
   immunoregulatory role of, 417–421
   interferon effect on
      in lysis susceptibility, 414, 415
      stimulatory, 393–396
   interleukin-1 regulation of, 398
   interleukin-2 stimulation of, 393–394, 396–400
   laminin/laminin receptors in tumor cell recognition by, 423–428
   large granular lymphocytes and, 403
   in macrophage microbicidal activity, 417–421
   met-enkephalin effect on, 207–209, 211
   in metastasis control, 425
   monensin effect on, 418
   surface phenotype of, 394, 396, 398, 399
   from T lymphocyte lines, 403
   tumoricidal activity of, 433
   tumorigenic distribution and phenotypic changes in, 438
   in viral infection, 404–406, 408
Nematode infection, 350, 360
Neoplasma. *See* Cancer, Tumors
Nerve cells
   astrocytes and oligodendrocytes
      interleukin effect on, 221–225

prostaglandin effect on, 222, 224
glial, immunoreactivity molecules in growth of, 221–225
Nerves
   plasma cells and, in tear gland, 227–232
   repair of, mast cells in, 350
Nervous system
   autonomic
      in immune system modulation, 227
      in tear gland innervation, 230–231
   central
      in chronic inflammation, 225
      immune system and, 188, 193–194, 197
      mast cell role in, 352
      opioid peptides of, 206
      thymosin effect on, 193
Neurofibromata, 349
Neutrophils
   adenylate cyclase activation in, 374, 377
   in arachidonate metabolism, 367–369
   capping phenomenon in, 373, 375–376
   chemiluminescence with bacterial killing by, 385–390
   chemoattractants for, 379–384
   collagen damage response of, 379
   connective tissue breakdown and, 383
   GTP-binding proteins in regulation of, 373–378
   growth factor for, 235
   in leukotriene synthesis, 367
   platelet interactions with, in eicosanoid pathway, 365–370
   receptor regulation of, 374–378
   transduction mechanisms of, 377

Oligodendrocytes
   interleukin effect on, 221–225
   prostaglandin effect on, 222, 224
Onchocera volvulus, 360
Oncogenes
   c-abl
      amplification of, 162
      in chronic myelogenous leukemia, 159–160, 163
   c-erbA, in acute promyelocytic leukemia, 160–161
   c-erbB, 158, 162

c-*ets*, 158
c-*mos*, in acute myelogenous leukemia, 160
c-*myc*
 amplification of, 161-162
 in Burkitt's lymphoma, 155-156, 163
 induction of, cell cycle for, 84
 interleukin-2 stimulation of, 84, 85, 89, 93
 lectin mitogen stimulation of, 85
 in T cell proliferation regulation, 83
 transferrin receptors in expression of, 85
c-*src*, 158
 cellular protein changes with, 168-174
 expression of, cell behavior with, 168
 interleukin-2 activity and, 76, 80
 phorbol ester stimulation of, 80
 protein kinase C activation effect on, 80
 proto-oncogenes, 167
 retroviral. *See* Retroviral oncogenes
 in T lymphocyte proliferation, 83
 tropomyosin synthesis in cells transformed by, 169-172
 tumor promoters and, 76
Oncogenesis
 biochemical changes leading to, 167-174
 cell growth behavior in, 168
 chromosomal changes in, 154
 immune surveillance and, 433-438
 macrophage growth factor in, 239
 retroviral oncogenes in. *See* Retroviral oncogenes
Opioids, endogenous
 action of, 205
 dinorphins, 205, 206
 endorphins
  localization of, 206
  in lymphocyte function modification, 213
  mast cell responsiveness to, 348, 349
  precursor for, 205
  structure of, 205
  thymosin effect on, 191-193
 enkephalins
  leu-enkephalin, 205, 206
  localization of, 206
  methionin. *See* Methionin-enkephalin

 precursor for, 205
 structure of, 205
 naloxone effect on, 206
Osteoporosis, 349

Pactamycin, 63
Parasitic infection
 eosinophils in, 357, 360-361
 lymphocyte proliferation around site of, protection from, 434-435
 macrophage interactions in, 316-322
Pergolide, 213-218
Pertussis toxin, 373-378
Philadelphia chromosome in chronic myelogenous leukemia, 154 158-160
Phorbol esters
 accessory cell signals from, 137
 in interferon transcription regulation, 79
 in oncogene stimulation, 80
 protein kinase C as receptor for, 76
Phosphatidylinositol, 76-77
Pichinde virus, 405
Pig
 sodium influx in T cell proliferation in, 123-129
 T cell activation requirements for, 137-142
Plasma cells and nerves in tear gland, 227-232
Plasminogen activator, 239
Platelet-activating factor
 mast cell synthesis of, 347
 neutrophil receptors for, 373
Platelets
 in leukotriene formation, 368
 lipoxygenase pathway of, 367
 neutrophil interactions with, in eicosanoid pathway, 365-370
Polyoma virus, 171
Potassium
 interleukin-2 effect on conductance of, 89
 in lymphocyte proliferation, 124-127
Prolactin
 gonadotropin levels in relation to, 218
 macrophage inhibition from pharmacologic blockade of, 213-218
 thymosin modulation of, 188-189

tumor cell inoculation effect on, 201
Promyelocytic leukemia
    chromosomal translocation in, 160-161
    gene amplification in, 161-162
Prostaglandin
    in adenylate cyclase activation, 243
    in AIDS, 179, 183
    astrocyte production of, 221, 222
    in B lymphocyte inhibition, 350
    macrophage growth factor effect on, 239
    macrophage synthesis of, 243
    mast cell synthesis of, 350
    monocyte synthesis of, 285
    in T lymphocyte inhibition, 350
Protease
    cytolytic, 449-450
    in macrophage cytotoxicity activation, 257-258
    in macrophage tumoricidal reaction, 448
    macrophage Fc receptor binding effect on, 247-248
Protein kinase C
    interleukin activation of, 76-77, 89
    oncogene stimulation from activators of, 80
    phosphatidylinositol activation of, 76-77
    phosphoprotein substrates of, 77-78
    as receptor for phorbol esters, 76

Quercetin, 349

Rats
    cell surface markers of T lymphocytes of, 47
    mast cell heterogeneity in, 347-349
    pulmonary fibrosis of, 351
Renal carcinoma chemoimmunotherapy, 457-463
Respiration inhibitory factor, 450
Retroviral oncogenes
    definition of, 167
    growth factors and, 275
    v-Ha-*ras*, 169-170
    v-Ki-*ras*, 168-169
    v-*myc*
        in Burkitt's lymphoma, 155

    in macrophage cell line establishment, 275-280
    v-*raf*, in macrophage cell line establishment, 275-280
Retroviruses
    AIDS from, 175
    HLTV-III
        in AIDS, 175, 181-182
        B cell infection by, 176
        carriers of, 176
        HTLV-I and HTLV-II vs, 175
    bone marrow cell infection with, 275-280
    tropomyosin synthesis in cell transformed by, 170, 171
Rheumatoid arthritis, 350
RNA in macrophage cytotoxicity activation, 253-258
RNA viruses. *See* Retroviruses

Salmonella typhimurium, 338, 339, 342
Scar formation, 349
Schistosoma mansoni, 357-358, 360, 361
Schistosomula, 350
Scleroderma, 328, 350
Sodium
    in lymphocyte proliferation, 123-129
    in repair of lymphocyte DNA strand breaks, 128
Sparsomycin, 63
Spectrin, 51
Staphylococcus aureus, 417-421
Stromal cells, thymic
    heterogeneity of, 26
    MHC-antigen bearing, 22
    monoclonal antibodies to, 26
    in ontogeny, 26-27
    in T cell restriction specificities, 21-27
Substance P
    in lymphocyte activity, 227
    mast cell responsiveness to, 348, 349
    in salivary gland stimulation, 231
Succinate-coenzyme Q reductase, 266, 269
Surgical removal of tumors, 461-462
SV-40 virus, 171

T cell growth factor. *See* Interleukin-2

Index

T cell leukemias
  chromosomal translocations in, 158–159
  interleukin-2 receptor in, 101
  tropomyosin synthesis in, 172
T lymphocytes
  AIDS infection of, 175–183
  accessory cell signals for activation of, 137–139
  activation requirements for, 137–142
  amplification of clones of, 11
  autoreactive, induction of, 325–330
  cell cycle progression of, 137–142
  cell surface markers of
    activation state and, 49–51
    capped spectrin as, 51
    differentiated state and, 49–50
    in effector-target interaction, 50
    function of, 50–51
    identification by, 49–50
    for initial contact with antigens, 50–51
    intrathymic vs gut-associated, 49
    lineages mapped by, 52
    precursor identification by, 51–52
    subset identification by, 49
    thymocytes and, 48
  clonotypic antibody stimulation of clones of, 331–336
  cytotoxic
    in adoptive immunotherapy, 462–463
    in AIDS, 175
    cell surface markers of, 49–51
    large granular lymphocyte morphology of, 403, 404
    tumor response of, 433–434
    virus-specific, 404, 405–408
  development and differentiation of
    catecholaminergic receptors in, 194
    cell surface maerks of, 47–52
    dendritic cells in, thymic, 23–25
    epithelial cells in, thymic, 22–23
    in fetal thymus organ cultures, 29–34
    MHC phenotype in, 21–27
    prothymocyte differentiating activity in, 51
    thymic cell interactions in, 11
    from thymic epithelial matrix grafts, 16–17
    thymocytes in, mature vs immature, 3–8
  in eosinophil control, 357–358
  gut-associated, cell surface markers of, 49
  helper cells
    in AIDS, 175
    autoreactive, clones of, 327
    cell surface markers of, 49, 50
    protein synthesis patterns with stimulation of, 89–93
  histamine effect on, 351
  interleukin-2 regulation of, 75–88
  interleukin-2 specificity for, 131
  MHC phenotype of, 21
    cell surface markers of, 49–50
    differentiation pathways for, 21
    in thymic epithelial matrix grafts, 17
    in thymic vs extrathymic environment, 21
    thymic stromal cells in development of, 21–27
    thymus MHC type effect on, 21, 29
  mast cells derived from, 348, 349
  met-enkephalin effect on, 206–208, 211
  met-enkephalin receptors on, 206–207, 210
  mitogen activation of, 137
    autoreactive clones of, 325–328
    hybridomas of, 328–330
  in mycobacterial infection, 325–330
  natural killer cell conversion from, 403
  progression of, from resting state into cell cycle, 109
  proliferation of
    independent of interleukin-2, 103–108
    interleukin-2 in, 75–88
  receptors of, antigen
    antigen binding of, 40, 43
    biochemical properties of subunits of, 42
    components of, 37–43
    concanavalin A activation of, 40
    endoglycosaminidase F treatment of, 39–40
    mechanism of action of, 43
    mitogen stimulation of, 40, 43, 85

monoclonal antibodies to, 37, 38, 41
peptides of, 37
phosphorylation of, 40-41
polypeptides precipitated with, 40-41, 43
SDS-PAGE analysis of, 38-39
T3 complex associated with, 37, 43
receptors of, genes for, 159
in spontaneous autoimmune thyroiditis, 69-73
suppressor
   in AIDS, 175, 177
   histamine effect on, 351
   leukotriene effect on, 350
   tumor induction of, 465
thymocyte receptors for, development of, 29-34
transferrin receptors in activation of, 85
tumoricidal activity of, 433
tumorigenic distribution and phenotypic changes in, 438
in viral infection, 407-408
T2 toxin, 63
Tear gland nerve and plasma cell association, 227-232
Testosterone, 203
Thymidine, 448
Thymocytes
   cell surface markers of, 47-49
   classification of, 3, 7
   development of T cell receptors on, 29
   epithelial cell association of, 7-8
   growth requirements for, 473-477
   immune function of, 6-7
   interleukin-2 receptors on, 107, 474
   location of, intrathymic, 4-7
   MHC antigens of, in T cell development 23
   macrophage interactions with, 52
   mature vs immature, 3-8
   nurse cells and, 7-8
   ontogenic appearance of, 473
   phenotypic properties of, 3-8, 473-477
   stromal cell interaction of, 22
   subset identification of, 473
Thymosin
   central nervous system function of, 193
   corticosterone responsiveness to, 191
   cortisol increase with, 190
   endorphin responsiveness to, 191-193
   growth hormone responsiveness to, 188
   as immunotransmitter, 194
   luteinizing hormone responsiveness to, 188, 189
   in pituitary-adrenal axis modulation, 190-194
   prolactin responsiveness to, 188-189
   sites of action of, 191-192
   in T cell rosette formation, 206-207
Thymus
   adoptive transfer of rudiments of, 11-19
   amplification of T cell clones in, 11
   dendritic cells of
      as antigen bearing cells, 23, 24
      MHC antigens of, in T cell development, 23-25
   development of, 473
   environmental effects of, on T cell differentiation, 52
   epithelial cells of. *See* Epithelial cells, thymic
   fetal, T cell receptor expression in, 29-34
   MHC antigens of, in T cell development, 23-25
   MHC phenotype of, 21, 29
   regeneration of, 475
   stromal cells of
      heterogeneity of, 26
      MHC-antigen bearing, 22
      monoclonal antibodies to, 26
      in ontogeny, 26-27
      in T cell restriction specificities, 21-27
   thymocyte location in, 4-7
Thyroiditis, 69-73
Thyroxine, 202-203
Toxoplasma gondii, 389
Transferrin receptors
   interleukin-2 in induction of, 89, 93
   in T cell activation, 85
Trichinella spiralis, 360, 361
Tripalmitoyl pentapeptide
   as immunoadjuvant, 338-343
   molecular structure of, 337
Tropomyosins from oncogene expression, 169-172

Trypanosoma cruzi, 421
Tumor necrosis factor
    in macrophage tumoricidal reactions, 448
    gene cloning for, 441
    in monocyte tumoricidal reactions, 451–452
    in tumor growth inhibition, 445
Tumor promoters
    interleukins and, 76
    in oncogene expression, 76, 170
    phorbol esters
        accessory cell signals from, 137
        in interferon transcription regulation, 79
        in oncogene stimulation, 80
        protein kinase C as receptor for, 76
Tumor-associated antigens, 433
Tumorigenesis. *See* Oncogenesis
Tumors
    cancer. *See* Cancer
    cell replication and growth in, 168, 436–437
    in cell-mediated immunity suppression, 465–470
    crowding of cells in, 436–437
    cytotoxins in monocyte/macrophage cytotoxicity against, 447–457
    development of, 435–437
    feedback differentiation pressures in, 435–436
    immunosuppression in promotion of, 433, 435
    laminin receptors in cell surfaces of, 423–428
    lymphocyte cytostatic factor synthesis in response to, 441–445
    mast cell hyperplasia in, 349
    natural killer cell recognition of, 423–428
    sneaking-through phenomenon of, 433–435

Ulcerative colitis, 349

Vaccination
    bacterial, adjuvant enhancement of, 338
    clonotypic antibodies for, 331, 336
    against listeriosis, 334–336
    with live organisms, 331
    tripalmitoyl pentapeptide enhancement of, 338–339, 342–343
Vaccinia virus, 405
Vasculitis, 385
Viral infections
    large granular lymphocytes in, 403–408
    retroviruses. *See* Retroviruses

DATE DUE

DEMCO 38-297